Ceramics in Orthopaedics

12th BIOLOX® Symposium
Proceedings

Edited by
JUN-DONG CHANG
KARL BILLAU

JUN-DONG CHANG
KARL BILLAU
Editors

Ceramics in
Orthopaedics

Bioceramics and Alternative Bearings in Joint Arthroplasty

12th BIOLOX® Symposium

Seoul, Republic of Korea
September 7 - 8, 2007
Proceedings

with 146 Figures in 259 separate Illustrations
and 47 Tables

STEINKOPFF VERLAG

JUN-DONG CHANG, M.D.
Department of Orthopaedic Surgery
Hangang Sacred Heart Hospital,
Hallym University College of Medicine
Youngdungpo-dong 2-ga, Youngdungpo-gu
150-719 Seoul, Korea

KARL BILLAU
CeramTec AG
Medical Products Division
Fabrikstrasse 23-29
73207 Plochingen, Germany

ISBN 978-3-7985-1782-0 Steinkopff Verlag

Cataloging-in-Publication Data applied for
A catalog record for this book is available from the Library of Congress.
Bibliographic information published by Die Deutsche Bibliothek
Die Deutsche Bibliothek lists this publication in the Deutsche Nationalbibliografie,
detailed bibliographic data is available in the Internet at <http://dnb.ddb.de>.

Steinkopff Verlag
a member of Springer Science+Business Media

http://www.steinkopff.springer.de

© Steinkopff Verlag, 2007
   Printed in Germany

Cover Design: TOP DESIGN, Thomas Schuster, Waiblingen

Production and Typesetting: druckerei justus kuch GmbH, Nürnberg

SPIN 12119837   105/7231-5 4 3 2 1 0 - Printed on acid-free paper.

Preface

Dear Colleague and Participant of the 12ᵗʰ International BIOLOX® Symposium

It is an honor for CeramTec to have the BIOLOX® Symposium in Asia. The selection of Seoul, Korea as the site was a difficult one due to the fact that there are many wonderful location options in this dynamic and fast growing region of the world. The selection was made easier by the outstanding support of our Symposium Chairman, Prof. Chang, as well as the excellent airline service and meeting facilities present in Seoul.

We hope that conducting the Symposium in this region will serve as a foundation for the increased recognition of the potential patient benefits to be derived from the use of ceramics and other alternative bearing technologies in Korea, China, India, Japan and the rest of the countries of the region.

We are convinced that the high quality of the program organized by the scientific committee, the prestigious faculty assembled and your contributions as participants will serve as a catalyst in order to make this Symposium a very enlightening and worthwhile personal experience for all. In order to enhance the value of the experience we are pleased to include this proceedings book as an integral part of your registration materials. We hope that this written more complete version of the scientific program will allow you to carry home a more concise view of the Symposium presentations.

Beginning in 2008, we have decided to modify our past practice by holding the meeting bi-annually instead of on an annual basis. We have elected to do this for two reasons. The most important reason is to allow both clinical and scientific knowledge to evolve further and secondly because the global leaders who form our speakers platform are simply confronted with so many meetings and Symposiums that their availability is very limited at times.

This year, we are very pleased to honor the lifelong contributions of Professor Heinz Mittelmeier by renaming the BIOLOX® Award normally granted to young clinicians and scientists in his honor. The Heinz Mittelmeier BIOLOX® Award will be granted in recognition of outstanding research work in the field of orthopaedics.

We welcome you to our Symposium in this wonderful country. We hope that you find the program we have put together to be of high value to you.

Best Regards,

Karl Billau
President, CeramTec Medical Products

Preface

I am very pleased to open the 12th International BIOLOX® Symposium in Seoul, Korea as a symposium president of this honorable meeting.

International BIOLOX® Symposium is a meeting for Bioceramics and alternative bearings in joint arthroplasty, which is carried out every year by CeramTec Company. I would like to express my deep gratitude to the CeramTec Company for its great support. This symposium has been prestigious for its informative and productive contents. From the beginning, the 11 previous meetings have been held in very attractive cities, including Rome last year. Symposium in Seoul marks the first time that this international ceramics forum for scientist and surgeons has ever been held in Asia. September is one of the best seasons in Korea, and just after our meeting, the 15th Triennial Congress of Asia Pacific Orthopaedic Association will be consecutively held here in Seoul.

Asia is the most populated continent consisting of nearly half of the world population living here in Asia. With its growing economical power and changing pattern of life, arthroplasty is increasingly performed at a phenomenal rate. Asian researchers are also very sensitive to adopt the recent technical and qualitative issues. Among the recent developments in the arthroplasty field, bearing surface occupies one of the most important positions. In Asian culture, sitting with crossed legs and squatting positions are more common compared to the Western culture. Because of such a different cultural background, in arthroplasty, impingement and wearing of liner are more important problems. With this point of view, the interest about bioceramic and alternative bearing is increasing.

The symposium is composed of 10 sessions and plenary lectures of the most current knowledge available in the use of Bioceramics and alternative bearings. We have invited more than 50 speakers with world-famous reputations from 12 countries. They joyfully accepted our invitation in spite of their busy schedule.

A total of 52 topics on recent developments in Bioceramic and alternative bearings in arthroplasty will be presented in this meeting. The scientific committee paid a lot of attention to make an academic and well-balanced scientific program. At a plenary lecture session, we will have three memorable lectures: 'Tribute to Heinz Mittelmeier', a respectable pioneer of bioceramic, by Professor K. Knahr, 'The Essential of Self-Locking THR with ceramic components. Basic Developments and Results.', by Professor H. Mittelmeier, and 'The Bearing of the Future: Delta Ceramics - Highly Crosslinked Polyethylene' by Professor R. H. Rothman. Just after plenary lecture, the symposium dinner is scheduled. I hope to spend our special time together for friendship sharing knowledge and experiences.

Finally, I would like to express my deep gratitude to all the speakers and attendants; the President of CeramTec, Ulf D. Zimmermann for his excellent vision and firm support; and also to all the CeramTec staff who have been involved to organize this symposium.

All this engagement will make the BIOLOX® Symposium in Seoul to a very successful meeting, and our cumulative effort will make the future of Arthroplasty more promising.

Jun-Dong Chang, MD, PhD
Symposium President
Hangang Sacred Heart Hospital
Hallym University College of Medicine
Seoul, Korea

List of contents

SESSION 1A

Tribology

**1A.1 Differences and Opportunities of THA
in the USA, Asia and Europe** 3
H. Kiefer

**1A.2 Influence of the Wear-Couple and Patient Activity
on Linear Wear in Total Hip Replacement** 9
Ch. Hendrich, N. Wollmerstedt, S. Goebel and J. M. Martell

**1A.3 Roles of Cellular and Molecular Targets
of Wear Debris in Periprosthetic Osteolysis** 19
S.-S. Lee, J.-D. Chang, P. E. Purdue, B. J. Nestor, T. P. Sculco and E. A. Salvati

SESSION 1B

Tribology

**1B.1 Wear Performance of 36mm BIOLOX® forte/delta
Hip Combinations Compared in Simulated
'Severe' Micro-Separation Test Mode** 33
I. C. Clarke, D. Green, P. Williams, G. Pezzotti and T. Donaldson

**1B.2 In-Vitro and In-Vivo Ceramic Debris
with Ceramic Prosthesis** 45
A. Toni, F. Traina, M. De Fine, E. Tassinari, F. Biondi, A. Galvani, F. Pilla and S. Stea

**1B.3 Surface Roughness of Ceramic Femoral Heads
after In-Vivo Transfer of Metal Correlation
to Polyethylene Wear** 49
Y.-H. Kim

**1B.4 Hydrothermal Stability of Ceramic
Femoral Heads** 59
V. Corfield, I. Khan and R. Scott

SESSION 2

Ceramic/Polyethylene

2.1 Ceramic on highly cross-linked Polyethylene
in cementless Total Hip Arthroplasty 67
J.-S. Kang and K.-H. Moon

2.2 Comparative Analysis of Ceramic to Ceramic
Bearing with Metal to Electron Beam-Irradiated
highly cross-linked UHMWPE Bearing 71
S.-K. Kim, J.-W. Park, J.-H. Wang and J.-G. Kim

2.3 Comparison of Uncemented Total Hip Arthroplasty
between Metal on Metal and Ceramic on
Polyethylene Bearing Surfaces in Young Patients 73
Y.-H. Kim

2.4 Comparison of Polyethylene Wear against
Alumina and Zirconia Heads in Cemented
Total Hip Arthroplasty 83
K. Kawanabe, B. Liang, K. Ise and T. Nakamura

SESSION 3

Large Diameter Wear Couples

3.1 Wear of large Ceramic Bearings 91
T. Pandorf

3.2 Evolution for Diameters Features and Results 99
P. Dalla Pria, M. Pressacco, F. Benazzo and S. Fusi

3.3 Design Rationale for Acetabular Cups with
alternative Bearings and large Diameter Heads 107
J. Oehy and M. Shen

3.4 Use of Modular Femoral Stem combined with
large Diameter Femoral Head in Alumina-on-Alumina
Total Hip Arthroplasty 117
Y.-S. Park, Y.-W. Moon and S.-J. Lim

SESSION 4

Ceramic Knee Implants

4.1 Ceramic Femoral Prosthesis in TKA
– Present and Future 123
M.-C. Lee and J.-W. Ahn

4.2 Finite-Element-Analysis of a Cemented Ceramic
Femoral Component in Total Knee Arthroplasty 133
Ch. Schultze, D. Klüß, A. Lubomierski, K.-P. Schmitz, R. Bader and W. Mittelmeier

4.3 Advanced Testing of Ceramic Femoral Knee
Components 137
T. Pandorf and M. Kuntz

4.4 Reasons using a Ceramic Femoral Component
and First Clinical Experience 145
F. Benazzo, P. Dalla Pria, W. Mittelmeier, D. Tigani, C. Zorzi, D. Ganzer,
C.H. Lohmann, E.G. Cimbrelo, C.R. Merchan, E.M. Saura, A.U. Lizaur,
J.F. Couceiro and S. Burelli

4.5 Comparison of In-Vivo Wear between Polyethylene
Inserts articulating against Ceramic and Cobalt-
Chrome Femoral Components in Total Knee Prostheses 149
H. Oonishi, S.-C. Kim, H. Oonishi, M. Kyomoto, M. Iwamoto and M. Ueno

SESSION 5A

Hard on Hard Bearings

5A.1 Toughening vs. Environmental Aging
in BIOLOX® *delta*: A micromechanics study 163
G. Pezzotti

5A.2 Clinical Experience with Ceramic on Ceramic
in the USA 169
J. P. Garino

5A.3 Why use an all Ceramic Tripolar THR ?
– clinical and experimental data 173
J.-Y. Lazennec, H. Sari Ali, M. Gorin, B. Roger, A. Baudoin and A. Rangel

5A.4 Lessons from 1st generation
Ceramic on Ceramic THA 179
Y.-J. Cho

5A.5 Nine-Year Experience with a Contemporary
Alumina-on-alumina THA Implant 181
H.-J. Kim and J.-J. Yoo

5A.6 Ceramic on Ceramic Bearing
in Coren® Hip System 187
J. - M. Lee

SESSION 5B

Hard on Hard Bearings

5B.1 Metallosis in Metal-on-Metal
PPF Total Hip Arthroplasties 193
R. Legenstein, W. Huber and P. Boesch

5B.2 Results of 10 Years' Follow-Up of Ceramic-
Ceramic Couples in Total Hip Replacement 205
M. Azizbaig Mohajer, F. Plattner and R. Graf

5B.3 Mid-Term Results of Ceramic-on-Ceramic
Bearing Extensively Porous Coated AML®
Total Hip Arthroplasty 211
K.-H. Moon, J.-S. Kang, D.-J. Lee, S.-H. Lee and K.-H. Kim

5B.4 Alumina-on-Alumina Total Hip Arthroplasty in
Patients with Osteonecrosis less than
50 Years Old 219
S.-Y. Kim

5B.5 Total Hip Arthroplasty using third Generation
Alumina-on-Alumina Articulation 221
K.-H. Koo

5B.6 Ceramic on Ceramic in Hybrid THR
(Cemented Femoral Stem)
– A five to seven year evalution 223
S.-J. Yim

5B.7 Mechanical Effect of the Articulating Materials
on the Proximal Femur and the Femoral Stem
in Total Hip Arthroplasty 229
Y.-Y. Won, K.-H. Moon, Y.-S. Yu, L.-S. Hyup and W.-Q. Cui

SESSION 6

Market Trends and Future Applications

6.1 Surface Characteristics and Biocompatibility
of Micro Arc Oxidized (MAO) Titanium Alloy 239
S.-Y. Kwon, Y.-S. Kim, D.-H. Sun, S.-S. Kim and H.-W. Kim

**6.2 Reasons for our Preference for Ceramic
over Metal Bearing –
clinical, radiological and biological evidences** 249
J.-Y. Lazennec, P. Boyer, J. Poupon, M. A. Rousseau,
F. Laude, Y. Catonné and G. Saillant

6.3 Spine: Ceramic Disc – what you should know 261
M. Grässel

6.4 Trend: Bigger Ball Heads: Is Bigger Really Better? 269
K.-H. Widmer

SESSION 7

Hip Revision

**7.1 Strategies for Head and Inlay Exchange
in Revision Hip Arthroplasty** 275
K. Knahr and M. Pospischill

7.2 Live-Time Prediction of BIOLOX® delta 281
M. Kuntz

**7.3 Revision Total Hip Arthroplasty with
Sandwich-type Ceramic on Ceramic Liner** 289
S.-H. Lee, J.-H. Hwang, B.-K. Kim and S.-H. Hong

**7.4 Revision Surgery of Acetabular Polyethylene Wear
– cup retention or revision?** 295
T.-C. Yu

SESSION 8

Tips and Tricks

**8.1 Tragedy of Polyethylene Back
Ceramic on Ceramic Articulation** 299
K. Kawate, T. Ohmura, I. Kawahara, H. Kataoka,
K. Tamai, T. Ueha and Y. Takakura

**8.2 Breakage of Alumina Ceramic Head
and Clinical Failure after Minor Modification
of Tapered Junction** 303
M. Ishii, M. Takagi, H. Ida, S. Kobayashi,
H. Kawaji and M. Hamasaki

8.3 Tips and Tricks: Fracture of a Ceramic Insert
with modern Ceramic Total Hip Replacement 311
B.-W. Min, K.-S. Song, C.-H. Kang, K.-J. Lee,
K.-C. Bae, C.-H. Cho and Y.-Y. Won

8.4 Minimally Invasive Two-Incision
Total Hip Replacement using large Diameter
Ceramic-on-Ceramic Articulation 319
T.-R. Yoon, C.-I. Hur, S. Diwanji and D.-S. Lee

8.5 MIS and the Demands on Bearing Couples 329
S. Junk-Jantsch and G. Pflüger

8.6 Computer Navigation: Improving Outcomes
with Hard on Hard Bearings 341
R. G. Middleton, C. Olyslaegers and T. W. Wainwright

Podium presenters and chairmen

FRANCESCO BENAZZO, M.D.
Fondazione I.R.C.C.S.
Policlinico San Matteo
Università di Pavia
27100 Pavia, Italy

KARL BILLAU
CeramTec AG
Medical Products Division
Fabrikstrasse 23-29
73207 Plochingen, Germany

JUN-DONG CHANG, M.D.
Department of Orthopedic Surgery
Hangang Sacred Heart Hospital
Hallym University
Yeongdeungpo-dong 2-ga
Yeongdeungpo-gu
150-719 Seoul, Korea

YOON-JE CHO, M.D.
Department of Orthopaedic Surgery
Kyunghee University Medical center
#1 Hoegi-dong, Dongdaemun-gu
130-702 Seoul, Korea

IL-YONG CHOI, M.D.
Department of Orthopedic Surgery
Hanyang University Hospital
Haengdang 1-dong 17, Seongdong-gu
133-792 Seoul, Korea

IAN CLARKE, M.D.
LLU Orthopedic Research Center
Dept of Orthopedics
Loma Linda University Medical Center
14606 Loma Linda Drive
Loma Linda CA 92354, USA

VICKI CORFIELD
Biomet UK Ltd.
Dorcan Industrial Estate
Swindon, Wiltshire SN3 5HY, UK

PAOLO DALLA PRIA
LIMA Lto spa
Via Nazionale
33038 Villanova (UD), Italy

JONATHAN P. GARINO, M.D.
Department of Orthopedic Surgery
Cupp building first floor
University of Pennsylvania
51 North 39th Street
Philadelphia, PA 19104, USA

MATTHIAS GRÄSSEL
CeramTec AG
Medical Products Division
Fabrikstrasse 23 - 29
73207 Plochingen, Germany

CHANG-DONG HAN, M.D.
Department of Orthopedic Surgery
Severance Hospital
Yonsei University
Sinchon-dong 134, Seodaemun-gu
120-752 Seoul, Korea

CHRISTIAN HENDRICH, M.D.
Orthopädisches Krankenhaus
Schloss Werneck
Balthasar-Neumann-Platz 1
97440 Werneck, Germany

SUNG-KWAN HWANG, M.D.
Department of Orthopedic Surgery
Wonju Christian Hospital
Yonsei University
Ilsan-dong, Wonju-si
220-701 Gangwon-do, Korea

MASAJI ISHII, M.D.
Yamagata Saisei Hospital
Dept of Orthopaedic Surgery
79-1 Okimachi, Yamagata
990-8545 Yamagata, Japan

SABINE JUNK-JANTSCH, M.D.
Evangelisches Krankenhaus Wien
Hans Sachs Gasse 10 - 12
1180 Vienna, Austria

JOON-SOON KANG, M.D.
Department of Orthopedic Surgery
Inha University Hospital 7-206
3-Ga Shinheung-Dong, Jung-Gu
400-103 Incheon, Korea

KEIICHI KAWANABE, M.D., PHD
Orthopedic Surgery, Kyoto University
54 Kawahara-cho, Shogoin, Sakyo-ku
606-8507 Kyoto, Japan

KENJI KAWATE, M.D.
Department of Orthopedic surgery
Nara Medical University
840 Shijo-cho, Kashihara
634-8522 Nara, Japan

HARTMUTH KIEFER, M.D., PHD
Department of Orthopaedic
and Trauma Surgery
Lukas Hospital
Hindenburgstraße 56
32257 Buende, Germany

HEE-JOONG KIM, M.D.
Department of Orthopedic Surgery
Seoul National University Hospital
28 Yongon-dong, Chongno-gu
110-744 Seoul, Korea

SHIN-YOON KIM, M.D.
Department of Orthopedic Surgery
Kyungpook National University Hospital
50 Samduk-2ga, Chung-Gu
700-721 Daegu, Korea

SUNG-KON KIM, M.D.
Department of Orthopedic Surgery
Korea University Anam Hospital
126-1, 5-ga, Anam-dong, Sungbuk-ku
136-075 Seoul, Korea

YONG-SIK KIM, M.D.
Department of Orthopedic Surgery
St. Mary's Hospital
The Catholic University of Korea
62 Yoido-dong, Youngdeungpo-ku
150-110 Seoul, Korea

YOUNG-HO KIM, M.D.
Department of Orthopedic Surgery
Hanyang University Kuri Hospital
249-1 Gyomun-dong, Guri-si
471-701 Gyunggido, Korea

YOUNG-HOO KIM, M.D.
The Joint Replacement Center of Korea
at Ewha Womans University
Dong Dae Mun Hospital, 70
ChongRo 6-Ga, ChongRo-Gu
110-783 Seoul, Korea

YOUNG-MIN KIM, M.D.
Department of Orthopedic Surgery
Seoul National University Bundang Hospital
Gumi-dong 300, Bundang-gu
Seongnam-si
463-707 Gyeonggi-do, Korea

KARL KNAHR, M.D.
Orthopedic Hospital Vienna - Speising
Speisingerstrasse 109
1130 Vienna, Austria

KYUNG-HOI KOO, M.D.
Department of Orthopedic Surgery
Seoul National University Hospital
28 Yongon-dong, Chongno-gu
110-744 Seoul, Korea

MEINHARD KUNTZ
CeramTec AG
Fabrikstrasse 23 - 29
73207 Plochingen, Germany

SOON-YONG KWON, M.D.
Department of Orthopedic Surgery
St. Mary's Hospital
The Catholic University of Korea
62 Yoido-dong, Youngdeungpo-ku
150-110 Seoul, Korea

JEAN-YVES LAZENNEC, M.D., PHD
Groupe Hospitalier La Pitié Salpetrière
Pavillon Gaston Cordier
83 bd de l'Hôpital
75013 Paris, France

MYUNG-CHUL LEE, M.D.
Department of Orthopedic Surgery
Seoul national University Hospital
28 Yongon-dong, Jongno-gu
110-744 Seoul, Korea

JOONG-MYUNG LEE, M.D.
Department of Orthopedic Surgery
National Medical Center
243 Euljiro Joong-gu
100-799 Seoul, Korea

SANG-SOO LEE, M.D.
Orthopedic Surgery
Hallym University
Chuncheon Sacred Heart Hospital
153 Kyo-dong, Chuncheon
200-704 Gangwon, Korea

SOO-HO LEE, M.D.
Department of Orthopedic Surgery
Asan Medical Center
388-1 Pungnap-2dong, Songpa-gu
138-736 Seoul, Korea

ROBERT LEGENSTEIN, M.D.
Orthopaedic Clinic
Hospital Wiener Neustadt
Corvinusring 3-5
2700 Wiener Neustadt, Austria

ROBERT G. MIDDLETON, MA, FRCS, ORTH
Royal Bournemouth Hospital
Castle Lane East
Bournemouth
Dorset BH7 7DW, UK

BYUNG-WOO MIN, M.D.
Department of Orthopaedic Surgery
Keimyung University, Dongsan Hospital
194 Dongsan-dong, Joong-gu
700-712 Daegu, Korea

WOLFRAM MITTELMEIER, M.D.
Department of Orthopaedics
University of Rostock
Ulmenstrasse 44/45
18055 Rostock, Germany

MOHAMMAD AZIZBAIG MOHAJER, M.D.
LKH-Stolzalpe
Department of Orthopaedics
8852 Stolzalpe, Austria

KYOUNG HO MOON, M.D.
Department of Orthopedic Surgery
Inha University Hospital, 7-206
3dr ST, Sinheung-dong, Jung-gu
400-711 Incheon, Korea

JÜRG OEHY
Zimmer Orthopedics
Sulzer Allee 8 / PO Box
8404 Winterthur, Switzerland

HINOROBU OONISHI, M.D., PHD
H. Oonishi Memorial Joint Replacement
Institute 4-48
Tominaga Hospital
1-4-48, Minato-Machi
Naniwa-Ku Osaka-Shi 556-0017, Japan

THOMAS PANDORF
CeramTec AG
Medical Products Division
Fabrikstrasse 23 - 29
73207 Plochingen, Germany

MYUNG-SIK PARK, M.D.
Department of Orthopedic Surgery
Jeonbuk National University Hospital
Geumam 2-dong, Deokjin-gu, Jeonju-si
561-712 Jeollabuk-do, Korea

SANG-WON PARK, M.D.
Department of Orthopedic Surgery
Korea University Anam Hospital
Anam-dong 5-ga 126-1, Seongbuk-gu
136-705 Seoul, Korea

YOUN-SOO PARK, M.D.
Department of Orthopedic Surgery
Samsung Medical Center
50 Ilwon-Dong, Kangnam-Ku
135-710 Seoul, Korea

GIUSEPPE PEZZOTTI
Kyoto Institute of Technology
Ceramics Physics Laboratory &
Research Institute for Nanoscience
Hashigami-cho
Matsugasaki, Sakyo-ku
Kyoto shi, Kyoto 606-8585, Japan

GERALD PFLÜGER, M.D.
Evangelisches Krankenhaus Wien
Hans Sachs Gasse 10 - 12
1180 Vienna, Austria

CHRISTINE SCHULTZE
Institute for Biomedical Engineering
University of Rostock
Ernst-Heydemann-Strasse 6
18057 Rostock, Germany

WON-YONG SHON, M.D.
Department of Orthopedic Surgery
Korea University Guro Hospital
Guro 2-dong, Guro-gu
152-703 Seoul, Korea

LUCIAN B. SOLOMON, M.D.
Royal Adelaide Hospital
Department of Orthopaedics
Adelaide SA 500, Australia

ALDO TONI, M.D.
First Department of Orthopaedic Surgery
Medical Technology Laboratory
Istituti Ortopedici Rizzoli
Via di Barbiano 1/10
40136 Bologna, Italy

KARL-HEINZ WIDMER, M.D.
Kantonsspital Schaffhausen
Geissbergstrasse 81
8208 Schaffhausen, Switzerland

YE-YEON WON, M.D.
Department of Orthopedic Surgery
Ajou University School of Medicine
San 5, Wonchond-Dong
Youngtong-gu, Suwon city
443-749 Kyung-Ki-Do, Korea

SOO-JAE YIM, M.D.
Department of Orthopedic Surgery
College of Medicine
University of Soonchunhyang
Bucheon Hospital
1174 Jung-Dong Wonmi-Gu Bucheon-Si
420-767 Gyeonggi-Do, Korea

MYUNG-CHUL YOO, M.D.
East-West Neo Medical Center
Kyunghee University
Sangil-dong 149, Gangdong-gu
134-727 Seoul, Korea

TAEK-RIM YOON, M.D.
Center for Joint Disease
Chonnam National University
Hwasun Hospital
160 Ilsimri, Hwasuneup, Hwasungun
519-809 Jeonnam, Korea

TZAI-CHIN YU, M.D.
Department of Orthopedics
Buddhist TzuChi MedicalCenter
707, Sec.3, Chung-Yang Rd.
Hualien, Taiwan

Scientific Committee

JUN-DONG CHANG, M.D.
Department of Orthopaedic Surgery
Hangang Sacred Heart Hospital
Hallym University College of Medicine
94-200 Youngdungpo-dong
Youngdungpo-gu
150-719 Seoul, Korea

YONG-SIK KIM, M.D.
Department of Orthopedic Surgery
St. Mary's Catholic University of Korea
62 Yoido-dong, Youngdeungpo-ku
150-713 Seoul, Korea

YOUN-SOO PARK, M.D.
Department of Orthopedic Surgery
Samsung Medical Center
50 Ilwon-Dong, Kangnam-Ku
135-710 Seoul, Korea

PAUL SILBERER
CeramTec AG
Medical Products Division
Fabrikstrasse 23 – 29
73207 Plochingen, Germany

YE-YEON WON, M.D.
Department of Orthopedic Surgery
Ajou University School of Medicine
San 5, Wonchond-Dong
Youngtong-gu, Suwon City
443-749 Kyung-Ki-Do, Korea

SESSION 1A

Tribology

1A.1 Differences and Opportunities of THA in the USA, Asia and Europe

H. Kiefer

Summary

There are several differences for total hip arthroplasty in USA, Asia and Europe. Primary osteoarthritis is the mean indication for hip replacement in Europe and USA, while in Asia secondary osteoarthritis encounters for most hip diseases and elective THA. Different needs for implant sizes have been solved for Asian countries since many developments of the 90s respected the needs for smaller patients and different bone morphology. However, the challenges with younger patients and an increased number of revision surgeries are the same for all orthopaedic surgeons. Consequent result documentation as it is in European hip registers in Scandinavia, is not yet established in other countries. Differences in implant selection and surgeon's preference are still obvious and influenced by education and experience. Different approval processes and the economic environment influence the availability of new implants or material and technology developments.

Introduction

Hip arthroplasty has proven to be a reliable and suitable surgical procedure to return patients back to function [1]. Patient selection, surgical procedures and the use of appropriate implant systems are comparable in many countries with well developed healthcare. Peer-reviewed literature and review articles dealing with country specific aspects of hip arthroplasty [2,3] (others than the USA's) are hardly available. In addition, these articles are disregarded, especially if "only" published in country-specific journals and language [4,5]. Hip registers only exist in some countries, as mentioned above.

However, this overview tries to summarize the differences of hip joint replacement in leading countries of Europe, Asia and the USA. Improved conditions for joint replacement and health care in less developed areas of Eastern Europe, many Asian countries and Middle or South America, are future challenges. Despite all differences, orthopedic communities can learn from each other in order to improve implants, surgical techniques [6] and individual skills [7] for the increasing number of procedures for primary and revision hip arthroplasty [8].

Hip Replacement in Europe, USA and Asia

From a population of 6,100,000 in Europe, 3,800,000 live in the European Union. More than 650,000 hip joint replacements and hip revision surgeries were performed in 2006. The incidence of primary THA and revision was 2.2 per 1000 inhabitants in some countries of Central Europe compared to 1.4 in the USA with a population of 2,910,000 and an estimated 420,000 hip joint arthroplasties. The number of procedures in Asian countries is significantly lower. Independent from the socio-economic aspects mentioned above, the etiology and incidence for hip replacements is different. Japan and Korea show comparable incidence of hip arthroplasty surgeries. Table 1 demonstrates the estimated numbers of hip arthroplasties in 2006 in selected countries and regions.

Country	Population (Millions)	Hip Arthroplasties	Ratio / 100.000 people
Germany	82	190,000	2.2
France	59	100,000	1.7
United Kingdom	60	90,000	1.5
Italy	58	70,000	1.2
Austria and Switzerland	15	32,000	2.1
Benelux	27	40,000	1.5
Scandinavia	24	35,000	1.5
USA	291	420,000	1.4
Japan	127	55,000	0.4
Korea	48	15,000	0.3

Table 1:
Hip replacement procedures and incidence per inhabitant in selected countries.

Different Origins of Implant Design

Experience, education, reimbursement, regulatory conditions and regional market situations all influence the available options of hip implants. There are substantial regional variations in Europe, mainly caused by the surgeons' education and experience, and less by approval restrictions as in the USA and some Asian countries.

Thanks to international well known joint registers in Scandinavia, the amount of different implant systems is reduced compared to other regions in Europe. The Scandinavian countries contributed excellent hip register data surveillance from Sweden since 1979, followed by Norway 1987, Finland 1993 and Denmark 1995. The results of these hip registers supported the use of several leading cemented implant designs. Cementless THA was not used to this extend. At present, there are no comparable hip registers available in Asia, the USA or the European countries with the highest number of implantations (Germany, France, Italy and the United Kingdom). However, improved reporting systems of early implant failures have been established in these countries and the efforts for hip register data collections are ongoing.

The United Kingdom is well known as the origin of classic cemented hip implant designs and recently metal on metal surface replacements. At present, these THA concepts in the UK represent the highest worldwide share of THA therapy. The success of cementless acetabular pressfit components, introduced in the USA more than two decades ago, lead to an increased use of hybrid THA. This is common in many countries with prevalence to cemented hip stems, such as Scandinavia and the UK, but also in many Asian countries.

Central Europe is the origin of contemporary cementless tapered straight stems, introduced in the mid 1980s. The leading European designs were flat and tapered, the bone preparation was similar to the basic principle of the cemented Müller straight stem which was developed in Switzerland. However, most of the USA hip designs from that time were rounded, distally more filling, porous or hydroxyapatite coated. Bone preparation was mostly based on an initial distal reaming procedure.

Many European cementless acetabular implant designs of the 1970s and 1980s were developed as screw cup designs either in conical or spherical shape. Up to the late 1980s, most of these screw cup sockets were used in Europe, until the introduction of cementless pressfit cup designs became more popular. Today, screw cup acetabular implants are only used in a minority of European countries.

The use of ceramic modular heads increased in Europe since this material was introduced and femoral heads were implanted in the mid 1970s in France and Germany. The 28 mm modular metal on metal THA was introduced in the late 1980s in Switzerland followed by larger head metal on metal THA in the 1990s.

In the 1980s, the development of specific Asian implant designs started for cemented THA, in the 1990s for cementless implants with a greater focus on the morphological differences and specific sizing needs for smaller patients' anatomy.

Differences in Ethnology and Morphology

Primary osteoarthritis is the mean indication for hip replacement in Europe and the USA while in Asia secondary osteoarthritis encounters for most hip diseases. The incidets of hip fractures are comparable in many countries, but the preferred therapy and surgical treatment differs. Dysplastic deformities play a major role for THA in Japan and avascular femoral necrosis in Korea. The aging population in Asian countries leads to a higher risk for hip fractures requiring increasing hip arthroplasties compared to the lower increase of indications for elective total hip replacement. The aging population in western countries increases the demand for THA in primary osteoarthritis. As the total number of implanted hip joints in the western world is rising, the risk of periprosthetic fractures in elderly people is getting more and more challenging. This is an essential part of the increasing number of hip revisions.

Differences in the morphological anatomy of Asian and Caucasian population are well known. Today many implants are size adapted towards smaller implants, different CCD angles and femoral offset characteristics. However, smaller bone morphology in Asian countries differs according to ethnology and regions. Therefore, the so-called standard western hip implants are also used and are necessary to cover at least all the cases with appropriately sized implant components. Size limits of femoral components limit the possibilities of modular hip revision systems as the material strength of some modular couplings decrease with size. Even if the widespread use of cementless reconstructive revision implants is somehow at a beginning phase in Asia, options for implant sizing for revision procedures can be improved.

Implants designed for the Asian population are also beneficial for patients in Europe and the USA. Western patients cover the complete etiology of indications and surgeons appreciate the availability of smaller implants for dysplastic and narrow bone conditions. Heavy patients and high BMI characterize the daily THA routine in the western world and the trend of increasing weight is ongoing. This trend is also reported in Asia. Current discussions for gender adapted implant components add more parameters to the so called "optimal implant design discussion" with even more THA variability and complexity of implant selection.

Differences of Surgical Approaches

As improved implant fixation methods decreased the rate of early revisions due to loosening, early revisions due to instability increased substantially during the same time. Dislocation after primary hip replacement continues to be a prevalent complication which diminishes an otherwise very successful surgical procedure. Improved techniques to perform posterior hip approaches and larger head diameters have decreased dislocation. The use of larger head sizes represents one of the key criteria of current implant selection.

As the head size is dependent on the acetabular cup dimension and not on the material selection for joint articulation, there are obvious differences between the USA, Europe and Asia. The use of ceramic heads for THA is common in Central and Southern Europe, in Japan and Korea, and less common in the USA. Today, metal on metal THA solutions are preferred as high demand options in the UK and USA and are less widespread in Asia. Highly crosslinked polyethylene is used in many countries, mostly in combination with metal heads.

The direct lateral and antero-lateral approach in supine patient position is very common in Central Europe and has shown lower dislocation rates. In the USA and Asia, lateral approaches are performed in the lateral decubitus position but in these countries and some other European countries the posterior approach is the golden standard.

Preferences for different approaches were recently influenced by the introduction of less invasive surgical techniques. Under this aspect, the usage of the posterior approach seems to decline slowly. Also, the direct anterior approach has slowly spread from its origin in France to the USA, Japan and Germany. However, lighter weight Asian patients allow for this minimal invasive surgical THA technique without additional hardware on the surgical table. The author prefers this THA approach by using a special extension device.

Challenge Hip Revision

Although most patients experience a success rate higher than 90% after total hip arthroplasty, others require revision surgery within the first 5 years. Some of these failures could be avoided if all aspects of the complex THA treatment could be considered. Quality aspects, patient behavior and other individual and case specific circumstances influence the outcome in addition to the choice of implant components.

Many attempts are made to improve the outcome for younger patients with new implant design and the significant improvement of hip articulation. The obvious trend to reduce patients' age for the first THA surgery might work against patients' expectation and long term results. Direct-to-patient advertising has become an influential factor in all countries and only the direct communication between surgeons and patients can influence patients' demands and surgeons' recommendations.

Revision of implant components with severe bone loss represents the most challenging problem associated with joint reconstruction. As the burden of hip revision interventions is mostly given as a percentage of all reconstructive hip interventions, the growing number of cases and individual patients' fates should not be underestimated. The number of revision interventions is reported at a level of 15% of all reconstructive hip interventions and seems to be at a comparable level in many countries. With the absolute increasing number of patients who have primary or multiple revision hip arthroplasties, the additional number of experienced surgeons and hospital resources will challenge the future of THA also.

Challenge Younger Patients

In all countries the preservation of muscle and bone tissue during THA intervention is challenging, at least independent from patients' age and indications.

In order to find dedicated implant solutions for an increasing number of younger and more active patients, contemporary resurfacing implants have been introduced in Europe. These are emerging to the USA, but are rarely used in Asian countries. Based on the experience of McMinn and Amstutz, metal on metal technology has been used since the early 1990s. Potential disadvantages of surface replacements are the risk of femoral head fractures, contraindications of metal on metal material, the unknown long-term fate of the increased rate of circulating metal ions, and limitations in some indications of secondary osteoarthritis. Surface replacement is appropriate for primary hip osteoarthritis

The proven concept of cementless proximal implant fixation aims for the treatment of younger patients, too. Different shorter hip stem designs are in a status of early clinical evaluation. Except for the reported result of Morrey, no clinical data is available for cementless shorter hip stem implant designs yet. Despite the fact that the most popular short hip stem was developed in the USA, these implants are mainly used in Germany, Italy and some other European countries today. Short hip stems also have potential disadvantages as the implant positioning might be different from straight standard stems. Varus alignment might cause unexpected periprosthetic bone remodeling and implant failure.

In Asia, the high incidence of secondary osteoarthritis limits indications for shorter hip stems especially in dysplastic and narrow femoral canal and valgus conditions. Limited femoral head necrosis without involvement of the femoral canal is no contraindication for shorter hip stems, as it is the case for most surface replacements.

Challenge Surgery Procedures

Beside all efforts to improve implants and materials, the performance of the surgical procedure is a key factor of success for the surgeon, his team and the patient's outcome. This aspect remains a challenge every day, in every surgery, and for every decision to indicate a hip replacement procedure.

The number of interventions in a hospital, a department and at least for the individual surgeon has been discussed and will be a subject of the future, when increased numbers of joint replacements are expected. This aspect is present everywhere where joint replacement is performed.

The use of navigation technology supports implant positioning for the acetabular component and recently also for the femoral implant. Hip navigation has followed the developments of knee navigation and is also useful in less invasive hip surgery procedures. However, THA navigation is much easier in supine patient positioning, and more information is needed for an optimal alignment for individual patient anatomy conditions. This seems to be the major reason that hip navigation is much more common in countries where supine patient position is selected for THA.

Conclusion

At least most so-called current trends or new developments in hip replacement are found in European countries and to a smaller extent in the USA or Asia. Different patient needs in Asia, and a strong economic and approval environment in the USA influence the situation of hip reconstruction. In Germany, most new hip arthroplasty procedures have been introduced, as the German health system allows for the use of all commercially available and CE approved implants for hip replacement. This leads to the availability of many implant options for the majority of patients.

References

1. Ethgen O, Bruyere O, Richy F, Dardennes C, Reginster JY. Health-related quality of life in total hip and total knee arthroplasty. A qualitative and systematic review of the literature. J Bone Joint Surg Am. 2004 May;86-A(5):963-74.
2. Sanfilippo JA, Austin MS. Implants for total hip arthroplasty. Expert Rev Med Devices. 2006 Nov;3(6):769-76.
3. Rosenberg AG. Fixation for the millennium: the hip. J Arthroplasty. 2002 Jun;17(4 Suppl 1):3-5.
4. Effenberger H, Imhof M, Richolt J, Rehart S. [Cement-free hip cups. Current status][Article in German] Orthopade. 2004 Jun;33(6):733-50; quiz 751.
5. Effenberger H, Imhof M, Witzel U, Rehart S. [Cementless stems of the hip. Current status] [Article in German] Orthopade. 2005 May;34(5):477-500.
6. Zhan C, Kaczmarek R, Loyo-Berrios N, Sangl J, Bright RA.Incidence and short-term outcomes of primary and revision hip replacement in the United States. J Bone Joint Surg Am. 2007 Mar;89(3):526-33.
7. Katz JN, Losina E, Barrett J, Phillips CB, Mahomed NN, Lew RA, Guadagnoli E, Harris WH, Poss R, Baron JA. Association between hospital and surgeon procedure volume and outcomes of total hip replacement in the United States medicare population. J Bone Joint Surg Am. 2001 Nov;83-A(11):1622-9.
8. Kurtz S, Ong K, Lau E, Mowat F, Halpern M. Projections of primary and revision hip and knee arthroplasty in the United States from 2005 to 2030. J Bone Joint Surg Am. 2007 Apr;89(4): 780-5.

1A.2 Influence of the Wear-Couple and Patient Activity on Linear Wear in Total Hip Replacement

Ch. Hendrich, N. Wollmerstedt, S. Goebel and J. M. Martell

In total hip replacement different factors have a major impact on wear behaviour and long-term durability. Beside the wear-couple the influence of patient activity is relatively undefined. Aim of this studies was to examine the wear behaviour of alumina heads in combination with conventional polyethylene (PE) (n=99) vs. CoCr heads (n=109), the wear behaviour of alumina heads in combination with highly-crosslinked PE (n=70), and the influence of patient activity in the groups with alumina heads. Linear wear was analyzed using Martell's method and activity was assessed using electronic step-watch monitors. Compared to CoCr heads the use of alumina significantly reduced linear wear. A further reduction was observed with the combination of alumina and highly-crosslinked PE after a certain period of higher wear during bedding-in. In spite of being nearly 20 years younger the activity in the patients with the highly-crosslinked PE differed only about 20% compared to the patients with conventional PE. In conclusion the selection of the wear-couple has a significant influence on linear wear while patient activity in our study groups was in the same magnitude.

Introduction

In total hip replacement polyethylene wear with its associated pelvic and femoral osteolysis has been proven to limit the longevity of modern type arthroplasty [4,10,22,23,25]. Several prosthetic and patient factors have been shown to influence the amount of polyethylene wear [1,8,11,18]. Today most studies try to focus on one particular effect, e.g. the sterilization process of polyethylene. A comprehensive view which factor contributes to what extent is still missing.

When factors influencing wear are discussed there are stronger and weaker factors. The strongest prosthetic factor is definitely the wear couple. Other factors prosthetice design, implant position (difficult to measure), femoral offset, implantation technique etc. are difficult to show to have any influence unless catastrophic failures of an implant has an extraordinary strong effect, e.g. the Hylamer series or third-body-wear of additional hardware.

The strongest patient-related factor is patient activity. However patient activity is the most difficult factor to describe. Patient weight and patient age have shown conflicting results. Other patient-related factors like range-of-motion and lifestyle are supposed to have minor influence or are extremely difficult to assess.

Also the results of different studies are hardly comparable. There are different experimental systems (e.g. Livermore's method) and different ways to report results. New digital measuring methods for analyzing wear made it possible to evaluate a high number of hip prosthesis in a short time and with high accuracy. With the method of Martell a repeatability coefficient of 0.004 mm for the same and 0.006 mm for different observers. [13] However the modern software systems can be used in different conditions and results may be interpreted in different ways. Another experimental drawback may be limited by patient numbers in some studies. Altogether if different factors influencing wear shall be discussed, a similar experimental setup, sufficient patient numbers and a system to describe patient activity is needed.

In this book chapter we highlight three clinical studies of our group which have been conducted using the same system. In study I the effect of 28 mm CoCr ball heads is compared to that of 28 mm BIOLOX heads. Study II compares the effect of crosslinking polyethylene in conjunction with 28 mm BIOLOX heads to the results of study I. In study III the measurement of patient activity in different age and patient groups is reported.

From the comparison of the results we try to discuss the strength of the most important prosthetic and patient-related factors on polyethylene wear.

Study I – CoCr vs. BIOLOX®

Alumina ceramic femoral heads were introduced in the early seventies. Ceramic femoral heads have been shown to be harder than metal ones, which makes them more resistant to damage by third body wear particles. Additionally, ceramic bearing surfaces have increased wetability, which improves lubrication and decreases friction and wear [7,9]. Unfortunately, the literature has few clinical studies investigating the wear performance of alumina on polyethylene. The few available studies are show both, reduction and an increase in wear [2,21].

A retrospective series of patients with type I and II of Harris-Galante (Zimmer) with either 28 mm BIOLOX or CoCr femoral heads were analyzed for linear polyethylene wear using a computerized edge detection technique (Fig. 1) [13]. The conventional UHMWE-poly was gamma-in-air irradiated. 109 CoCr implants were compared to 89 hips with BIOLOX-heads.

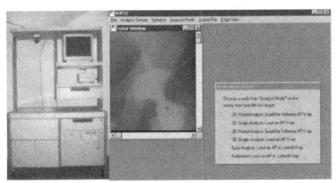

Figure 1:
12-bit CCD-Scanner and the method of Martell [13] for clinical wear measurement.

In both groups there were certain demographic differences (e.g. the BIOLOX-patients was significantly older (p < 0.0001), had an higher body-mass-index (p = 0.001) and osteoarthritis was more prevalent (72% vs. 60%) among the alumina patients. However there was no statistical influence on the linear wear rate of one of those demographic factors in both patient groups. The linear rate of wear among the CoCr metal bearings was 0.14 ± 0.11 mm per year (Fig. 2). The alumina heads had an annual wear rate of 0.088 ± 0.11 mm (Fig. 3). The Mann-Whitney-U-test showed significant difference between the two groups (p = 0.0102).

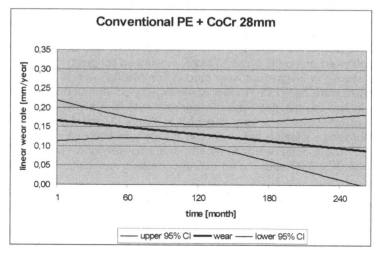

Figure 2:
Regression analysis of the linear wear rate of conventional PE in combination with 28mm CoCr heads over time.

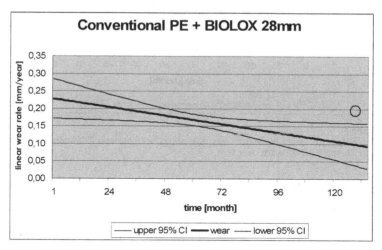

Figure 3:
Regression analysis of the linear wear rate of conventional PE in combination with 28mm BIOLOX® heads over time.

Study II – Crosslinked Polyethylene

In total hip replacement one of the most promising developments during the last years was the introduction of new types of polyethylene (PE) [4]. The use of irradiation in combination with heat treatment results in highly cross-linked polyethylenes with no measurable wear under *in vitro* conditions [14]. The clinical results are limited to short-sterm studies yet which were performed in combination with metal femoral heads. Already in the 80ies one study with irradiated PE in combination with alumina femoral heads was performed showing reduced wear rates [24]. The effect of the combination of the new highly crosslinked PE with alumina heads has not been investigated, yet.

The linear wear rates of two groups of patients with primary total hip arthroplasty was investigated using the identical method like in study I. In the crosslinked group (58 patients) highly crosslinked Longevity® (Zimmer, Warsaw, IN, USA) liners in Trilogy-cups were used in combination with 28 mm BIOLOX® heads. Results were compared to that of the BIOLOX-patients of study I (Fig. 3).

To illustrate the decrease of wear rate over time the regression for the linear wear rate over time are depicted in Figure 3 and Figure 4. Also the 95% confidence intervals are shown. In the crosslinked-PE group the 0.1 mm/year wear rate is achieved at 53 months. Using conventional PE in combination with 28mm BIOLOX® heads the 0.1 mm/year treshold is calculated at 129 months.

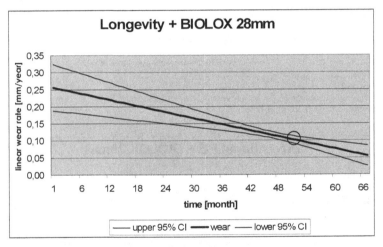

Figure 4:
Regression analysis of the linear wear rate of highly crosslinked PE in combination with 28mm BIOLOX® heads over time.

Study III – patient activity

Hip simulator analyses show that polyethylene wear is predominantly governed by the number of load cycles per year [17,18]. The standardized ISO-testing for artificial joints considers 1 million load cycles per year. In a study performed in the US, the rate of individual activity showed a range from 395 to 17718 cycles per day [19]. One American study found an average of 5275 cycles per day (range 1737 to 11805 cycles) of patients with a mean age of 72 years, which showed an average of 1.9 million load cycles per year [18]. The aim of this study was to measure the activity of patients with osteoarthritis of the hip pre- and postoperatively with an electronic pedometer in different patient groups. For representative results all patients had to wear the StepWatch for 5 to 7 days (Fig. 5, 6).

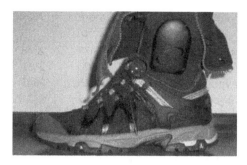

Figure 5:
StepWatch® Activity Monitor (Firma CymaTech, Mountlake Terrace, WA).

StepWatch Activity Statistics

Step Activity as Step Rates Per Minute

Day	Date	Total	Step incl.	Min. Incl.	Min. None	Min. Low	Min. Med	Min. Hi	Step Low	Step Med	Step Hi
8 incl.	Average	5821	5464	1256	71,12%	17,46%	9,84%	1,57%	1403	3071	990
Thu	27.6.02	4290	0	0	0	0	0	0	0	0	0
Fri	28.6.02	3127	906	529	438	69	21	1	357	502	47
Sat	29.6.02	6191	6191	1440	1079	183	166	12	1296	4309	586
Sun	30.6.02	5587	4953	880	519	228	121	12	1576	2847	530
Mon	1.7.02	7502	7502	1440	893	340	197	10	2327	4728	447
Tue	2.7.02	2350	2350	1440	1209	177	51	3	1006	1205	139
Wed	3.7.02	7611	7611	1440	931	330	138	41	1990	3488	2133
Thu	4.7.02	7875	7875	1440	1074	169	128	69	980	3313	3582
Fri	5.7.02	6330	6330	1440	1004	259	167	10	1692	4182	456
Sat	6.7.02	54	0	0	0	0	0	0	0	0	0
Sun	7.7.02	0	0	0	0	0	0	0	0	0	0
Mon	8.7.02	1	0	0	0	0	0	0	0	0	0

Figure 6:
Example of a StepWatch® daily activity count.

The following patient groups were examined

- patients with osteoarthritis of the hip and scheduled for THR in 1 to 4 months, 329 days analyzed, mean age 65 years (range 50 to 79)
- after THR and a follow-up of 1 year, 173 analyzed days, mean age 67 years (52 to 80)
- after a follow-up of 4 years, 414 days analyzed, mean age 59 years (range 37 to 77)
- after a follow-up of 10 years, 433 days analyzed, mean age 69 years (range 48 to 86).

Patients suffering from osteoarthritis had the lowest activity. One year after surgery and even more 4 years after surgery the number of steps increased significantly. After a follow-up of 10-years the number of steps decreased again (Table 1).

Patient group	Mean steps	SD	Steps/ year (calculated)	Days analyzed	Variance analysis
pre-surgery	5479	2348	1.928.608	329	
1-year post surgery	6020	2653	2.119.040	173	p < 0,001
4-years post surgery	6565	2645	2.310.880	414	
10-years post surgery	5159	2421	1.815.968	433	

Table 1

To examine the influence of age the patients post-surgery were grouped (Table 2). Using a variance analysis for each ten years difference in age between 15 and 20% decrease in activity were found.

Age groups of patients post surgery	Mean steps	SD	Difference per age decade	Days analyzed	Variance analysis
51 - 60 years	7037	2892		266	
61 - 70 years	5934	2464	15,7%	380	p <0,001
71 - 80 years	4738	2057	20,1%	271	

Table 2

Regarding the question to what extent the activity of the patients is influenced by their age regression analyses demonstrated that in patients after surgery 7% of the activity is determined by age and in patients prior to surgery 14.4% (Fig. 7, 8).

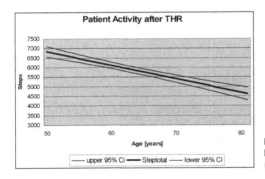

Figure 7:
Regression analysis of patient activity (Stepwatch®) after THR vs. patient age.

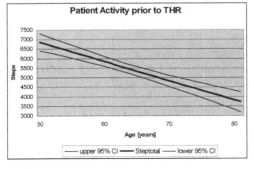

Figure 8:
Regression analysis of patient activity (Stepwatch®) prior to THR vs. patient age.

Discussion

In this book chapter we highlight three clinical studies of our group which have been conducted using the same system of wear measurement. From the comparison of the results we try to discuss the strength of the most important prosthetic and patient-related factors on polyethylene wear.

From the prosthetic factors the wear couple is thought to the most important factor governing polyethylene wear. In study I the effect of 28 mm CoCr ball heads was compared to that of 28 mm BIOLOX heads. Compared to the CoCr metal bearings (0.14 ± 0.11 mm per year) in the alumina group a significantly reduced annual wear rate of 0.088 ± 0.11 mm was found. Previous studies with 32 mm heads had found conflicting results. While the German experience using conventional measuring methods [26] stated a similar reduction an US-study found nearly no difference between CoCr and alumina [20]. For 28 mm heads to our knowledge no study comparing both heads with adequate patient numbers is published, yet. As mentioned earlier the systems of wear measurement and even more the way of reporting results differs and makes the comparison of study results difficult. In most studies a steady-state wear-rate after different times of service is reported to avoid the influence of the bedding-in period. True long-term results using modern measurement systems are missing so far. If results are depicted as regression lines the influence of follow-up is obvious. The wear-rate seems to decrease constantly. This makes comparison of results even more confusing especially when comparing new wear couples with conventional ones. In Study II the effect of crosslinking polyethylene in conjunction with 28 mm BIOLOX heads was compared to the results of study I. We demonstrated that the mean linear wear rates declined over a 5-year period. The regression analysis showed an earlier reduction of wear compared with the groups of conventional PE. A linear wear-rate of 0.1 mm/y is observed after 52 months usning crosslinked PE, and after 126 months for conventional PE vs. alumina and after 240 months with CoCr heads. Meanwhile some short- and mid-term results for different highly crosslinked UHMWPEs are available. After different follow-up times of >2 years various crosslinked PEs have shown reduced wear rates compared to conventional ones [3,5,12]. However all studies so far have used metal heads.

The most important patient-related factor for wear is activity. Activity is always mentioned when results are difficult to explain. The most favorized concept is that of Schmalzried et al.(18) In this concept the patient acts like a wear simulator in which a certain number of steps results in a specific wear rate. Consqently the wear-rates are normalized to a model patient with a given activity [6]. For the measurement of activity dedicated accelerometers (StepWatch®) were used. The same method was used in our study. Our results show that the mean activity of different patient groups varies significantly. We found that the activity of the preoperative patients and the patients 10 years after surgery was only 1.8 million load cycles per year in each group and therefore lower compared to the load cycles of the group 4-year after surgery, which were 2.4 million cycles per year. All patient groups exceeded the generally accepted test standard for total joint replacement of 1 million load cycles per year by far. Also in a study by Schmalzried et al., the average load cycles of patients after THR and a mean age of 72 years were 1.9 million per year [16]. Most other authors [15,20] use the age as a surrogate parameter for activity. However the correlation of age to wear is weak and varies in different studies. We therefore analyzed our results in different age groups. Generally there is a decrease in activity with increasing age. As a rule of thumb for each decade the activity decreases between 15 and 20%. In contrast the regression analysis shows that age contributes only to 7% in postoperative patients and to 14% in patients with osteoarthritis to their activity. The use of age for the description of patient activity therefore is not sufficient.

Taken together different wear couples show extreme differences in their wear behaviour. With the use of the same cup and an identical measurement system the strongest reduction of the linear wear-rate can be obtained by the use of alumina instead of a CoCr head. A further reduction may be obtained by crosslinking of polyethylene. All wear couples show a decrease of wear over time which has not been investigated extensively so far. It is tempting to speculate that this is due a decreased activity of the patients. In fact we were able to show that patient activity decreases with time. However this explanation might be to simple. Up to now it has never been shown that a reduced activity results in decreased wear. A study that a patient behaves like a wear-simulator is still missing. It is also unclear to which extent the activity in comparison to the wear couple contributes to the wear-rate. Looking on the facts from another point of view could act as a future work hypothesis: In Germany between the age of 60 and 70 the mean patient activity decreases by about 15% within this decade. During this time the standard deviation is relatively constant. Given this as a baseline the wear-rate can mainly be changed by the wear couple in an otherwise similar prosthesis. Changing the head from metal to alumina or crosslinking the PE make the biggest differences.

References

1. Bankston AB, Faris PM, Keating EM and Ritter MA. Polyethylene wear in total hip arthroplasty in patient-matched groups. A comparison of stainless steel, cobalt chrome, and titanium-bearing surfaces. J Arthroplasty 8: 315-322, 1993.
2. Devane PA and Horne JG. Assessment of polyethylene wear in total hip replacement. Clin Orthop Relat Res 59-72, 1999.
3. Digas G, Karrholm J, Thanner J, Malchau H and Herberts P. Highly cross-linked polyethylene in cemented THA: randomized study of 61 hips. Clin Orthop Relat Res 126-138, 2003.
4. Harris WH. The problem is osteolysis. Clin Orthop 311: 46-53, 1995.
5. Heisel C, Silva M and Schmalzried TP. In vivo wear of bilateral total hip replacements: conventional versus crosslinked polyethylene. Arch Orthop Trauma Surg 125: 555-557, 2005.
6. Heisel C, Silva M, Skipor AK, Jacobs JJ and Schmalzried TP. The relationship between activity and ions in patients with metal-on-metal bearing hip prostheses. J Bone Joint Surg Am 87: 781-787, 2005.
7. Izquierdo-Avino RJ, Siney PD and Wroblewski BM. Polyethylene wear in the Charnley offset bore acetabular cup. A radiological analysis. J Bone Joint Surg Br 78: 82-84, 1996.
8. Jasty M, Goetz DD, Bragdon CR, Lee KR, Hanson AE, Elder JR and Harris WH. Wear of polyethylene acetabular components in total hip arthroplasty. An analysis of one hundred and twenty-eight components retrieved at autopsy or revision operations. J Bone Joint Surg Am 79: 349-358, 1997.
9. Jazrawi LM, Kummer FJ and DiCesare PE. Alternative bearing surfaces for total joint arthroplasty. J Am Acad Orthop Surg 6: 198-203, 1998.

10. Joshi AB, Markovic L and Ilchmann T. Polyethylene wear and calcar osteolysis. Am J Orthop 28: 45-48, 1999.
11. Livermore J, Ilstrup D and Morrey B. Effect of femoral head size on wear of the polyethylene acetabular component. J Bone Joint Surg Am 72: 518-528, 1990.
12. Martell J, Berkson E, Berger R and Jacobs J. Comparison of two and three-dimensional computerized polyethylene wear analysis after total hip arthroplasty. J Bone Joint Surg Am 85: 1111-1117, 2003.
13. Martell JM and Berdia S. Determination of polyethylene wear in total hip replacements with use of digital radiographs. J Bone Joint Surg Am 79: 1635-1641, 1997.
14. Muratoglu OK, Greenbaum ES, Bragdon CR, Jasty M, Freiberg AA and Harris WH. Surface analysis of early retrieved acetabular polyethylene liners: a comparison of conventional and highly crosslinked polyethylenes. J Arthroplasty 19: 68-77, 2004.
15. Orishimo KF, Claus AM, Sychterz CJ and Engh CA. Relationship between polyethylene wear and osteolysis in hips with a second-generation porous-coated cementless cup after seven years of follow-up. J Bone Joint Surg Am 85-A: 1095-1099, 2003.
16. Schmalzried TP, Shepherd EF, Dorey EJ, Jackson WJ, Rosa M, Fa'vae F, McKellop HA, McClung CD, Martell J, Moreland JR and Amstutz HC. Wear Is a Function of Use, Not Time. Clin Orthop Relat Res 381: 36-46, 2004.
17. Schmalzried TP and Callaghan JJ. Wear in total hip and knee replacements. J Bone Joint Surg Am 81: 115-136, 1999.
18. Schmalzried TP, Shepherd EF, Dorey FJ, Jackson WO, dela RM, Fa'vae F, McKellop HA, McClung CD, Martell J, Moreland JR and Amstutz HC. The John Charnley Award. Wear is a function of use, not time. Clin Orthop Relat Res 36-46, 2000.
19. Schmalzried TP, Szuszczewicz ES, Northfield MR, Akizuki KH, Frankel RE, Belcher G and Amstutz HC. Quantitative assessment of walking activity after total hip or knee replacement. J Bone Joint Surg Am 80: 54-59, 1998.
20. Sychterz CJ, Orishimo KF and Engh CA. Sterilization and polyethylene wear: clinical studies to support laboratory data. J Bone Joint Surg Am 86-A: 1017-1022, 2004.
21. Urban JA, Garvin KL, Boese CK, Bryson L, Pedersen DR, Callaghan JJ and Miller RK. Ceramic-on-polyethylene bearing surfaces in total hip arthroplasty. Seventeen to twenty-one-year results. J Bone Joint Surg Am 83-A: 1688-1694, 2001.
22. Wan Z and Dorr LD. Natural history of femoral focal osteolysis with proximal ingrowth smooth stem implant. J Arthroplasty 11: 718-725, 1996.
23. Willert HG, Bertram H and Buchhorn GH. Osteolysis in alloarthroplasty of the hip. The role of ultra-high molecular weight polyethylene wear particles. Clin Orthop Relat Res 95-metal-polyethylene in clinical trials. Clin Orthop Relat Res 86-94, 1992.
24. Wroblewski BM. Direction and rate of socket wear in Charnley low-friction arthroplasty. J Bone Joint Surg Br 67: 757-761, 1985.
25. Zicat B, Engh CA and Gokcen E. Patterns of osteolysis around total hip components inserted with and without cement. J Bone Joint Surg Am 77: 432-439, 1995.
26. Zichner LP and Willert HG. Comparison of alumina-polyethylene and metal-polyethylene in clinical trials. Clin Orthop Relat Res 86-94, 1992.

1A.3 Roles of Cellular and Molecular Targets of Wear Debris in Periprosthetic Osteolysis

S.-S. Lee, J.-D. Chang, P. E. Purdue, B. J. Nestor, T. P. Sculco and E. A. Salvati

Wear-generated particulate debris is the main cause of initiating this destructive process. We present recent advances in understanding of how wear debris causes osteolysis in the aspect of cellular and molecular biological levels. Macrophages, the most important cellular target for wear debris, respond to particle challenge in two distinct ways of pro-inflammatory signaling and inhibition of the protective actions of anti-osteoclastogenic cytokines, finally leading to suppression of osteogenic activity as well as increased osteoclast activity. At a molecular level, such alterations of cellular activities occur through MAP kinase, transcription factors including NF-κB, Wnt/β-catenin signaling and cytokine signaling cascades in various kinds of cells.

However, in spite of complex researches concerning periprosthetic osteolysis, no approved treatments are yet available. In addition, research to find new articulation materials that can minimize the production of wear debris is ongoing. Therefore, it will be of immense interest to see what will make rapid progress to the solution of periprosthetic osteolysis in the future.

Introduction

The most common reason for revision THA is aseptic loosening, and a substantial percentage of these failures occur secondary to osteolysis and periprosthetic bone loss [25]. Periprosthetic osteolysis ultimately develops in approximately 20% of patients and in younger patients failure rates of 13% for the femoral component and 34% for the acetabular component have been reported [36]. Osteolysis is initiated by wear debris and corrosion products from prosthetic implants. Wear debris can be generated from various prosthesis components and bone cement. Higher wear rates are seen in patients with osteolysis [13]. Design of implants profoundly can affect the composition, size, and shape of generated particles and influences cellular responses. Therefore choice of implant design may have a substantial impact on the potential for development of osteolysis.

Once macrophages are activated by particulate debris, they secrete various kinds of mediators to incite a complex cascade for osteoclast maturation [15]. Other main cells mainly involved in this process include osteoblast (OB), fibroblast, and osteoclast (OC). Several cytokines and inflammatory mediators are secreted by macrophages and other cells, including tumor necrosis factor (TNF)-α, interleukin (IL)-1β, IL-6, IL-10, and prostaglandins (PG)[10]. Matrix degradative enzymes and chemokines also released [35,61]. Another important critical step for OC differentiation and activation involves Receptor activator of NF-κB ligand (RANKL)-RANK axis for osteoclast precursor (OCPs), resulting in their differentiation and maturation. This article presents novel insights into the current knowledge regarding how wear debris participates in the cellular and molecular level to cause periprosthetic osteolysis.

Cellular Targets of Particles in Periprosthetic Osteolysis

Various kinds of cells have been implicated in the mechanisms of periprosthetic osteolysis in response to wear debris, indicative of a complex network of cellular pathogenesis (Fig.1) [12]. Studies on retrieved implants, animal models, *in vitro* studies on particle bioreactivity, suggest that wear-mediated periprosthetic osteolysis is unlikely to be caused solely by one particular cell type or particulate species, but is rather the cumulative consequence of a number of biological reactions [70].

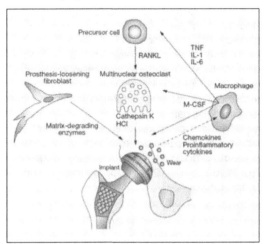

Figure 1:
Wear debris induces interplay between prosthesis-loosening fibroblasts, multinucleated osteoclasts and macrophages. Wear debris particles released at the cement–bone interface attract macrophages, which, in turn, are stimulated to produce proinflammatory mediators and proteolytic enzymes. In particular, RANKL, TNF, IL-1, IL-6, IL-17, and M-CSF mediate the differentiation of myeloid precursor cells into multinucleated osteoclasts, which release cathepsin K and acid and cause resorption lacunae. Mesenchymal cells [prosthesis-loosening fibroblasts] present at the bone surface contribute actively to bone resorption (Courtesy of Dr. Philipp Drees, University Hospital Mainz, Germany).

Macrophages

Recent advances in osteoclast (OC) biology indicated that bone marrow-derived macrophages may play a dual role in osteolysis associated with total joint replacement. Firstly, as the major cell in host defense they respond to particles through cytokine production. Secondly macrophages have a role as precursors for the OCs [33]. Activation of macrophages by particulate debris is a critical event in this process. Particles of 0.3-10.0 μm in diameter are phagocytosed, but cannot be digested by cells [59]. However phagocytosis of particles was not always necessary for induction of the release of TNF-α or IL-6 in macrophages [44]. Recently this phenomenon can be explained with the role of tall-like receptor (TLR). Takaki M *et al.* reported that TLRs on macrophages respond to particle debris in vitro [62]. Once macrophages, cellular orchestrators of osteolysis, are activated by particulate debris, they secrete various kinds of mediators to incite a complex cascade for OC maturation [15].

Cytokines and inflammatory mediators secreted by macrophages of the osteolytic infiltrate include TNF-α, IL-1β, IL-6 and PGs. The specific nature of this response depends on numerous parameters including the composition [26,58], size [22], shape [73], volume, and surface area [59] of wear debris. Macrophages and giant cells in the interfacial membranes of osteolysis patients have also been reported to express RANKL [27], despite the fact that macrophage lineage cells are generally thought not to express RANKL under normal conditions. Expression and secretion of matrix metalloproteinases (MMPs) also are elevated in macrophages exposed to wear debris in vitro [44]. Elevated levels of degradation enzymes in periprosthetic osteolysis tissues were also observed [37]. This array of chemokines, growth factors, pro-inflammatory and anti-inflammatory cytokines, and mediators demonstrate a potent ability of periprosthetic tissues to recruit and stimulate cells capable of propelling osteoclastic bone resorption and fibrous tissue formation [65].

Recently, Sabokbar A et al. reported that human arthroplasty–derived macrophages are capable of osteoclastic differentiation in vitro in the presence of M-CSF and TNF-α [33,52]. Although recruitment of osteoclast precursor (OCP)s from the blood is more important as their source, roles of macrophage as OCPs in the periprosthetic space of osteolysis should be more clarified.

Ability of prosthetic wear debris to induce pro-inflammatory responses in macrophages is widely appreciated, but little is known about the molecular mechanisms involved in particle recognition concerning the cell surface receptors that can interact with wear debris. Role of macrophage complement receptors (CR)-3 in particle up-take has been reported [9,55]. Rakshit DS et al. reported the involvement of opsonization, complement, and integrin receptors, including CR-3 and fibronectin receptors, in PMMA action, and an involvement of scavenger receptors in responses to Ti [49]. It suggests different particles may use different surface receptors. However opsonization is not essential (although it may be involved) in responses of human monocytes and macrophage cell lines to Ti [45,46].

Osteoclast and Pre-Osteoclast

The final cellular consequence of particle action is an excess of OC activity, which results in unchecked bone erosion. Osteoclasts (OCs) are multinucleated cells derived from circulating osteoclast precursor cell (OCPs) of the monocyte/macrophage lineage, and represent the only cell type capable of bone resorption [3]. OCPs are supplied from the periprosthetic space or recruitment from the blood [52]. Wear debris probably increases OCP recruitment to periprosthetic tissues via activation of chemokine (macrophage chemoattractant protein-1, MCP-1; IL-8) expression by macrophages and fibroblasts [14,43,75]. In addition, macrophage lineage cells isolated from these tissues display a greatly increased propensity to differentiate to OCs [52,54].

OCs can be differentiated under two critical cytokines, RANKL and M-CSF. TNF-α also promotes osteoclastogenesis, particularly in states of inflammatory osteolysis such as rheumatoid arthritis and periprosthetic osteolysis. RANKL and TNF-α seem to play roles in the OC activation with collaboration. However periprosthetic osteolysis is a kind of inflammatory osteolysis, researches concerning wear debris induced osteoclastogenesis have focused mainly on TNF-α and IL-1 in the past. Overexpression of TNF-α is sufficient to induce calvarial osteolysis even in the absence of added particles, emphasizing its pro-resorptive characteristics in mice [57]. However, it should be clarified whether these inflammatory cytokines are elevated in end-stage osteolysis, suggesting other mechanisms may be at work [48].

Once differentiated, newly formed OCs polarizes and forms a ruffled membrane that adheres to the bone matrix. This reaction occurs via the αvβ3 integrin, which transmits matrix-derived, cytoskeleton-organizing signals. These integrin-transmitted signals include activation of the associated proteins, c-src, syk, Vav3, and Rho GTPases [66]. Organized cytoskeleton generates an isolated microenvironment between the cell's plasma membrane and bone surface. In this isolated microenvironment, matrix mineral is mobilized by the acidic milieu and lysosomal protease cathepsin K, leading to extensive resorption lacunae.

Cathepsin K is a serine–threonine protease that cleaves the helical and telopeptide regions of collagen at the appropriate pH; the expression of this protease is regulated by RANKL [6]. The production of acid is mediated by osteoclastic H+-ATPase in vacuolar proton pump. As the vacuolar proton pump is structurally distinct from the P-type gastric H+-K+-ATPase, it is not inhibited by the conventional proton-pump inhibitors such as Omeprazole [56]. Molecular targets descried above will be focused soon in the pathogenesis of periprosthetic osteolysis and serve as candidate anti-resorptive therapeutic targets.

Osteoblasts

Research has been limited to in vitro models of osteoblast (OB) cell-particle interactions. PE and metal particles can be phagocytosed by OBs [41]. Particles less than 5 μm can also undergo phagocytosis by mature OBs [18], leading to potential adverse effects on cellular viability, proliferation and function. Wear particles can inhibit bone formation by altering cell differentiation and decreasing matrix synthesis: particles inhibit bone cell viability and proliferation, and down-regulate markers of bone formation at the mRNA and protein level. Addition of PE particles to cultured OB-like cells reduces matrix production, alkaline phosphatase and TGF-β produced by these cells [8]. PMMA particles also reduce OB differentiation of bone marrow osteoprogenitor cells [4]. Metallic particles also decrease expression of collagens by OBs [67,68]. Ti reduces OB viability by inducing apoptosis [47]. However metal and polymer particles in non-toxic doses stimulate pro-inflammatory factor release more than ceramic particles of a similar size [20].

Therefore it is clear that suppressive effects are also dependent on particle size, composition and dosage: different particle types can differentially affect OB proliferation and activity [40]. The size and degree of clumping of particles are also important variables determining the biological response especially in OB. The nanophase [agglomerated] particles were associated with increased cell viability, more normal cellular morphology and spreading compared to conventional particles [23]. Thus, decreasing particle diameter to the nanometer range, which results in particle clumping into a nanophase, may facilitate OB survival.

On the other hand, besides suppressed osteoblastic activity, OBs can also affect on production of RANKL and OPG by particle. OB lineage cells can induce RANKL, OPG, IL-1, TNF, IL-6, IL-11, and TGF-β [28]. UHMWPE increased the release of RANKL from human OB, while OPG were significantly inhibited. There was inductive effect of on the osteoclastogenesis with UHMWPE human OB-conditioned medium. Interestingly these changes could not be observed with treatment of Al_2O_3, indicating wear debris of Al_2O_3 are less active [20,21,23]. Although insufficient attention has been paid to the involvement of OB the cell type responsible for bone formation, more researches should be recommended to delineate the potentially critical role of OBs in particle induced osteolysis.

Mesenchymal Stem Cells and Osteoprogenitors

Mesenchymal stem cell(MSCs) and osteoprogenitors are also profoundly affected by wear particles [12,18]. Differentiation of OBs from MSCs is also down-regulated by Ti particles [69]. PMMA particles also reduce OB differentiation of bone marrow osteoprogenitor cells [4]. Ti and zirconium oxide induce MSC apoptosis [71]. Since MSCs and osteoprogenitors from the bone marrow are the precursors of OBs, the reaction of these cells to wear particles is critical to both initial osseo-integration of implants and ongoing regeneration of the periprosthetic bed [18]. Future studies should delineate the molecular mechanisms by which particles adversely affect MSCs and the bone cell lineage and provide strategies to modulate these effects [18].

Fibroblasts

Fibroblasts are abundant within the interfacial membrane of osteolysis. Particles can also induce production in cultured fibroblasts of pro-inflammatory mediators, collagenase and stromelysin [74], which could contribute to the development of osteolysis, and chemokines, which could contribute to the recruitment of increased numbers of OCPs to periprosthetic tissues [75]. Recent studies report that fibroblasts within the interfacial membrane can express RANKL [31]. Likewise, fibroblasts isolated from arthroplasty membranes of osteolysis patients were able to support generation of OCs from human monocytes [53]. Therefore periprosthetic fibroblasts exposed to wear and/or pro-inflammatory mediators may be a major source of the RANKL required to drive osteoclastogenesis in osteolysis patients.

Lymphocyte

Activated T-cells not only positively (i.e., RANKL) regulate but also negatively (i.e., interferon gamma) control osteoclastogenesis. T-cell derived RANKL plays a central role in inflammatory bone loss. However involvement of lymphocytes in osteolysis remains controversial. Perhaps the strongest evidence for the involvement of lymphocytes in aseptic loosening are two recent reports correlating a metal-specific lymphocyte response to poor implant performance [24] and characterizing lymphocytic infiltration around metal-on-metal arthroplasties [7]. More research will be necessary to determine whether lymphocytes are substantially involved in osteolysis or not.

Molecular Targets in Periprosthetic Osteolysis

Although it is generally accepted that wear debris and activated macrophages have a key role in particle induced osteolysis, molecular pathophysiology of this condition is not well characterized. We will present the molecular target that are responsible for periprosthetic osteolysis and deserve to be a target for research and therapeutic approaches for this devastating complication [12].

Mitogen-Activated Protein (MAP) Kinases

MAP kinases are important kinases for differentiation and growth of all kind of cells. The three major MAP kinase subgroups (p38, ERK, and JNK) also are involved in macrophage and OB for inflammatory response [44,50] and in particle-induction of OCs [1]. JNK pathway is also essential for basal and PMMA-stimulated osteoclastogenesis [72]. In cultured OCPs, Ti and PMMA induce rapid activation of MAP kinase family members to induce pro-inflammatory cytokine induction [50]. In addition, MAP kinases mediate the ability of PMMA and Ti wear debris to induce expression of SOCS3, a suppressor of anti-osteoclastogenic cytokine signaling [50].

p38 inhibition in OCPs protects against inflammatory bone destruction [42]. MAPK also mediate particles induce expression of IL-8 in OB [14]. However when the oral p38 MAPK inhibitor was given with the bone harvest chamber in rabbits, there was a suppression of bone ingrowth and alkaline phosphatase staining [19]. This might represent low possibility for MAP kinase inhibition as a target for therapies.

Transcription and other Factors related to Particle-Induced Osteolysis

Efforts to find out signaling targets by particles at a level of transcription are very important because it can make more effective target for therapeutics. The most notable transcription factor implicated in wear debris action is Nuclear factor (NF)-κB. This protein complex, long known as a key regulator of inflammatory gene expression, is also emerging as an important player during osteoclastogenesis. Mice lacking NF-κB are osteopetrotic, resulting from an inability to generate functional OCs.Ti or PMMA wear debris can activate NF-κB in cultured macrophages and OCPs [1]. Inhibition of NF-κB blocks PMMA induction of osteoclastogenesis in vitro [5].

Activating Protein 1 (AP-1: a heterodimer of c-Fos and c-Jun) is an important transcription factor acting downstream of RANKL. c-fos is considered an essential regulator of the OC differentiation: the up-regulation of c-fos corresponds to the passage from macrophages into the OC lineage. AP-1 become activated after Ti treatment of macrophages and fibroblast [20,39]. By an as yet unknown mechanism, RANKL induces the expression of the proto-oncogene c-Fos [32,63].

The expression of the c-fms gene, which encodes the receptor for M-CSF, is directly linked to the activation of the receptor for the granulocyte/macrophage colony-stimulating factor (GM-CSF). The binding of M-CSF to the 'c-fms' receptor triggers a signal transduction pathway which promotes the growth and survival of the committed OCPs, and up-regulates the RANK expression, thus making them available for the RANKL stimulus [20]. However, little is know about c-fms concerning particle induced osteolysis. Src protein, a tyrosine-specific kinase, is required for cytoskeleton rearrangements, polarization of newly formed OCs, motility, and cell survival [66]. Although, the relevance of these factors in particle-induced osteolysis remains unclear, these will provide new insight into the molecular basis of particle-induced osteoclastogenesis.

RANKL-OPG-RANK Axis

Although multiple hormones and cytokines regulate various aspects of OC formation, the final two effectors are Receptor Activator of NF-κB (RANK) ligand/osteoclast differentiation factor (ODF), a recently cloned member of the TNF superfamily, and macrophage colony stimulating factor (M-CSF). RANKL is the key cytokine regulator of OC generation and activation: interaction between RANK and RANKL constitutes a pivotal signaling pathway in the formation of OCs. RANKL is expressed on the surface of activated T cells, marrow stoma cells, and OBs as a 45-kDa transmembrane protein. It binds to RANK expressed on the surface of OCs and OCPs and is necessary for the differentiation of OCPs to mature and functional OCs in the presence of the survival factor M-CSF. By binding RANKL, RANK receptor recruit TNFR(TNF receptor)-associated cytoplasmic factors (TRAF): in particular TRAF6 acts as a key adaptor to assemble signaling proteins that direct OC-specific gene expression leading to differentiation and activation [64].

The molecular basis of increased RANKL in osteolysis is likely downstream of pro-inflammatory cytokines such as TNF-α and IL-1β, which are known to increase RANKL expression in several cell types [48]. Activation of NF-κB signaling pathways also regulates the secretion of TNF, which acts on the secreting cell itself as well as on various cell types present in the periprosthetic membrane [12]. Therefore, TNF-α and IL-1, acting in concert with RANKL, can powerfully promote OC recruitment, activation, and osteolysis in RA [51]. Interaction between RANKL-RANK can be inhibited by osteoprotegrin (OPG; osteoclastogenesis inhibitory factor), a member of the TNF-receptor superfamily. OPG is a naturally occurring decoy receptor for RANKL and secreted by stromal cells including OBs as a soluble 110 kDa disulfide-linked homodimer. It down-regulates osteoclastogenesis by binding RANKL. OC formation may be determined principally by the relative ratio of RANKL/OPG in the bone marrow microenvironment, and alterations in this ratio has been correlated with various bone disorders [29]. Particulate debris induces OC generation and activation by modulation of the RANKL/OPG ratio. This most likely involves direct effects of particles on cells in the periprosthetic tissue and indirect effects mediated by particle-mediated perturbations of cytokines, which can modulate RANKL/OPG ratios [2].

WNT/β-catenin signaling in Osteoblast and Osteoclast

In the past several years, studies have revealed that Wnt signaling occurs downstream of additional signaling cascades that involve BMPs: the Wnt signaling pathway thus serves as a master controller of bone formation [17]. Activation of the canonical pathway by Wnt and nuclear translocation of β-catenin interact with T-cell factor (Tcf)/lymphoid-enhancing factor (Lef) transcription factors to control the expression of target genes

In two recent breakthrough studies, Wnt signaling in OBs through the canonical β-catenin pathway has also been implicated unexpectedly in regulating the formation of OCs, the cells that resorb bone. One study provided evidence that the Wnt pathway positively regulates OB expression of OPG [16]. Another study took a slightly different approach and came to a similar conclusion: the Wnt pathway can suppress OC mediated bone resorption—this suppression seems to occur through down-regulation of RANKL and up-regulation of OPG in OB lineage cells [30]. Early B cell factor (EBF)-2 is expressed in OB progenitors. Kieslinger M. et al. reported that EBF2, downstream of WNT/β-catenin, play central roles in regulating OB-dependent differentiation of OCs by down-regulation of OPG [38]. Thus, it seems that the Wnt pathway not only boosts bone formation by fostering OB activity, but it can also inhibit bone resorption by affecting OCs.

As the pivotal role of the Wnt/β-catenin pathway in the regulation of bone remodeling became clear, attention should turn to approaches for manipulating this system to treat bone-remodeling disorders, including the bone loss in particle-induced osteolysis and rheumatoid arthritis. As wear particles induce various kind of cellular response to contribute to periprosthetic osteolysis: we speculate that particles may modulate OB and OC through Wnt/β-catenin signaling, resulting increased RANKL/OPG ratio and decreased osteoblastic activity.

Perspectives and Conclusions

Periprosthetic osteolysis is a complex phenomenon by various kinds of cellular activities which a lot of molecular networks are involved with. For that reasons, to date, there is no approved medical therapy to prevent or inhibit periprosthetic osteolysis yet, in spite of a lot of progression in researches understanding of it. However, molecular biological, tribological, or clinical researches to find better articulation that can minimize the production of wear debris have also been ongoing.

The incidence of osteolysis can increase as the rate of wear increases. Fortunately osteolysis occurs very rarely at a wear rate of <0.1 mm/y after THA [11,60]. Dumbleton JH et al. suggested that a practical wear rate threshold of 0.05 mm/y would eliminate osteolysis following THA [13]. In addition, smaller particles with nanophase size have less detrimental effect on the functions of OBs, compared to conventional particles [20,23]. Nanometer particulate wear debris may result from friction between articulating components of orthopedic implants composed of novel nanophase ceramic materials.

Such reports provide additional evidence that nanophase ceramics may become the next generation of bone prosthetic materials with increased efficacy and, thus, deserve further testing [23]. Therefore to blow up periprosthetic osteolysis, multi-disciplinary researches forward minimal wear articulation should be essential as well as extensive in-vivo molecular and cellular studies.

References

1. Abbas S, Clohisy JC, Abu-Amer Y [2003] Mitogen-activated protein [MAP] kinases mediate PMMA-induction of osteoclasts. J Orthop Res, 21, 1041-8.
2. Baumann B, Rader CP, Seufert J, et al. [2004] Effects of polyethylene and TiAlV wear particles on expression of RANK, RANKL and OPG mRNA. Acta Orthop Scand, 75, 295-302.
3. Boyle WJ, Simonet WS, Lacey DL [2003] Osteoclast differentiation and activation. Nature, 423, 337-42.

4. Chiu R, Ma T, Smith RL, Goodman SB [2006] Polymethylmethacrylate particles inhibit osteoblastic differentiation of bone marrow osteoprogenitor cells. J Biomed Mater Res A, 77, 850-6.

5. Clohisy JC, Hirayama T, Frazier E, Han SK, Abu-Amer Y [2004] NF-kB signaling blockade abolishes implant particle-induced osteoclastogenesis. J Orthop Res, 22, 13-20.

6. Corisdeo S, Gyda M, Zaidi M, Moonga BS, Troen BR [2001] New insights into the regulation of cathepsin K gene expression by osteoprotegerin ligand. Biochem Biophys Res Commun, 285, 335-9.

7. Davies AP, Willert HG, Campbell PA, Learmonth ID, Case CP [2005] An unusual lymphocytic perivascular infiltration in tissues around contemporary metal-on-metal joint replacements. J Bone Joint Surg Am, 87, 18-27.

8. Dean DD, Schwartz Z, Liu Y, et al. [1999] The effect of ultra-high molecular weight polyethylene wear debris on MG63 osteosarcoma cells in vitro. J Bone Joint Surg Am, 81, 452-61.

9. DeHeer DH, Engels JA, DeVries AS, Knapp RH, Beebe JD [2001] In situ complement activation by polyethylene wear debris. J Biomed Mater Res, 54, 12-9.

10. Dorr LD, Bloebaum R, Emmanual J, Meldrum R [1990] Histologic, biochemical, and ion analysis of tissue and fluids retrieved during total hip arthroplasty. Clin Orthop Relat Res, 82-95.

11. Dowd JE, Sychterz CJ, Young AM, Engh CA [2000] Characterization of long-term femoral-head-penetration rates. Association with and prediction of osteolysis. J Bone Joint Surg Am, 82-A, 1102-7.

12. Drees P, Eckardt A, Gay RE, Gay S, Huber LC [2007] Mechanisms of disease: Molecular insights into aseptic loosening of orthopedic implants. Nat Clin Pract Rheumatol, 3, 165-71.

13. Dumbleton JH, Manley MT, Edidin AA [2002] A literature review of the association between wear rate and osteolysis in total hip arthroplasty. J Arthroplasty, 17, 649-61.

14. Fritz EA, Jacobs JJ, Glant TT, Roebuck KA [2005] Chemokine IL-8 induction by particulate wear debris in osteoblasts is mediated by NF-kappaB. J Orthop Res, 23, 1249-57.

15. Glant TT, Jacobs JJ, Molnar G, Shanbhag AS, Valyon M, Galante JO [1993] Bone resorption activity of particulate-stimulated macrophages. J Bone Miner Res, 8, 1071-9.

16. Glass DA, 2nd, Bialek P, Ahn JD, et al. [2005] Canonical Wnt signaling in differentiated osteoblasts controls osteoclast differentiation. Dev Cell, 8, 751-64.

17. Goldring SR, Goldring MB [2007] Eating bone or adding it: the Wnt pathway decides. Nat Med, 13, 133-4.

18. Goodman SB, Ma T, Chiu R, Ramachandran R, Smith RL [2006a] Effects of orthopaedic wear particles on osteoprogenitor cells. Biomaterials, 27, 6096-101.

19. Goodman SB, Ma T, Spanogle J, et al. [2006b] Effects of a p38 MAP kinase inhibitor on bone ingrowth and tissue differentiation in rabbit chambers. J Biomed Mater Res A, 81A, 310-316.

20. Granchi D, Amato I, Battistelli L, et al. [2005] Molecular basis of osteoclastogenesis induced by osteoblasts exposed to wear particles. Biomaterials, 26, 2371-9.

21. Granchi D, Ciapetti G, Amato I, et al. [2004] The influence of alumina and ultra-high molecular weight polyethylene particles on osteoblast-osteoclast cooperation. Biomaterials, 25, 4037-45.

22. Green TR, Fisher J, Stone M, Wroblewski BM, Ingham E [1998] Polyethylene particles of a 'critical size' are necessary for the induction of cytokines by macrophages in vitro. Biomaterials, 19, 2297-302.

23. Gutwein LG, Webster TJ [2004] Increased viable osteoblast density in the presence of nanophase compared to conventional alumina and titania particles. Biomaterials, 25, 4175-83.

24. Hallab NJ, Anderson S, Stafford T, Glant T, Jacobs JJ [2005] Lymphocyte responses in patients with total hip arthroplasty. J Orthop Res, 23, 384-91.

25. Harris WH [1995] The problem is osteolysis. Clin Orthop Relat Res, 46-53.

26. Haynes DR, Boyle SJ, Rogers SD, Howie DW, Vernon-Roberts B [1998] Variation in cytokines induced by particles from different prosthetic materials. Clin Orthop Relat Res, 223-30.

27. Haynes DR, Crotti TN, Potter AE, et al. [2001] The osteoclastogenic molecules RANKL and RANK are associated with periprosthetic osteolysis. J Bone Joint Surg Br, 83, 902-11.

28. Hofbauer LC, Khosla S, Dunstan CR, Lacey DL, Boyle WJ, Riggs BL [2000] The roles of osteoprotegerin and osteoprotegerin ligand in the paracrine regulation of bone resorption. J Bone Miner Res, 15, 2-12.

29. Hofbauer LC, Schoppet M [2004] Clinical implications of the osteoprotegerin/RANKL/RANK system for bone and vascular diseases. Jama, 292, 490-5.

30. Holmen SL, Zylstra CR, Mukherjee A, et al. [2005] Essential role of beta-catenin in postnatal bone acquisition. J Biol Chem, 280, 21162-8.

31. Horiki M, Nakase T, Myoui A, et al. [2004] Localization of RANKL in osteolytic tissue around a loosened joint prosthesis. J Bone Miner Metab, 22, 346-51.

32. Ikeda F, Nishimura R, Matsubara T, et al. [2004] Critical roles of c-Jun signaling in regulation of NFAT family and RANKL-regulated osteoclast differentiation. J Clin Invest, 114, 475-84.

33. Ingham E, Fisher J [2005] The role of macrophages in osteolysis of total joint replacement. Biomaterials, 26, 1271-86.

34. Iotsova V, Caamano J, Loy J, Yang Y, Lewin A, Bravo R [1997] Osteopetrosis in mice lacking NF-kappaB1 and NF-kappaB2. Nat Med, 3, 1285-9.

35. Jacobs JJ, Roebuck KA, Archibeck M, Hallab NJ, Glant TT [2001] Osteolysis: basic science. Clin Orthop Relat Res, 71-7.

36. Keener JD, Callaghan JJ, Goetz DD, Pederson DR, Sullivan PM, Johnston RC [2003] Twenty-five-year results after Charnley total hip arthroplasty in patients less than fifty years old: a concise follow-up of a previous report. J Bone Joint Surg Am, 85-A, 1066-72.

37. Kido A, Pap G, Nagler DK, et al. [2004] Protease expression in interface tissues around loose arthroplasties. Clin Orthop Relat Res, 230-6.

38. Kieslinger M, Folberth S, Dobreva G, et al. [2005] EBF2 regulates osteoblast-dependent differentiation of osteoclasts. Dev Cell, 9, 757-67.

39. Lee SS, Woo CH, Chang JD, Kim JH [2003] Roles of Rac and cytosolic phospholipase A2 in the intracellular signalling in response to titanium particles. Cell Signal, 15, 339-45.

40. Lohmann CH, Dean DD, Koster G, et al. [2002] Ceramic and PMMA particles differentially affect osteoblast phenotype. Biomaterials, 23, 1855-63.

41. Lohmann CH, Schwartz Z, Koster G, et al. [2000] Phagocytosis of wear debris by osteoblasts affects differentiation and local factor production in a manner dependent on particle composition. Biomaterials, 21, 551-61.

42. Mbalaviele G, Anderson GD, Jones AL, et al. [2006] INHIBITION OF p38 MAPK PREVENTS INFLAMMATORY BONE DESTRUCTION. J Pharmacol Exp Ther.

43. Nakashima Y, Sun DH, Trindade MC, et al. [1999a] Induction of macrophage C-C chemokine expression by titanium alloy and bone cement particles. J Bone Joint Surg Br, 81, 155-62.

44. Nakashima Y, Sun DH, Trindade MC, et al. [1999b] Signaling pathways for tumor necrosis factor-alpha and interleukin-6 expression in human macrophages exposed to titanium-alloy particulate debris in vitro. J Bone Joint Surg Am, 81, 603-15.

45. Palecanda A, Kobzik L [2001] Receptors for unopsonized particles: the role of alveolar macrophage scavenger receptors. Curr Mol Med, 1, 589-95.

46. Palmbos PL, Sytsma MJ, DeHeer DH, Bonnema JD [2002] Macrophage exposure to particulate titanium induces phosphorylation of the protein tyrosine kinase lyn and the phospholipases Cgamma-1 and Cgamma-2. J Orthop Res, 20, 483-9.

47. Pioletti DP, Leoni L, Genini D, Takei H, Du P, Corbeil J [2002] Gene expression analysis of osteoblastic cells contacted by orthopedic implant particles. J Biomed Mater Res, 61, 408-20.

48. Purdue PE, Koulouvaris P, Potter HG, Nestor BJ, Sculco TP [2007] The cellular and molecular biology of periprosthetic osteolysis. Clin Orthop Relat Res, 454, 251-61.

49. Rakshit DS, Lim JT, Ly K, et al. [2006a] Involvement of complement receptor 3 [CR3] and scavenger receptor in macrophage responses to wear debris. J Orthop Res, 24, 2036-44.

50. Rakshit DS, Ly K, Sengupta TK, et al. [2006b] Wear Debris Inhibition of Anti-Osteoclasto-genic Signaling by Interleukin-6 and Interferon-{gamma} Mechanistic Insights and Implications for Periprosthetic Osteolysis. J Bone Joint Surg Am, 88, 788-99.

51. Romas E, Gillespie MT, Martin TJ [2002] Involvement of receptor activator of NFkappaB ligand and tumor necrosis factor-alpha in bone destruction in rheumatoid arthritis. Bone, 30, 340-6.

52. Sabokbar A, Fujikawa Y, Neale S, Murray DW, Athanasou NA [1997] Human arthroplasty derived macrophages differentiate into osteoclastic bone resorbing cells. Ann Rheum Dis, 56, 414-20.

53. Sabokbar A, Itonaga I, Sun SG, Kudo O, Athanasou NA [2005] Arthroplasty membrane-derived fibroblasts directly induce osteoclast formation and osteolysis in aseptic loosening. J Orthop Res, 23, 511-9.

54. Sabokbar A, Kudo O, Athanasou NA [2003] Two distinct cellular mechanisms of osteoclast formation and bone resorption in periprosthetic osteolysis. J Orthop Res, 21, 73-80.

55. Santavirta S, Konttinen YT, Bergroth V, Eskola A, Tallroth K, Lindholm TS [1990] Aggressive granulomatous lesions associated with hip arthroplasty. Immunopathological studies. J Bone Joint Surg Am, 72, 252-8.

56. Schlesinger PH, Mattsson JP, Blair HC [1994] Osteoclastic acid transport: mechanism and implications for physiological and pharmacological regulation. Miner Electrolyte Metab, 20, 31-9.

57. Schwarz EM, Lu AP, Goater JJ, et al. [2000] Tumor necrosis factor-alpha/nuclear transcription factor-kappaB signaling in periprosthetic osteolysis. J Orthop Res, 18, 472-80.

58. Sethi RK, Neavyn MJ, Rubash HE, Shanbhag AS [2003] Macrophage response to cross-linked and conventional UHMWPE. Biomaterials, 24, 2561-73.

59. Shanbhag AS, Jacobs JJ, Black J, Galante JO, Glant TT [1994] Macrophage/particle interactions: effect of size, composition and surface area. J Biomed Mater Res, 28, 81-90.

60. Sychterz CJ, Engh CA, Jr., Young AM, Hopper RH, Jr., Engh CA [2000] Comparison of in vivo wear between polyethylene liners articulating with ceramic and cobalt-chrome femoral heads. J Bone Joint Surg Br, 82, 948-51.

61. Takagi M, Santavirta S, Ida H, Ishii M, Mandelin J, Konttinen YT [1998] Matrix metalloproteinases and tissue inhibitors of metalloproteinases in loose artificial hip joints. Clin Orthop Relat Res, 35-45.

62. Takagi M, Tamaki Y, Hasegawa H, et al. [2007] Toll-like receptors in the interface membrane around loosening total hip replacement implants. J Biomed Mater Res A, 81, 1017-26.

63. Takayanagi H, Kim S, Matsuo K, et al. [2002] RANKL maintains bone homeostasis through c-Fos-dependent induction of interferon-beta. Nature, 416, 744-9.

64. Takayanagi H, Ogasawara K, Hida S, et al. [2000] T-cell-mediated regulation of osteoclastogenesis by signalling cross-talk between RANKL and IFN-gamma. Nature, 408, 600-5.

65. Talmo CT, Shanbhag AS, Rubash HE [2006] Nonsurgical management of osteolysis: challenges and opportunities. Clin Orthop Relat Res, 453, 254-64.

66. Teitelbaum SL [2007] Osteoclasts: what do they do and how do they do it? Am J Pathol, 170, 427-35.

67. Vermes C, Chandrasekaran R, Jacobs JJ, Galante JO, Roebuck KA, Glant TT [2001] The effects of particulate wear debris, cytokines, and growth factors on the functions of MG-63 osteoblasts. J Bone Joint Surg Am, 83-A, 201-11.

68. Vermes C, Roebuck KA, Chandrasekaran R, Dobai JG, Jacobs JJ, Glant TT [2000] Particulate wear debris activates protein tyrosine kinases and nuclear factor kappaB, which down-regulates type I collagen synthesis in human osteoblasts. J Bone Miner Res, 15, 1756-65.

69. Wang ML, Nesti LJ, Tuli R, et al. [2002] Titanium particles suppress expression of osteoblastic phenotype in human mesenchymal stem cells. J Orthop Res, 20, 1175-84.

70. Wang ML, Sharkey PF, Tuan RS [2004] Particle bioreactivity and wear-mediated osteolysis. J Arthroplasty, 19, 1028-38.

71. Wang ML, Tuli R, Manner PA, Sharkey PF, Hall DJ, Tuan RS [2003] Direct and indirect induction of apoptosis in human mesenchymal stem cells in response to titanium particles. J Orthop Res, 21, 697-707.

72. Yamanaka Y, Abu-Amer Y, Faccio R, Clohisy JC [2006] Map kinase c-JUN N-terminal kinase mediates PMMA induction of osteoclasts. J Orthop Res, 24, 1349-57.

73. Yang SY, Ren W, Park Y, et al. [2002] Diverse cellular and apoptotic responses to variant shapes of UHMWPE particles in a murine model of inflammation. Biomaterials, 23, 3535-43.

74. Yao J, Glant TT, Lark MW, et al. [1995] The potential role of fibroblasts in periprosthetic osteolysis: fibroblast response to titanium particles. J Bone Miner Res, 10, 1417-27.

75. Yaszay B, Trindade MC, Lind M, Goodman SB, Smith RL [2001] Fibroblast expression of C-C chemokines in response to orthopaedic biomaterial particle challenge in vitro. J Orthop Res, 19, 970-6.

SESSION 1B

Tribology

1B.1 Wear Performance of 36mm Biolox® forte/delta Hip Combinations Compared in Simulated 'Severe' Micro-Separation Test Mode

I. C. Clarke, D. Green, P. Williams, G. Pezzotti and T. Donaldson

Introduction

Ceramic-polyethylene (CPE) and ceramic-on-ceramic (COC) total hip replacements (THR) have now been in use for 37 years (Table 1). Alumina was the first ceramic considered for hip-bearings by virtue of its extreme wear-resistance and bio-inertness (Table 2). The second ceramic type coming into the medical field by 1985 was the yttria-stabilized zirconia (Y-TZP) with fracture toughness and strength more than double that of alumina. However, this zirconia revealed an enigmatic clinical history with an uncertain risk due to its 'metastable' characteristics, i.e. under certain conditions the Y-TZP could undergo adverse phase changes (Clarke et al, 2003). An unfortunate manufacturing change by one company produced very high fracture rates in one brand of Y-TZP and this was abandoned circa 2000-2001 (Table 1). The third ceramic type coming into the market was a composite of alumina and zirconia (Table 1: trade name BIOLOX-delta™). This alumina-matrix composite (AMC) virtually doubled the

YEAR	CERAMIC	DIAMETER	DETAILS
1970	alumina	32	non-modular ceramic ball and 1-piece cemented ceramic cup (Ceraver Inc: Boutin MD)
1973	alumina	28, 32, 35	modular ceramic balls (Feldmühle Inc: Griss; Mittelmeier MD)
1977	alumina	28,32	modular ceramic balls (Ceraver Inc: Sedel MD)
1985	zirconia (Y-TZP)	22, 26, 28, 32	modular zirconia balls (JMMC-Japan, Metoxic-Switzerland, Morgan Matroc-UK, NGK -Japan, Saint Gobain-France)
1989	alumina	28, 32	modular ceramic cup, threaded with hydroxyapatite coating (JRI Inc; Furlong MD)
1989	alumina - zirconia	26, 28, 32	various alumina and Y-TZP zirconia approved by FDA (for use with PE bearings)
1999	zirconia (Y-TZP)	28, 32	manufacturing and major fracture problem begins (Prozyr™, Saint Gobain Desmarquest Inc, France)
1997	alumina	36	large ball (Biolox-forte™; CeramTec) approved by FDA (for use by Wright Medical with PE cups)
2000	alumina- zirconia	28, 32	Biolox-delta™ and forte™ ceramic balls and liners (CeramTec) marketed in Europe
2000	alumina- zirconia	28, 32	Biolox-delta™ ball (CeramTec) approved by FDA (with PE cups)
2003	alumina	28, 32	ceramic liners FDA approved (Biolox-forte™ cup inserts)
2006	alumina - zirconia	36	large ball of Biolox-delta™ (CeramTec) approved by FDA (for use with PE cups)

Table 1:
History of ceramic innovations with timing of FDA approvals for US.
Companies and names of pioneering surgeons are indicated in parenthesis (Clarke et al, 2007a).

strength and fracture toughness of the pure alumina. BIOLOX-*delta*™ was introduced to the marketplace in year 2000 (Willmann, 2000). Another ceramic innovation was the 36mm alumina femoral head, introduced to the US in 1997 (Table 2: Wright Medical Inc).

FEATURE	PERFORMANCE
Benefit	Clinical studies span 37 years
Benefit	Ultra-low wear
Benefit	No adverse biological reactions
Benefit	Ball diameters 28, 32, 36mm
Risk	Timing of FDA approval uncertain
Risk	Alumina fracture rate 0.01% to 0.1%
Risk	Revision options limited after a fracture
Risk	Cup design limitations (deformation, inadequate insertion, impingement, fretting, disassociation)
Risk	Metal-backed ceramic cups may not fit the smaller hip joints
Risk	Squeaking (impingement; other)

Table 2:
Perceived risks and benefits of ceramic THR.

Surgeon Pierre Boutin (1972) was the pioneer who first described COC run-in wear as only a few microns over the first million load cycles and the COC steady-state wear was undetectable. This ultra-low wear performance of ceramics has since been confirmed in many simulator and clinical studies (Clarke et al, 2007a). Wear rates of all-alumina bearings would typically average 0.5 and 0.05mm^3/Mc for run-in and steady-state phases, respectively (Table 3). Alumina bearings have also proved to be well accepted biologically with no evidence of adverse effects over thee decades of use (Sedel et al, 2003). The remaining disadvantage of alumina ceramic appeared to be uncertainty involving some albeit small risk of fracture (Heros and Willlman 1998; Tateiwa et al, 2006)).

PARAMETERS	WEAR (mm^3/MC)
Run-in range	0.02 to 1
Typical Run-in	0.5
steady-state range	0.02 to 0.05
Typical steady-state	0.05

Table 3:
Ceramic wear parameters taken from simulator studies running under standard test modes, indicating steady-state wear decreased by factor of 10-fold from run-in (Clarke et al, 2007a).

Stewart et al (2003) introduced "micro-separation" (MSX) as a simulator test mode and successfully demonstrated peripheral stripe wear as seen on retrieved ceramic implants (Nevelos et al, 1999; Shishido et al, 2003). Their simulator studies compared the wear with the high-strength Biolox-*delta*™ (D) to the control Biolox-*forte*™ (F) in three combinations all 28mm diameter (ball:cup: FF, DF and DD). They demonstrated 'stripe' wear in all implants at 1 million (1Mc) cycles duration. There was greater surface disruption evident with stripe wear compared to the mild polishing evident in the main-wear zone (Fig. 1). The 28mm control FF-combination had run-in and steady state wear of 4 mm^3/Mc and 1.3 mm^3/Mc, respectively. Overall the 28mm AMC combination showed wear reduced 12-fold compared to 28mm FF controls whereas the AMC/alumina hybrid wear was reduced some 3-fold overall.

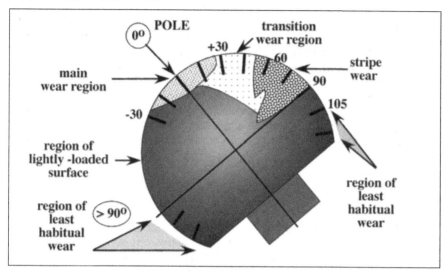

Figure 1:
Schematic of wear mapping sites on ceramic ball showing approximate positions of main-wear zone, transition and stripe wear zones.

The purpose of our study was to evaluate the wear performance of the high-strength Biolox-*delta*™ in large diameter (36mm) implants using our 'severe' microseparation test mode. We ran detailed analyses during run-in and steady-state wear phases, mapped surface topography looking for wear-stripe formation, identify any monoclinic phase transformation in zirconia grains and also examine the morphology of the ceramic wear debris. Our controls were the all-alumina combination (36mm) run simultaneously with the AMZ combinations.

Method

We studied 36mm diameter bearings using the Biolox forte™/delta™ ball:cup combinations; FF, FD, DF and DD (N=3 each). All implant combinations were diametrically matched and compared to alumina as the historical control. A 12-station, hip simulator (Shore Western Manufacturing, Monrovia CA) was modified for micro-separation test mode. On heel-strike loading, the ceramic ball made contact with the superior cup bevel producing a stress point on the rotating ball as it re-reduced into normal cup position. The second peak load came from the toe-off position in the gait cycle. Cups were set up in the anatomical position, positioned at 50° to the horizontal axis. The lubricant was alpha-calf serum (Hyclone™, Utah, USA) diluted to protein concentration 10mg/ml with filtered, de-ionized water and EDTA added (20ml/l). The chamber volume was 400ml and adding de-ionized water compensated for lubricant evaporation. All lubricants were replaced at each weighing event and stored frozen for analysis. Test duration was 5 million cycles (5Mc), wear was detected by weight change and wear trends were quantified by linear regression technique. Run-in and steady-state wear were each assessed with 10 events with 100k cycle and 500k cycle intervals, respectively. At completion of each wear event the implants were cleaned by standard protocol. Components were weighed and the weights averaged for weight-loss assessment (Sartorius MC1 microbalance). Weight changes for alumina and AMC were converted to volumetric using the specific gravities of 3.98 and 4.36, respectively. The ceramic implants were mapped in degrees from 0° (pole) to beyond +90° (equator) for comparative analyses (Fig. 1). Bearing surfaces were analyzed at 6 locations by scanning electron microscopy (Phillips FEG SEM XL-30) and surface roughness was measured at 1 and 5.0Mc duration by laser profilometer (Zygo New View 5000, CT USA). Since AMC implants contained 24% zirconia, possible transformations from tetragonal to monoclinic phase were studied by confocal Raman microprobe spectroscopy (RMS).

Results

At our initial wear assessment (0.1Mc) all implants had clear evidence of stripe wear. On the femoral heads, two prominent stripes appeared, a broad scar located at 75 to 90° and a narrow scar at 45 to 60° relative to the pole (Fig. 1). Over the 5.0Mc study, these two stripes converged forming a large wear scar spanning a 45 to 90° arc. Overall the FF combination had the largest scars and the DD the least (stripe areas varying 150-350 mm² range). Note the main wear zones were only identifiable by SEM (Fig. 1).

All ceramic liners showed stripes juxtaposed to the cup bevel by 0.1Mc duration. These stripes were narrow and located superiorly over a 10° to 90° arc. These stripes progressed gradually along the cup circumference (an arc of 180° for FF) and also expanded radially towards the MWZ during 5Mc test duration.

The SEM wear maps of the alumina and AMC balls showed three quite different regions. The habitual non-wear zone (Fig. 1: -60° to -30°) still had the original machine polish marks indicating minimal contact over 5Mc duration. The main wear zone (Fig. 1, 0° to +30°) had undergone mild relief polishing, the original machine marks had been removed revealing the grain structure and some minor pitting. In contrast, the stripe wear zones had undergone major surface disruption with intergranular fracture and grain pullout resulting in a greater loss of surface.

Surface roughness of non-wear zones did not change from the starting value (Ra ≤ 10 nm). The main wear zones also showed no change in roughness at 5Mc duration. As expected from SEM mapping, the stripe zones showed roughness increased up to 113nm. Also as expected the FF combination had the deepest stripe wear (40 μm), with overall stripe depth ranking as follows:

$$FF > FD > \{DF, DD\}.$$

THR control-FF revealed the highest run-in wear averaging 6.3 mm³/Mc whereas the DD combination was lowest with 0.5 mm³/Mc, a 12-fold reduction. The steady-state trends also showed that FF had the highest wear at 0.97 mm³/Mc whereas the DD combination had lowest at 0.13 mm³/Mc representing a 7-fold reduction. Comparing hybrid FD and DF combinations, there was little difference in wear; these approximately doubled that of the DD-combination (Fig. 2).

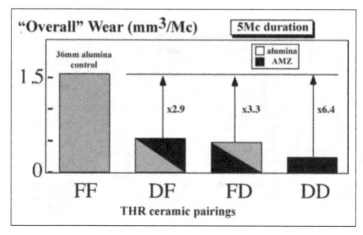

Figure 2:
Comparison of 'overall' wear rates for four 36mm ceramic combinations at 5 million cycles duration.

Tetragonal to monoclinic transformation was detected in all AMC implants by the end of the run-in phase (1Mc) and at the end of study (5Mc). The main wear zone on femoral heads had least transformation (14%) at 1Mc and this doubled by 5Mc duration (23%). In contrast the stripe regions showed higher transformation at 1Mc (24% monoclinic) and then only a modest gain to 5Mc duration (25-29%). The AMC cups showed modest monoclinic content (~15%) regardless of location. This was likely due to poor detection levels, given these intact hemispherical cup geometries.

The ceramic debris varied from very small globular, polygonal shapes to large sharp-edged fragments that had been chipped off the surface by the violence of the MSX wear mode (Fig. 3). Debris from all combinations were similar in size up to 5-Mc duration. At end of steady-state phase, the debris averaged an ECD size of 0.5 microns, unchanged from intervals 2.5Mc to 5Mc (Fig. 4).

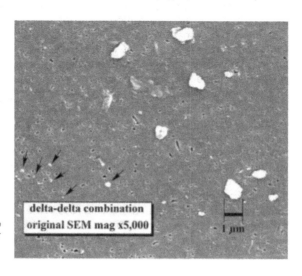

Figure 3:
Ceramic particles from microseparation wear study of 36mm AMC-AMC combination. Arrows contrast the sub-micron ceramic debris on filter paper to the appearance of much larger and irregular ceramic fragments.

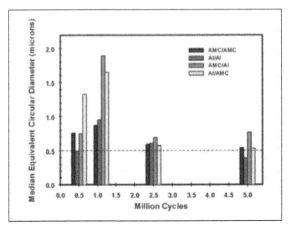

Figure 4:
Distribution of ceramic particles by size (median ECD) from microseparation wear study of 36mm AMC-AMC combination over 5 million cycles duration.

Discussion

This is the first simulator study of alumina and AMC in large-diameter, ceramic bearings. Compared to the 36mm control alumina, the AMC-AMC and AMC hybrids reduced wear by 6 and 3-fold, respectively. During our run-in phase we found a 12-fold reduction of wear in DD compared to FF combinations. The prior 28mm diameter microseparation study found that the AMC-AMC and AMC hybrids reduced wear by 12 and 4-fold, respectively (Stewart et al, 2003). Therefore we were in good agreement overall that the AMC/alumina combination averaged 3 to 4-fold less wear than the control combination. Thus, even given the evident differences in ball-diameter, test methods and incidence of stripe-wear formation, these data showed good inter-laboratory correlation. We also found a linear relationship between surface-roughness (Ra) of the femoral stripes and the overall ceramic wear-rates. This confirmed that the increased wear rates in our microseparation studies came predominantly from the stripe scars. It was therefore interesting that the AMC ceramic consistently conferred more resistance to stripe wear in each of the 3 combinations (DD, DF and FD). Thus the AMC was not only a stronger ceramic but also more resistant to stripe wear in our 'severe' microseparation test mode.

With the clinical evidence of Y-TZP femoral heads having transformed in-vivo (zirconia-polyethylene THR; Clarke et al, 2003) it is important to carefully examine the performance of new alumina-zirconia composites. A priori, it is to be expected that, given the right conditions, zirconia grains exposed on any free surface will tend to transform from tetragonal to monoclinic phase (Sato and Shimada, 1985; Chevalier 1999). We know that the transformation with Y-TZP from tetragonal to monoclinic phase can be triggered by certain environmental conditions that include moisture and heat (Brown et al, 2007). In the articulating hip joint, the lubricant provides the moisture, the dynamic hip-loading provides the stress and the sliding conditions provide frictional heating. Extensive monoclinic transformation has been observed with the zirconia-polyethylene hip combinations retrieved after 3 to 9 years use in the patient (Haraguchi et al, 2001; Clarke et al, 2003; Green et al, 2003). However this does not appear to have been duplicated in any hip simulator wear study (Brown et al, 2007; Clarke, 2007b).

With this 'severe' microseparation test mode, we appear to be the first reporting progressive monoclinic transformation in AMZ ceramics. From 1 to 5 million cycles under 'severe' microseparation test mode, the monoclinic content increased from approximately 15% to 30%, the latter plateau being reached in both stripe and main wear zones. A previous study stated that their alumina-zirconia composite ceramic ("CZTA") was apparently produced with 35% monoclinic phase on the surface and that with 'accelerated aging' there was no further transformation detected (Insley et al, 2004). However their ceramic processing and test conditions were not clarified and it was also not clear how their x-ray diffraction study would correlate with our Raman Spectroscopy data.

The articular surface of AMC ceramic contains agglomerates of both tetragonal and monoclinic zirconia interspersed in a dominant alumina matrix (Fig. 5a). In the sub-surface layers it can be assumed that the alumina matrix constrains the tetragonal zirconia grains, thereby maintaining the desired high-strength core. In contrast, on the articular surface some 10 to 15% tetragonal zirconia may already be transformed into monoclinic phase. Then with the in-vivo joint articulation effects of moisture, stress and frictional heating, further transformation of exposed tetragonal zirconia can be anticipated (Fig. 5b). The concomitant expansion of tetragonal grains to monoclinic grains and the formation of micro-cracks will lead to erosion of more zirconia grains. However the main alumina matrix will continue to transfer the hip loads and provide the ultra-low wear performance (Fig. 5c). In interpreting this behavior it would appear that the normal wear products will include tetragonal and monoclinic zirconia along with eroded alumina particles and the transformed zirconia phase appears to plateau at 30% monoclinic.

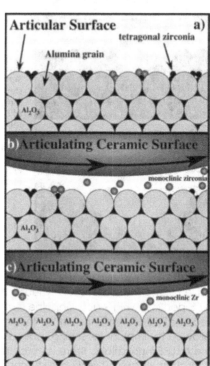

Figure 5:
Schematic cross section of articular surface showing steps in wear of articulating AMZ ceramic surface:
a) Pristine AMC bearing surface contains a small percentage of sub-micron tetragonal zirconia (small black circles) interspersed with the larger grains of the alumina matrix. Some tetragonal grains on the free surface will have already transformed into the monoclinic phase (small gray circle)
b) Hydrothermal effects created by mechanical stress and frictional heating during articulation will drive more exposed tetragonal grains (black) to monoclinic phase (gray). These will expand and likely be eroded from the surface.
c) Continuing wear process will release combinations of alumina, tetragonal and monoclinic grains. Subsequently the dominant, hard alumina matrix will control the wear process, identical to wear occurring in implants of pure alumina.

The transformation in Y-TZP zirconia implants (Fig. 6a) follows a very different pathway. With joint articulation the effects of shear stress and frictional heating will initiate transformation of exposed tetragonal grains to their monoclinic phase (Fig. 6b). In contrast to the AMZ material, there is no hard protective matrix of alumina grains to stabilize the sub-surface, zirconia grains. Thus the continued erosion of monoclinic phase reduces constraint on neighboring tetragonal grains that can then undergo the same transformation process. As a result, this progressive erosive process can produce deeply cratered surfaces (Fig. 6c). While in-vitro aging studies predicted worst-case < 10% monoclinic after 2 or more decades of use, we have measured monoclinic transformation > 80% on retrieved Y-TZP implants after only 9 years in vivo (Green et al., 2003). The resulting surface roughening can be over 200 µm (Ra). Such roughened ceramic surfaces running against softer polyethylene bearings are likely to be quite destructive (Clarke et al, 2003; Walters et al, 2005).

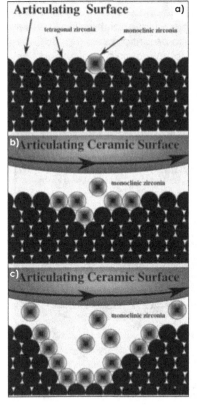

Figure 6:
Schematic cross section of articular surface showing steps in wear of a metastable Y-TZP zirconia ceramic surface:
a) Pristine matrix of predominantly sub-micron tetragonal grains (black) will contain a few transformed monoclinic grains (gray) on the free surface (2-3%).
b) Hydrothermal effects created by pressure and frictional effects of articulation starts to transform more tetragonal grains into monoclinic phase along zones of weakness in the surface.
c) Continuing articulation with wear and hydrothermal effects provokes more transformation of tetragonal grains with release of more transformed monoclinic grains resulting in extensive cratering of the bearing surface.

Each THR system confers both risks and benefits for the patient. The polyethylene cups are known debris shedders, capable of creating millions of XLPE particles with each step the patient takes (Clarke et al, 2007a). Over a period of 10-15 years the risk to the more active THR patients will be osteolysis followed by implant loosening, pain and revision. While more is hoped with the latest XLPE innovations, there is no credible proof that they are superior until the clinical results at > 10 years are demonstrated.

An alternate THR system of metal-on-metal bearings (MOM) was re-introduced in Europe in 1985. Since 1999 the FDA has approved many MOM brands in the 28-60mm diameter range (Clarke et al, 2005). However some types of MOM have recently demonstrated extensive joint effusions in cases revised at < 10 years. The associated metallosis and necrosis appeared to be associated with a hypersensitivity to metal debris, with published rates occurring at the 27 to 70 per 1,000 (2 to 7%: Milosev et al, 2006; Korovessis et al, 2006). In contrast, ceramic-on-ceramic bearings (COC) experience have shown no risk of adverse biological changes over their 37 year clinical history (Sedel et al, 2003). However with ceramic implants, the risk of fracture has always been uppermost in the mind of the surgeon. Overall fracture incidence has been quite small (Heck et al, 1995; Heros and Willmann, 1998; Tateiwa et al, 2006) and appears to lie between 1 per 1,000 and 1 per 10,000 cases (Clarke et al, 2007c). It is notable that the FDA-monitored experience with modular, metal-backed ceramic cups has over 2,700 cases enrolled. With follow-ups extending now to 10 years, there have been zero fractures reported in these carefully monitored series (D'Antonio et al, 2005). Thus the surgeon has to weigh the advantage of large diameter MOM bearings (benefit) with the possibility of 2-7% adverse biological reactions (published risk) against the 0.01% to 0.1% incidence of fractures (risk) with COC but a 35-year history with no adverse biological events (published benefit).

With every technical option given to the surgeon, it can be anticipated that some downside risks will appear. Modular, porous-coated metal shells contribute superior options and flexibility during surgery. However their greatly increased surfaces of metal may contribute greater concentrations of metal ions, assisted by fretting wear if not securely seated and may risk disassociation in some instances. Also it is now clear that the surgeon's press-fit technique inserting porous-coated acetabular components can deform metal shells. One study measured deformations up to 470 μm in type-A bone (Fig. 7) and found shells deformed in 90% of their surgical insertions (Squires et al, 2006). For a non-modular cup design, this has important implications for the tribology of MOM bearings, which typically have ball-cup clearances of 80 to 250 μm. For a modular cup design, this has implications for proper alignment and seating of the liner. A study of ceramic liners used in one modular cup design found that 16% of their cases were incompletely seated (Langdown et al, 2007). Thus inadequate seating and neck-cup impingement may play a major role (Table 3) in squeaking phenomenon (Eickmann et al, 2002; Walter et al, 2007).

From the history of total hip replacements (THR) it has been apparent that one of the most critical elements has been the design and materials used for the acetabular cup. The modern THR evolved from 1963 thanks to the pioneering efforts of the late Sir John Charnley. Some 44 years later we still have much to learn about the efficacy of polyethylene, CoCr and ceramic in contemporary modular cup designs. From the foregoing it is clear that the ultra-low wear performance of ceramic bearings has an important role to play in protecting the patient from the effects of wear debris and eliminating the risk represented by Co and Cr ions produced by MOM bearings. However there is still much to learn about the interactions of modular, porous-coated, metal-backings with the ceramic inserts. For now the only ceramic-on-ceramic bearings approved for use in the USA are the 28 mm and 32mm Biolox-forte™ combinations. The 36mm diameters of alumina and alumina-zirconia composite are only approved for use with XLPE cups and only with certain companies' products (Table 1).

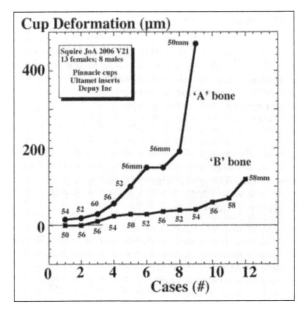

Figure 7:
Diametral deformations measured in titanium acetabular shells (porous) after insertion during surgery into bone ranked as either 'A' or 'B' type (shell diameters as indicated; graph drawn from tabulated data provided in Squire et al, 2006).

Acknowledgements

Our grateful thanks to CeramTec Inc (Plochingen, Germany) for funding the simulator wear study and to the Howard and Irene Peterson Fund of Loma Linda University for financial support of the laboratory.

References

1. Boutin P. [Total arthroplasty of the hip by fritted aluminum prosthesis. Experimental study and 1st clinical applications]. Rev Chir Orthop Reparatrice Appar Mot, 1972, 58(3): 229-46.
2. Brown, S. Green, D. Pezzotti G., Donaldson T. and Clarke IC. Possible Triggers for Phase Transformation in Zirconia Hip Balls. Submitted to J. Biomed. Mater. Res. 2007.
3. Chevalier, J., B. Cales, and J.M. Drouin, Low-temperature aging of Y-TZP ceramics. Journal of American Ceramic Society, 1999. 82(8): p. 2150-2154.
4. Clarke IC, Manaka M, Green DD, Williams P, Pezzotti G, Kim YH, Ries M, Sugano N, Sedel L, Delauney C and others. Current status of zirconia used in total hip implants. J Bone Joint Surg Am 2003;85-A Suppl 4:73-84.
5. Clarke IC, Donaldson T, Bowsher JG, Nasser S, Takahashi H. Current Concepts of metal-on-metal hip resurfacing. Orthop Clin Am 2005; 36: 143-162.
6. Clarke IC, Donaldson T. and Jobe, C. Impact of Wear Debris on Success of Total Hip Replacements. In 'Adult Reconstruction and Arthroplasty: Core Knowledge in Orthopedics, by Eds JP Garino and PK Beredjiklian, Mosby/Elsevier, In Press 2007A.
7. Clarke IC. Metastable nature of zirconia femoral heads from a 20-year perspective of clinical and simulator wear studies. In "Seminars in Arthroplasty", In press, Cadmus Pub., 2007B.
8. Clarke IC, Walter W., Donaldson T., Green D. and Williams PA. Status of alumina, zirconia and zirconia toughened alumina in the USA. Scientific Exhibit #12, AAOS, San Diego, 2007C.

9. D'Antonio J, Capello W, Manley M, Naughton M, Sutton K. Alumina Ceramic Bearings for Total Hip Arthroplasty: Five-year Results of a Prospective Randomized Study. Clin Orthop Relat Res, 2005, (436): 164-171.

10. Eickmann T, Manaka M, Clarke IC, Gustafson A: Squeaking and neck-socket impingement in a ceramic total hip arthroplasty. In Bioceramics-15, pp. 849-852. Edited by Sher, D., Sydney, Australia, Trans Tech Pub, 2002.

11. Green DD, Pezzotti G, Sakakura S, Ries DM, Clarke IC: Zirconia ceramic femoral heads in the USA. In 49th Annual Meeting of the Orthopaedic Research Society, pp. 1392. Edited, New Orleans, Louisiana, 2003.

12. Haraguchi, K., et al., Phase transformation of a zirconia ceramic head after total hip arthroplasty. J Bone Joint Surg Br, 2001. 83: p. 996-1000.

13. Heck D, Patridge, CM., Reuben, JD., Ianzer WL, Lewis CG and Keating EM. Prosthetic component failures – A 5-years review of 60,000 THA. J. Arthrop, 10(5)575-, 1995.

14. Heros RJ, Willmann G. Ceramic in total hip arthroplasty: history, mechanical properties, clinical results, and current manufacturing state of the art. In Seminars in Arthroplasty, Vol. 9, pp. 114-122. Edited, 1998.

15. Insley GM and Streicher RM. Surface analysis of explanted alumina-alumina bearings. In Bioceramics in Joint Arthroplasty, Eds. J.I. Lazennec and M. Dietrich, Pub. Stenkopff Verlag, Darmstadt (2004), 9-12.

16. Korovessis P, Petsinis G., Repanti M and Repanti T. Metalossis after contremporary metal-on-metal total hip arthroplasy five to nine-year follow-up. J. Bone Jt. Surg. Am. 88:1183-1191, 2006.

17. Langdown, AJ., Pickard, RJ., Hobbs CM., Clarke HJ., Dalton DJN and Grover ML. J. Incomplete seating fo the liner with the Trident acetabular system. Bone Jt. Surg. 89-B(3), 291-295, 2007.

18. Milosev, I, Trebse, R., Kovac, S, Cot, A. and Pisot, V. Survivorship and retrieval analysis of Sikomet metal-on-metal total hip replacements at a mean of seven years. J. bone Jt. Surg. Am. 88:1173-1182, 2006.

19. Nevelos JE, Ingham E, Doyle C, Fisher J, Nevelos AB. Analysis of retrieved alumina ceramic components from Mittelmeier total hip prostheses. Biomaterials, 1999, 20(19): 1833-1840.

20. Sato T. and Shimada M. Transformation of yttria-doped tetragonal ZrO2 polycrystals by annealing in water. J Amer Ceram Soc, 1985, 68(6): 356-359.

21. Sedel L, Hamadouche M, Bizot P, Nizard R. Long term data concerning the use of alumina on alumina bearings In total hip replacements. In Bioceramics-15, Vol. 15, pp. 769-772. Edited by Ben-Nissan, B.; Sher, D.; and Walsh, W., Enfield, New Hampshire, Trans Tech Publications, 2003.

22. Shishido T, Clarke IC, Williams P, Boehler M, Asano T, Shoji H, Masaoka T, Yamamoto K, Imakiire A. Clinical and simulator wear study of alumina ceramic THR to 17 years and beyond. J Biomed Mater Res, 2003, 67B(1): 638-47.

23. Squire M, Griffin WL, Mason JM, Peindl RD. and Odum, S. Acetabular Component deformation with press-fit fixation.J. Arthrop. 21(6), Sup-2, 72-77, 2006.

24. Stewart TD, Tipper JL, Insley G, Streicher RM, Ingham E, Fisher J. Long-term wear of ceramic matrix composite materials for hip prostheses under severe swing phase microseparation. J Biomed Mater Res B Appl Biomater, 2003, 66(2): 567-73.

25. T. Tateiwa, IC. Clarke, PA. Williams, J. Garino, M. Manaka, T. Shishido, K. Yamamoto and A. Imakiire. Ceramic THR in USA – safety and risk issues revisited.

26. Walter WL, Skyrme, AD, Richards S, Chai M, Green D., Walter WK Zicat B Polyethylene wear rates with zirconia and cobalt chrome heads. In 51st ORS, p1194, 2005.

27. Walter WL, et al. Hip Society, San Diego, February 2007.

28. Willmann G. New generation ceramics. In Bioceramics in Hip Joint Replacement, pp. 127-135. Edited by Willmann, G., and Zweymuller, K., Stuttgart, Georg Thieme Verlag, 2000.

1B.2 In-Vitro and In-Vivo Ceramic Debris with Ceramic Prosthesis

A. Toni, F. Traina, M. De Fine, E. Tassinari, F. Biondi, A. Galvani, F. Pilla and S. Stea

Introduction

Ceramic prostheses have had some promising long term results [1], and modern metal-back alumina cups have shown very good clinical results [2,3,4]. Alumina has excellent tribological properties, a very high Young's modulus that leads to very good compression strength, but it has poor bending strength: it has no way to deform [5]. This means that ceramic can break without warning. With modern ceramics, under normal physiologic conditions, the fatigue limit is never reached, therefore ceramic head fractures are seldom reported (0.004%[10] in one study). On the contrary, ceramic liner fractures are not well recognized and their frequency could be underestimated. Besides, it is difficult to identify those patients at risk, because liner fractures can be related to multiple causes: dislocation, impingement, malpositioning, microseparation [6,7]. When a ceramic fracture involves the liner and is the consequence of repeated micro-trauma, the diagnosis is rarely made early, except when ceramic fragments are visible on X-ray. Moreover, revision surgery decision making after a failed ceramic-on-ceramic prosthesis is troublesome: the ceramic fragments which have spread into the periarticular space are abrasive, and they can lead to early failure of the revision procedure. In a multicenter study on 105 total hip revisions due to ceramic head fracture, Allain et al. reported a second revision rate of 31% (33 hips) at 5 years follow up. The main cause of the repeat revisions was aseptic loosening due to metal and polymethyl methacrylate wear [8]. While ceramic head fractures are sudden and catastrophic events that usually can not be prevented, ceramic liner fractures are usually the consequence of repeated trauma due to head subluxation. The early diagnosis of a ceramic liner fracture is desirable and reasonable, to avoid a wide spread of ceramic particles in the periarticular space. The purpose of this study was to present our in-vivo ceramic debris findings with stable, unstable and failed ceramic prosthesis; we will correlate this findings with the experiences reported in vitro with hip simulators in order to correlate the presence and dimensions of ceramic fragments with a clinical situation.

Materials and Methods

Since during revision of the clinical files of ceramic liner fracture we have found that the only relevant early clinical sign was hip noise perceivable during walking, we have performed a study to correlate hip noise with a possible early diagnosis of ceramic failure.

554 patients were telephoned and asked if they ever felt noise in the ceramic THA. The 58 patients who answered in the affirmative were evaluated clinically to exclude a snapping hip: only 10 patients (1.8%) had a noise that could be related to the THA. In the those 10 patients, a computed tomographic scan (CT) to evaluate impingement or instability of the prosthesis, and a needle aspiration for

synovial fluid examination were performed. As a control a needle aspiration was also performed in 7 well performing total THAs. Since this patients recall we have routinely investigate hip noises during follow up clinical controls and we have found 10 more patients presenting a noise related to the ceramic THA.

Results

In the control group of normal ceramic THAs, ceramic fragments were either not detected upon synovial fluid examination (4 cases) or were less than 1 micron in major dimension (3 cases). In contrast, in all the noisy ceramic THAs the presence of ceramic fragments was shown. Scanning electronic microscopy showed that fragment dimensions (>2 µm) and shapes were not compatible with wear, but rather with an early stage of liner fracture. When fragments dimensions were larger then 5µm, a macroscopic liner fracture was found at revision surgery. While, when the fragments were smaller then 5µm and the CT scan showed prosthesis impingement, metal staining of the liner and a mark on the femoral neck were found at revision surgery.

Discussion and Conclusion

The purpose of this study was to present guidelines for the early recognition of clinical signs of ceramic liner fractures. We have found a possible correlation between ceramic liner fracture and an audible hip noise on clinical examination. After ruling out a snapping hip, we recommend performing a CT scan and a needle aspiration in all the patients with a noisy ceramic THA. In our experience, both procedures are helpful for early recognition of ceramic liner chipping/fracture, before wide dissemination of ceramic fragments into the periarticular space occurs. To our knowledge there are no published studies correlating hip noise with ceramic liner fractures.

The particular liner design under investigation (with the liner rim protruding from the metal back) could have increased the incidence of neck-liner impingement and thus of noisy THAs The liner rim did not always fracture at the impingement point with the neck, but it also occurred on the opposite side where there was impact with the dislocating ceramic head. This means that, apart from ceramic liner design, dislocation or subluxation is a major factor causing liner fractures. In this regard, important factors are probably neck design and head diameter and their ratio. In the present series all the THAs had a modular neck [9] and a 28mm head.

Our clinical findings could be also correlated with the in vitro finding in hip simulator tests: Tipper et Al. [10] at SEM analysis report the presence of alumina particle smaller than 1µm after 400,000 cycles running hot isostatically pressed alumina-alumina prosthesis with a a microseparation simulator setting. This finding is in accord with our clinical findings in stable clinically well performing implants.

In conclusion, a noisy ceramic THA can be an early clinical sign of liner chipping or fracture. In presence of a noisy ceramic THA, clinical and radiographic signs of hip instability should be sought so that timely remedial measures can be taken. A needle aspiration could be useful, in presence of ceramic fragments bigger than 1µm a closer follow up is advise, if fragments are bigger than 5µm a ceramic fracture could be suspected.

References

1. Hamadouche, M.; Boutin, P.; Daussange, J.; Bolander, M. E.; and Sedel, L.: Alumina-on-alumina total hip arthroplasty: a minimum 18.5-year follow-up study. J Bone Joint Surg Am, 84-A(1): 69-77, 2002.

2. Bizot, P.; Hannouche, D.; Nizard, R.; Witvoet, J.; and Sedel, L.: Hybrid alumina total hip arthroplasty using a press-fit metal-backed socket in patients younger than 55 years. A six- to 11-year evaluation. J Bone Joint Surg Br, 86(2): 190-4, 2004.

3. D'Antonio, J.; Capello, W.; Manley, M.; Naughton, M.; and Sutton, K.: Alumina ceramic bearings for total hip arthroplasty: five-year results of a prospective randomized study. Clin Orthop Relat Res, (436): 164-71, 2005.

4. Garino, J. P.: Modern ceramic-on-ceramic total hip systems in the United States: early results. Clin Orthop Relat Res, (379): 41-7, 2000.

5. Hannouche, D.; Hamadouche, M.; Nizard, R.; Bizot, P.; Meunier, A.; and Sedel, L.: Ceramics in total hip replacement. Clin Orthop Relat Res, (430): 62-71, 2005.

6. D'Antonio, J.; Capello, W.; Manley, M.; and Bierbaum, B.: New experience with alumina-on-alumina ceramic bearings for total hip arthroplasty. J Arthroplasty, 17(4): 390-7, 2002.

7. Nevelos, J.; Ingham, E.; Doyle, C.; Streicher, R.; Nevelos, A.; Walter, W.; and Fisher, J.: Microseparation of the centers of alumina-alumina artificial hip joints during simulator testing produces clinically relevant wear rates and patterns. J Arthroplasty, 15(6): 793-5, 2000.

8. Allain, J.; Roudot-Thoraval, F.; Delecrin, J.; Anract, P.; Migaud, H.; and Goutallier, D.: Revision total hip arthroplasty performed after fracture of a ceramic femoral head. A multicenter survivorship study. J Bone Joint Surg Am, 85-A(5): 825-30, 2003.

9. Traina, F., Baleani M, Viceconti M, Toni A . Scentific Exhibit SE23: Modular neck primary prosthesis: eperimental and clinical outcomes. In 71st AAOS Annual Meeting. Edited, San Francisco, 2004.

1B.3 Surface Roughness of Ceramic Femoral Heads after In-Vivo Transfer of Metal Correlation to Polyethylene Wear

Y.-H. Kim

Abstract

Background: A dark metallic-appearing smear resembling a lead pencil mark may be seen on the ceramic femoral head component at revision total hip surgery. The purpose of this study was to investigate the hypothesis that such a mark on a retrieved ceramic femoral head is associated with increased surface roughness of the head, and increased polyethylene liner wear in total hip arthroplasty.

Methods: Fifteen ceramic prosthetic femoral heads retrieved from fifteen patients at revision arthroplasty were examined in this study. Thirteen heads had been in vivo for an average of 10.8 years (range, 7.8 to 14.2 years). The remaining two heads had been in vivo for less than one month. The surface roughness characteristics of the explanted ceramic heads, the linear wear of the polyethylene liner, and the patient activity levels after primary replacement before revision were determined.

Results: Four of thirteen ceramic heads which had been in vivo more than 7.8 years had severe (greater than 6% at the surface area) smears and the remaining nine heads had slight smears (less than 6% at the surface area). The two heads which had been in vivo less than one month had severe smears. The mean Ra and Rpm, surface roughness values, in the hips with slightly smeared regions were 26.38 nm and 323.82 nm, respectively and they were 180.77 nm and 1245.88 nm, respectively in the hips with severely smeared regions (P=0.002). The mean linear liner wear rate in the hips with slightly smeared heads was 0.10 mm per year and 0.19 mm per year in the hips with severely smeared heads (P=0.002). The activity score for all patients was 5 or 6 points on a 6 point scale.

Conclusions: The results of this study confirmed the hypothesis that a visual dark metallic-appearing smear on the ceramic femoral head correlates with increased surface roughness of the head and increased polyethylene wear. These findings imply that contact of a ceramic femoral head with a metallic material, such as may occur with femoral head reduction or dislocation of a total hip arthroplasty, is best avoided to prevent this metallic smear phenomenon.

Introduction

Wear-related complications have been a major cause of revision following total hip arthroplasty. The surface roughness of the prosthetic femoral head plays an important role in generating polyethylene wear debris after total hip arthroplasty [1,2]. It has been reported that cobalt-chrome (Co-Cr) heads have rougher surfaces than ceramic heads3 and produce more wear than ceramic heads in studies using a hip simulator [4-7], but studies on the wear of polyethylene liners in vivo have conflicting results [8-17].

At revision surgery a dark metallic-appearing smear resembling a lead pencil mark may be seen on a ceramic femoral head. The purpose of this study was to investigate the hypothesis that ceramic femoral heads exhibiting a metallic-appearing smear, when compared to those that do not, will have a rougher surface and will be associated with greater in vivo polyethylene wear.

Materials and Methods

The study was approved by our institutional review board. All patients provided informed consent. We examined fifteen ceramic femoral heads retrieved at the time of revision operation from fifteen patients with a mean age at the time of the operation of 49.9 years (range, thirty-one to sixty-one years), a mean weight of 61.2 kg (range, 48 to 78 kg), and a mean height of 164.8 cm (range, 154 to 176 cm). The mean duration of implantation of thirteen heads was 10.8 years (range, 7.8 to 14.2 years) and that of two heads was less than one month. One of these two heads was retrieved at a primary total hip arthroplasty, because a ceramic head was scratched very much by a rim of metallic acetabular component during reduction of a femoral head. The other one was retrieved at open reduction of a dislocated total hip arthroplasty. All heads articulated with a polyethylene liner made of ram-extruded 415 GUR polyethylene. The polyethylene had been irradiated in a vacuum and was packaged in a vacuum state. All hips had a 28-mm femoral head.

Analysis of retrieved femoral heads
The surface characteristics of the fifteen explanted ceramic heads were evaluated using three different methods: visual assessment, interferometry (Wyko RST 500 interferometer, Wyko Corporation, Tucson, Arizona), and environmental scanning electron microscopy. Using visual assessment, the femoral head was defined as non smeared if there was no smeared region visible on the femoral head. The femoral head was defined as slightly smeared if the smeared region was less than 6% of the total head surface, and it was defined as severely smeared if the smeared region was more than 6% of the total head surface.

The interferometry measurements were undertaken at two different magnifications using x20 and x40 lenses. The areas of analysis were 125 by 125 microns and 64 by 64 microns, respectively. At each magnification, six measurements were taken on the smeared and non-smeared regions. The results are presented in terms of Ra and Rpm. The parameter Ra is defined as the mathematical average of all deviations (peaks and valleys) from the mean line of the surface profile. The parameter Rpm (the mean leveling depth) is defined as the distance between the mean line and a line parallel to it, which passes through the highest point. The intrinsic errors of the measurement of Ra and Rpm were 0.0219 nm and 0.157 nm, respectively. The measurement resolution of the interferometer is less than 1 angstrom in phase shift interferometry (PSI) mode and less than 1 nm in vertical shift interferometry (VSI) mode. Therefore, the phase shift interferometry mode is more accurate for highly polished surfaces. The vertical shift interferometry is appropriate for surfaces that are rough, or highly contoured, or sharp peaked surfaces typically greater than 0.6 microns in height [18].

The roughness values in the non-smeared region of each head were used to estimate the roughness values of each head before implantation. In addition, two nonimplanted ceramic heads were analyzed to confirm that the non-smeared regions of the retrieved specimens reflected the surface roughness of heads before implantation and thus were appropriate to use as controls.

Further analysis was completed by two scientists who had no knowledge of the clinical and experimental results using a Camscan 4 environmental scanning electron microscopy (Leeds University, Leeds, United Kingdom). Secondary and back scattered images were reviewed at various magnifications (particularly x250) to attempt to identify the composition and origins of the materials adherent to the head surfaces as well as to assess the pits and scratches on the head surfaces.

A Nikon stereoscopic zoom microscope (Nikon Incorporated, Melville, NY) was used to examine grossly the polyethylene liners corresponding to each femoral head for evidence of embedded particle debris. The evidence for particle embedding was examined qualitatively by a research associate who had no knowledge of the clinical and experimental results.

Radiographic analysis

We measured the linear wear of polyethylene radiographically by determining the migration of the center of the femoral head relative to the center of the cup, based on the computer-aided technique of Kim et al. [13]. The 95% confidence interval was taken as a measure of reproducibility. Intraobserver error was ±0.047 mm.

We compared the radiographic measurements with direct measurements of all fifteen cups to validate this wear measurement technique. The linear wear was measured directly from the retrieved polyethylene liners using a three-dimensional co-ordinate measuring machine (BHN 305; Mitutoyo Corporation, Tokyo, Japan). Validation testing revealed that the measuring machine tended to underestimate the true amount of penetration by a mean of 0.08 mm. Therefore, the radiographic measurements of penetration were felt to be reproducible.

Activity levels of patients

The level of activity of patients between primary and revision total hip arthroplasty was assessed with the activity score of Tegner and Lysholm [19]. The activity grading scale, where work and sport activities were graded numerically, was constructed as a complement to the functional score. The patients were given a score according to the activities in which they engaged in daily life. The score ranges from 0 points for a hip-related disability to 10 points for participation in competitive sports at a national level.

Statistics

The Student t test was used to determine possible correlations between the rate of penetration and several specific variables: age, gender, activity level, implantation duration, head type, stem type and cup type. Linear regression analysis was used to reveal any relationship between surface roughness values and age, gender, weight, activity, duration of implantation in vivo, head type, stem type and cup type. The Wilcoxon rank sum test was used to determine any statistical difference in surface roughness between heads articulating with liners that did or did not have embedded debris. P values of less than 0.05 was considered as statistically significant.

Results

Analysis of retrieved femoral heads
Eleven heads were alumina ceramic and four heads were zirconia ceramic. Patient demographics and component data are summarized in the Appendix. On visual evaluation, severe smear was observed on six components and slight smear on nine components (Fig. 1). Four of the thirteen heads which had been in vivo for more than 7.8 years had severe smears and the remaining nine heads had slight smears. Both of the heads which had been in vivo less than one month had severe smears. The area of smearing on the heads ranged from less than 1% to 10% of the total head surface. The results of the measurements by interferometer on the smeared and non-smeared regions on all heads are summarized in Table 1.

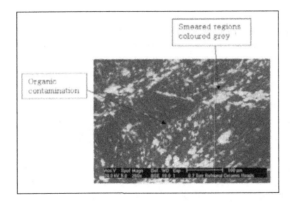

Figure 1:
Photographs of two ceramic femoral heads reveal the smeared area on the head is more than 6% of total head surfaces.

	RA (nm)	STANDARD DEVIATION	95% CONFI-DENCE LIMIT	Rpm (nm)	STANDARD DEVIATION	95% CONFI-DENCE LIMIT
Non-smeared region	Mean, 7.81 (range, 2.53-28.94)	10.05	2.54	Mean, 76.49 (range, 20.27-265.75)	107.43	27.18
Slightly smeared region	Mean, 44.95 (range, 11.44-200.80)	102.39	27.83	Mean, 571.15 (range, 86.94-1331.15)	695.01	188.90
Severely smeared region	Mean, 180.77 (range, 15.3-331.27)	147.81	64.78	Mean, 1245.88 (range, 920.31-1913.5)	986.69	432.43

Table 1:
The results of the interferometry measurements on the smeared and non-smeared regions on all heads (magnification x40).

The roughness values for non-smeared regions of ceramic heads compared well with the roughness values from two never implanted heads. The mean Ra and Rpm values for the never implanted ceramic heads were the same as the mean Ra and Rpm values for the non-smeared regions of the fifteen implanted ceramic heads (Ra: 7.81 nm, Rpm: 76.49 nm). The mean Ra and Rpm values for the slightly smeared regions (in nine heads) were 44.95 nm and 571.15 nm, respectively. The mean Ra and Rpm values for the severely smeared regions (six heads) were 180.77 nm and 1245.88 nm, respectively. The differences in Ra and Rpm values between the slightly smeared and severely smeared regions were significant (P=0.002) irrespective of magnification.

The surfaces roughness values for the slightly smeared regions in the nine ceramic heads without third-body debris embedded in the corresponding polyethylene liner were lower (Ra: 44.95 nm, Rpm: 571.15 nm) than those for the severely smeared regions in six ceramic heads associated with embedded debris (Ra: 180.77 nm, Rpm: 1245.88 nm). The differences in roughness values between two groups were statistically significant both (P=0.02). There was no correlation based on the numbers, however, between roughness parameters of ceramic heads (slightly or severely smeared) and the following parameters: age, gender, weight, activity, duration of implantation in vivo, head type, stem type, and cup type (P>0.05 by linear regression analysis).

Environmental scanning electron microscopic evaluation of the ceramic heads revealed small pits and scratches on the surfaces of ceramic heads in six of nine slightly smeared heads and in all of six severely smeared heads. The difference is not statistically significant based on the numbers (P=0.078) (Fig. 2).

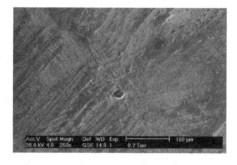

Figure 2:
Three bar graphs demonstrate mean Ra in non-smeared, slightly smeared, and severely smeared regions on the femoral heads. There is no statistical difference (P=0.15) in Ra between the slight smeared and non-smeared regions. On the contrary, there is a significant difference (P=0.002) in Ra between the non-smeared and severely smeared regions irrespective of magnification.

Environmental scanning electron microscopic evaluation of the smeared regions demonstrated a higher atomic number than the ceramic substrate in the back scattered image (Fig. 3). This is indicative of metal deposits on the surface of the ceramic head. However, confirmation of this was difficult because the film of deposited material was very thin (on the order of 3 microns). Therefore, complete chemical identification of the material with energy-dispersive x-ray spectrometry was not possible. Some regions also had particles with a lower atomic number than that of the ceramic substrate, perhaps attributable to organic contamination of the head surface.

Radiographic analysis
Validation testing of the measuring technique revealed a good correlation between the radiographic and direct measurements of polyethylene wear (R²=0.95), and that the radiographic measurement underestimated the direct

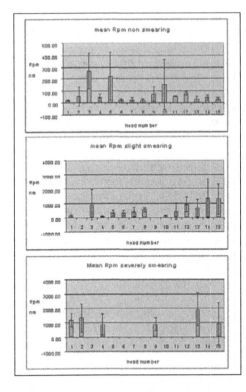

Figure 3:
Three bar graphs show mean Rpm in non-smeared, slightly smeared, and severely smeared regions on the femoral heads. There is no statistical difference (P=0.15) in Rpm between the slightly smeared and non-smeared regions. On the contrary, there is a significant difference (P=0.002) in Rpm between the non-smeared and severely smeared regions of irrespective of magnification.

measurement by a mean of 0.08 mm (Appendix). The mean linear wear rate in the hips with slightly smeared heads was 0.10 mm per year (range, 0.09 to 0.12 mm), and it was 0.19 mm per year (range, 0.16 to 0.24 mm) in the hips with severely smeared heads. This difference was statistically significant (P=0.002).

The mean linear wear rate of polyethylene in the hips with low Ra and Rpm (26.38 nm and 323.82 nm, respectively) was 0.10 mm per year (range, 0.09 to 0.12 mm), and it was 0.19 mm per year (range, 0.16 to 0.24 mm) in the hips with high Ra and Rpm (180.77 nm and 1245.88 nm, respectively). This difference was statistically significant (p=0.002).

The polyethylene linear wear rate for cups associated with third body embedded debris was 0.20 mm per year (range, 0.16 to 0.24 mm), and it was 0.09 mm per year (range, 0.08 to 0.12 mm) in the cups without third body embedded debris. This difference was statistically significant (P=0.03). The polyethylene linear wear rate associated with surface pits and scratches of the femoral heads was 0.21 mm per year (range, 0.16 to 0.24 mm), and it was 0.11 mm per year (range, 0.09 to 0.12 mm) in the heads without surface pits and scratches. This difference was statistically significant (P=0.002)

There was no correlation, based on the numbers, between the wear rate of polyethylene and the following parameters: age, gender, activity level, duration of implantation, head type, stem type, and cup type (P>0.05).

Activity Score
Many patients were quite active despite the usual cautions to avoid activities involving impact after total hip replacement. All patients had an activity score of

5 or 6 points before revision, indicating participation in strenuous farm work (a score of 5 points) or participation in tennis (a score of 6 points).

Discussion

The surface characteristics of the femoral head play an important role in generating polyethylene wear debris after total hip arthroplasty [1,2]. It has been reported that the adherence of third-body particles to the femoral head increases its surface roughness and the resultant abrasive wear process increases the wear rate of the polyethylene liner in the total hip arthroplasty [11]. In the current series, metallic-appearing smears on the ceramic head were found to be transferred metallic debris on the basis of findings of environmental scanning electron microscopic and energy-dispersive x-ray spectrometric examinations. This debris increased the surface roughness and consequently increased the wear of the polyethylene liner through either an abrasive or a third-body wear mechanism. An increase in surface roughness and wear as a result of transferred metal debris might be one of the explanations for the sporadic cases of excessive wear of alumina-on-alumina bearings and the poor results with alumina-on-polyethylene bearings [14-18,20-26]. We confirmed the hypothesis in our study that metallic transfer onto the ceramic femoral head increases surface roughness and consequently increases the wear rate of polyethylene liner.

The transfer of metal debris to the ceramic head occurs even with relatively minor scratching. Black discoloration of a ceramic head can occur simply by lightly scratching the head on a metal surface. Luchetti et al [27]. reported that metal was transferred to a zirconia head when the head was scratched on the metal shell during a closed reduction of a dislocated total hip prosthesis. Therefore, caution is require to avoid contact of the ceramic head with metallic materials during the operation. Because of the hardness of ceramic, one can expect more metal to be transferred to ceramic than to other materials used for a prosthetic head [28].

This study also found that the surface roughness of the ceramic head and an increased polyethylene wear rate were associated with the presence of embedded debris in the articulating polyethylene liner. Therefore, third body contamination should be avoided as much as possible.

Our study has several limitations. The surface characteristics and wear pattern of retrieved femoral heads at revision hip arthroplasty may not represent the surface characteristics and wear pattern of well functioning total hip replacements. The number of heads examined was small, limiting our conclusions. In addition, the examination was not performed in a population al having identical components; femoral heads from different manufacturers may have different initial roughness. However, we attempted to normalize the effect of manufacturing technique on initial surface roughness by using a non-smeared area of each head to estimate the preimplantation roughness of that head.

The results of this study demonstrate that the area of a visual smear resembling a lead pencil mark (metallic transfer) on the ceramic femoral head has increased surface roughness and that presence of a severe (>6% at surfaces area) visual smear correlates with increased polyethylene wear. These findings imply that contact of a ceramic femoral head with metallic material, such as may occur with femoral head reduction or dislocation of a total hip arthroplasty, is best avoided to prevent this metallic smear phenomenon.

Appendix: Tables presenting patient demographic and component data, a comparison of the direct and radiographic measurements of wear, and relationships between wear and demographic data, and figures graphically showing toughness of each femoral head can found on our web site at www.jbjs.org (go to the article citation and click on "Supplementary Material") and on our quarterly CD-ROM (call our subscription department, at 781-449-9780, to order the CD-ROM)

References

1. Cuckler JM, Bearcroft J. Asgian CM. Femoral head technologies to reduce polyethylene wear in total hip arthroplasty. Clin Orthop. 1995; 317: 57-63.
2. Weightman B, Light D. The effect of the surface finish of alumina and stainless steel on he wear rate of UHMW polyethylene. Biomaterials. 1986; 17: 20-4.
3. Davidson JA. Characteristics of metal and ceramic total hip bearing surfaces and their effect on long-term ultra high molecular weight polyethylene wear. Clin Orthop. 1993; 294: 361-78.
4. Saikko VA, Paavolainen PO, Slätis P. Wear of the polyethylene acetabular cup: metallic and ceramic heads compared in a hip simulator. Acta Orthop Scand. 1993; 64: 391-402.
5. Dowson D. A comparative study of the performance of metallic and ceramic femoral head components in total replacement hip joints. Wear 1995; 190: 171-83.
6. Cooper JR, Dowson D, Fisher J, Jobbins B. Ceramic bearing in total artificial joints: resistance to third body wear damage from bone cement particles. J Med Eng Technol. 1991; 15: 63-7.
7. Wroblewski BM, Siney PD, Dowson D, Collins SN. Prospective clinical and joint simulator studies of a new total hip arthroplasty using alumina ceramic heads and cross-linked polyethylene cups. J Bone Joint Surg Br. 1996; 78: 280-5.
8. Schuller HM, Marti RK. Ten-year socket wear in 66 hip arthroplasties: ceramic versus metal heads. Acta Orthop Scand. 1990; 61: 240-3.
9. Zichner LP, Willert H-G. Comparison of alumina-polyethylene and metal polyethylene in clinical trials. Clin Orthop. 1992; 282: 86-94.
10. Oonishi H, Igaki H, Takayama Y. Comparisons of wear of UHMW polyethylene sliding against metal and alumina in total hip prostheses. In: Oonishi H, Hideki A, Sawai K, eds. Bioceramics: vol. 1. St Louis: Ishiyaku Euro America, 1989: 272-7.
11. Tanaka K, Tamura J, Kwanabe K, Shimizu M, Nakamura T. Effect of alumina femoral heads on polyethylene wear in cemented total hip arthroplasty: old versus current alumina. J Bone Joint Surg Br. 2003; 85: 655-60.
12. Dowson D, Diab M, Gillis B, Atkinson J. Influence of countersurface topography on the wear of UHMWPE under wet or dry conditions: polymer wear and its control. Washington DC, American Chemical Society. 1985; 171-87.
13. Kim Y-H, Kim J-S, Cho S-H. A comparison of polyethylene wear in hips with cobalt-chrome or zirconia heads: a prospective, randomized study. J Bone Joint Surg Br. 2001; 83: 742-50.
14. Sychterz CJ, Engh CA Jr, Young AM, Hopper RH Jr, Engh CA. Comparison of in vivo wear between polyethylene liners articulating with ceramic and cobalt-chrome femoral heads. J Bone Joint Surg Br. 2000; 82: 948-51.
15. Sychterz CJ, Engh CA Jr, Swope SW, McNulty DE, Engh CA. Analysis of prosthetic femoral heads retrieve at autopsy. Clin Orthop. 1999; 358: 223-34.
16. Sychterz CJ, Engh CA Jr, Shah N, Engh CA Sr. Radiographic evaluation of penetration by the femoral head into the polyethylene liner over time. J Bone Joint Surg Am. 1997; 79: 1040-46.

17. Devane PA, Horne JG , Botsford D. Do ceramic femoral heads lower three dimensional polyethylene wear? A matched comparison with stainless steel femoral heads. Trans Orthop Res. 1997.

18. Lippold S, Podlesny J. RST Plus tehnical reference manual. 2nd ed. Tucson, AZ: Wyko Corporation; 1995.

19. Tegner Y, Lysholm J. Rating systems in the evaluation of knee ligament injuries. Clin Orthop. 1985; 198: 43-9.

20. Hasegawa M, Ohashi T, Tani T. Poor outcome of 44 cemented total hip arthroplasties with alumina ceramic heads: clinical evaluation and retrieval analysis after 10-16 years. Acta Orthop Scand. 2001; 72: 449-56.

21. Boehler M, Knahr K, Plenk H Jr, Walter A, Salzer M, Schreiber V. Long-term results of uncemented alumina acetabular implants. J Bone Joint Surg Br. 1994; 76: 53-9.

22. Garino JP. Modern ceramic-on-ceramic total hip systems in the United States: early results. Clin Orthop. 2000; 379: 41-7.

23. Mahoney OM, Dimon JH 3rd. Unsatisfactory results with a ceramic total hip prosthesis. J Bone Joint Surg Am. 1990; 72: 663-71.

24. Saito M, Saito S, Ohzono K, Takaoka K, Ono K. Efficacy of alumina ceramic heads fo cemented total hip arthroplasty. Clin Orthop. 1992; 283: 171-7.

25. Winter M, Griss P, Scheller G, Moser T. Ten-to 14-year results of a ceramic hip prosthesis. Clin Orthop. 1992; 282: 73-80.

26. Wirganowicz PZ, Thomas BJ. Massive osteolysis after ceramic on ceramic total hip arthroplasty. A case report. Clin Orthop. 1997; 338: 100-4.

27. Luchetti WT, Copley LA, Vresilovic EJ, Black J, Steinberg ME. Drain entrapment and titanium to ceramic head deposition: two unique complications following closed reduction of a dislocated total hip arthroplasty. J Arthroplasty. 1998; 13: 713-7.

28. Skinner HB. Ceramic bearing surfaces. Clin Orthop. 1999; 369: 83-91.

1B.4 Hydrothermal Stability of Ceramic Femoral Heads

V. Corfield, I. Khan and R. Scott

Introduction

Alumina ceramics have been used in total hip replacements for over 30 years with much success, although some *in-vivo* failures of early generation alumina ceramic heads were reported. This resulted in the introduction of zirconia (yttria-stabilised tetragonal zirconia, Y-TZP) as a ceramic femoral head, with its improved strength and fracture toughness. Zirconia, however, is known to undergo hydrothermal degradation. This hydrothermal degradation is due to the phase transformation from the metastable tetragonal phase into the monoclinic phase. This transformation starts from the surface and progresses into the bulk with a volume increase of approximately 3-4 %. This increase in monoclinic phase content may result in surface roughening of the ceramic head and is linked to a reduction in strength and increased UHMWPE wear [1,5].

To overcome the issue of hydrothermal instability of zirconia, a ZTA ceramic, Biolox Delta, was developed. Biolox Delta consists of an alumina matrix with a finely dispersed Y-TZP component (approximately 24%) and other oxides (Cr_2O_3 and SrO). It has been described as a material that "combines the excellent material properties of alumina ceramics in terms of chemical stability, hydrothermal stability, biocompatibility and extremely low wear and of zirconia ceramics with its superior mechanical strength and fracture toughness" [7].

The presence of Y-TZP within Biolox Delta suggests that hydrothermal degradation of this material may occur and the hydrothermal stability must be investigated fully. The resistance of Biolox Delta to artificial aging has been reported previously in terms of monoclinic content, flexural strength, burst strength and wear rate but surface roughening has not been investigated [3,9,10].

This current study investigated the monoclinic phase content, surface roughness and burst strength of Biolox Delta (ZTA) femoral heads in comparison with Biolox Forte (alumina) and Zyranox (zirconia) following artificial aging. A comparison has also been made with a Zyranox zirconia ceramic femoral head retrieved after 12 years implantation.

Materials and Methods

Zirconia (Zyranox, Morgan Advanced Ceramics, 32 mm diameter, Type 1, -3), alumina (Biolox Forte, CeramTec, 28 mm diameter, 12/14 taper, +3.5) and ZTA (Biolox Delta, CeramTec, 28 mm diameter, 12/14 taper, +3.5) ceramic femoral heads were investigated. The ceramic heads were cleaned and packaged in accordance with Biomet specifications. They were then irradiated at Isotron at an absorbed dose of 25 – 40 kGy. The ceramic heads were artificially aged within an autoclave at a temperature of 135 °C at a pressure of 2 bar for periods of 5, 10 and 50 hours. These autoclave time points correspond to approximately 10, 20 and 100 years *in-vivo* in accordance with ASTM standard F2345-03.

For each time point, the average surface roughness was measured using a non-contact Proscan 2000 profilometer and stylus Talysurf profilometer. The monoclinic content of zirconia-containing ceramic heads was measured using X-ray diffraction. Axial ultimate compression strength tests were also performed on the ceramic femoral heads in accordance with ISO 7206-10, 2003. The non-contact profilometry was carried out at the University of Bath, Bath, UK. X-ray diffraction analysis was undertaken at Cranfield University, Shrivenham, UK. Axial ultimate compression testing was performed at NPL, Teddington, UK. The surface roughness and monoclinic content of a Zyranox zirconia ceramic head retrieved after 12 years in vivo was also measured.

Results

Following artificial aging, visual inspection of the zirconia ceramic showed that surface roughening had occurred after 10 hours, as illustrated by the change in reflection shown in Figure 3.1. The zirconia femoral heads also changed colour from a purplish-grey following irradiation to off-white after artificial aging. The surface roughening of the zirconia ceramic was confirmed using profilometry measurements. The roughness values measured using non-contact profilometry were higher than those measured using stylus profilometry. Using non-contact profilometry, the average surface roughness (R_a) after 10 hours aging was nearly 7 times greater than the unaged zirconia samples. With stylus profilometry, an average surface roughness of 47.6 nm (±5.4 nm) was measured after 10 hours and appeared to decrease again after 50 hours to 35.4 nm (±0.1 nm). The alumina and ZTA ceramics did not undergo any surface roughening and the roughness values were approximately 15 nm at all time points. The average surface roughness value of the retrieved zirconia ceramic femoral head was measured as 36.4 nm (±3.9 nm) and is also plotted in Figure 1.

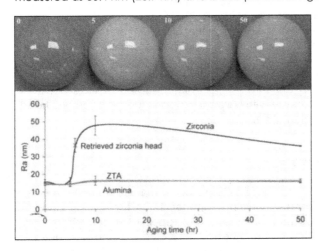

Figure 1:
Zirconia ceramic femoral heads at different aging time points (top). Average roughness (R_a) of ceramic femoral heads (bottom).

The monoclinic content of the zirconia containing ceramics was measured and the results are shown in Figure 2. For the artificially aged ceramic heads, the surface monoclinic content of zirconia increased from 2.9 wt.% to 66 wt.% after 50 hours. However, the surface monoclinic content within ZTA only increased from

3.4 wt.% to 5.5 wt.% after 50 hours. Phase transformation was also observed on the retrieved zirconia femoral head. The surface monoclinic content varied with location on the femoral head and ranged from 40 wt.% to 60.8 wt.% as shown in Figure 3. The greatest surface monoclinic phase content was noted at the pole of the femoral head.

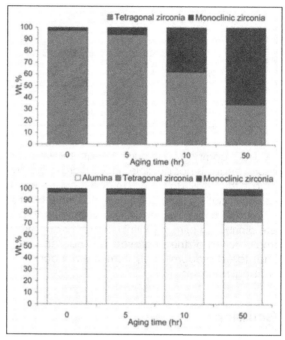

Figure 2:
Wt.% content of tetragonal and monoclinic zirconia phases within the articulating surface of (top) zirconia (Zyranox) and (bottom) ZTA (Biolox Delta).

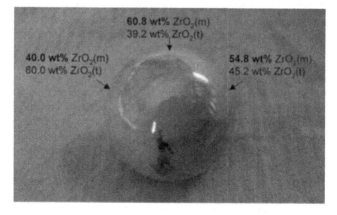

Figure 3:
Wt.% content of tetragonal and monoclinic zirconia phases at different regions on the retrieved Zyranox (zirconia) ceramic head.

The burst strength of the ceramic femoral heads was measured and the results are shown in Figure 4. For zirconia, the average burst strength appeared to increase with artificial aging time, however, a Welch's t-test was carried out at each aging time point in comparison with the unaged condition and no statistical significant differences were seen. Student's t-tests were performed on alumina and ZTA at each time point in comparison with the unaged condition and once again no statistical significant differences were seen.

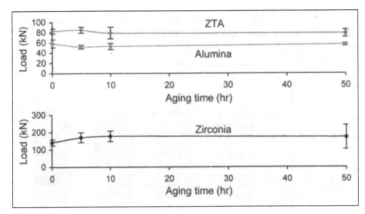

Figure 4:
Burst strength of ceramic femoral heads at different aging time points.

A direct comparison in burst strength between zirconia and the other ceramic femoral heads is not possible since a larger diameter head size for zirconia was tested in this study. However, ZTA had a burst strength in the region of 81 kN, which was significantly greater than alumina with a burst strength in the region of 55 kN. The fracture origin sites for all the ceramic femoral heads were investigated and were distributed primarily within the taper and around the taper mouth. Four ZTA samples failed at the engraved text near the mouth of the taper and zirconia heads failed predominately from internal pores or small cracks associated with hard agglomerates.

Discussion

In this study, the surface roughness and burst strength of Biolox Delta were unchanged by artificial aging in an autoclave for up to 50 hours. Rack and Pfaff also reported no change in the burst strength following artificial aging in a steam autoclave at 135 °C and a pressure of 2 bar for up to 20 hours [10].

The monoclinic content of Biolox Delta increased slightly from 3.4 wt.% to 5.5 wt.% after 50 hours aging. This increase is much lower than that observed by Burger and Richter where an increase to approximately 30% was seen following approximately 1 hour aging at 140 °C before remaining constant [3]. The requirement of Biolox Delta to undergo phase transformation as a toughening mechanism during severe loading conditions means that the initial monoclinic phase must be as low as possible, and Biolox Delta components are produced with a monoclinic content below the acceptable benchmark value of 10% [6]. The Biolox Delta investigated in this study remained below this benchmark value even after 50 hours' artificial aging.

Alumina was unaffected by artificial aging in a steam autoclave, even after 50 hours. However, artificial aging of zirconia ceramic heads resulted in increased surface roughness and monoclinic content. The increase in surface roughness measured using stylus profilometry was within the acceptable range, as stated by Clarke et al. [4]. The difference between the non-contact and stylus profilometry results could be attributed to optical irregularities with the non-contact measuring system caused by the highly polished ceramic surface. It is important to note that the average roughness values measured using different profilometry techniques cannot be compared directly.

Pfaff and Willmann have reported an increase in surface roughness of zirconia following artificial aging. Bumps were seen on the surface, corresponding with regions of increased monoclinic content. It was hypothesised that non-homogeneous surface phase transformation of zirconia results in a decrease in mechanical properties, which is a probable cause of *in vivo* failure [8]. In the current study, a high surface monoclinic content of 60.9 wt.% did not result in a change in average burst strength. This is in agreement with Blaise et al. who reported that the burst strength of zirconia ceramic heads with 60% surface monoclinic content was the same as unaged zirconia ceramic heads [2].

Mixed reports on the hydrothermal stability of retrieved zirconia ceramic femoral heads are available in the literature. In this study, a zirconia femoral head retrieved following 12 years implantation had undergone hydrothermal degradation. The Zyranox ceramic head had an increased average surface roughness value of approximately 36 nm and a high monoclinic phase content (40 wt.% to 60.8 wt.%). The surgeon who retrieved the component reported that the UHMWPE that had articulated against the zirconia head had excessively worn. This excessive wear could possibly be attributed to the increase in surface roughness of the zirconia head. However, the articulating UHMWPE component was manufactured during the period when gamma irradiation in air was used and it is probable that oxidation of the UHMWPE component occurred resulting in excessive wear, although the UHMWPE component was not available for analysis.

Conclusion

Biolox Delta ceramic femoral heads have improved burst strength in comparison to alumina. In addition, they do not appear to undergo the hydrothermal degradation, particularly surface roughening, reported with zirconia ceramic femoral heads following artificial aging or longterm implantation.

References

1. Allain J, Le Mouel S, Goutallier D, Voisin MC (1999) Poor eight-year survival of cemented zirconia-polyethylene total hip replacements. The Journal of Bone and Joint Surgery (British Edition) vol 81-B, no 5, pp. 835-842.
2. Blaise L, Villermaux F, Cales B (2001) Ageing of Zirconia: Everything You Always Wanted to Know. Key Engineering Materials vol 192-195, pp. 553-556.
3. Burger W, Richter HG (2001) High strength and toughness alumina matrix composites by transformation toughening and 'in situ' platelet reinforcement (ZPTA) - The new generation of bioceramics. Key Engineering Materials vol 192-195, pp.545-548.
4. Clarke IC, Green DD, Pezzotti G, Donaldson D (2005) 20 Years Experience of Zirconia Total Hip Replacements. In: D'Antonio JA, Dietrich M (eds) Ceramics in Orthopaedics 10th Biolox Symposium Proceedings, pp. 67-78.
5. Hernigou P, Bahrami P (2003) Zirconia and alumina ceramics in comparison with stainless-steel heads, polyethylene wear after a minimum ten-year follow-up. The Journal of Bone and Joint Surgery (British Edition) vol 85-B, pp. 504-509.

6. Kuntz M, Schneider N, Heros R (2005) Controlled Zirconia Phase Transformation in Biolox® delta – a Feature of Safety. In: D'Antonio JA, Dietrich M (eds) Ceramics in Orthopaedics 10th Biolox Symposium Proceedings, pp. 79-83.

7. Merkert P (2003) Next Generation Ceramic Bearings. In: Zippel H, Dietrich M (eds) Bioceramics in Joint Arthroplasty 8th BIOLOX Symposium Proceedings, pp. 123-125.

8. Pfaff H-G, Willmann G (1998) Stability of Y-TZP Zirconia. In: Puhl W (ed) Bioceramics in Orthopaedics – New Applications Proceedings of the 3rd International Symposium on Ceramic Wear Couple, pp. 29-31.

9. Rack R, Pfaff H-G (2000) A New Ceramic for Orthopaedics. In: Willmann G, Zweymuller KA (eds) Bioceramics in Hip Joint Replacement Proceedings 5th International CeramTec Symposium, pp. 141-145.

10. Rack R, Pfaff H-G (2001) Long-term Performance of the Alumina Matrix Composite Biolox® Delta. In: Toni A, Willmann G (eds) Bioceramics in Joint Arthroplasty Proceedings 6th International BIOLOX Symposium, pp. 103-108.

SESSION 2

Ceramic/Polyethylene

2.1 Ceramic on highly cross-linked Polyethylene in cementless Total Hip Arthroplasty

J.-S. Kang and K.-H. Moon

Abstract

Thirty six patients (42 hips) underwent cementless total hip arthroplasty using a porous-coated acetabular cup, highly cross linked polyethylene liner (Marathon™), and a extensively porous-coated femoral stem. One patient (1 hip) died and 2 patients (3 hips) were lost to follow-up. The remaining 33 patients (39 hips) were followed for 4 to 6 years. Their mean age at the index operation was 67 years. Clinical assessment was performed with use of the Harris hip score and radiographic analysis included measurements of acetabular component position, fixation, and osteolysis. The mean Harris hip score was 92 points at the time of final follow-up. Four patients (4 hips) had mild thigh pain. All acetabular and femoral components were bone-ingrown, and neither pelvic nor femoral osteolysis was identified. The subsequent head penetration, with elimination of the bedding-in wear, resulted in a linear wear rate of 0.032 +/- 0.02 mm per year. These early data support the continued use of this highly cross-linked polyethylene liner for total hip arthroplasty.

Introduction

Total hip arthroplasty is one of the most successful and cost effective surgical interventions in medicine, relieving pain and restoring function of hip joint. Improvements in septic prophylaxis, implant fatigue strength and osteointegration have made wear and the biologic response to the subsequent particulate debris the weak link in the long term success of total joint arthroplasty [1,8,14]. The annual wear rate in polyethylene articulation should be 0.1mm or less to avoid future osteolysis [2,8]. Highy crosslinked polyethylene demonstrates 80-90% wear reduction in hip simulating test [11]. We prospectively analyzed midterm results in patients who cementless total hip arthroplasty using a porous-coated acetabular cup, highly cross linked polyethylene liner (Marathon™).

Material and Method

Thirty six patients (42 hips) underwent cementless total hip arthroplasty using a porous-coated acetabular cup, highly cross linked polyethylene liner (Marathon™), and an extensively porous-coated femoral stem(Anatomic Medullary Locking, AML, Depuy, Warsaw, In, USA). A 28mm alumina head used in all hips. One patient (1 hip) died and 2 patients (3 hips) were lost to follow-up. The remaining 33 patients (39 hips) were followed for 4 to 6 years. Their mean age at the index operation was 67 years. The diagnosis was osteonecrosis for 22 hips, osteoarthritis secondary to developmental dysplasia for 10 hips and femoral neck fracture for 7 hips. Clinical assessment was performed with use of the Harris hip score and radiographic analysis included measurements of acetabular component position, fixation, and osteolysis. Two dimensional femoral head penetration was manually measured with use of Dorr and Wan method [3,4].

Results

Clinical results

The average Harris hip score was 92.3(range, 76-100) points at the final follow-up. Hip scores at last follow-up were; excellent in 28 out of 39 hips (71.8%), good in 8 (20.5%) hips and fair in 3(7.7%) hips. The prevalence of thigh pain was 23.7%(4 hips) initially and the pain disappeared 3 years after surgery in all hips.

Radiographic results

Thirty-five(89.75%) stems had good canal fill. All of these showed bone ingrowth. Four (10.5%) hips had a poor canal fill. Three of these showed bone ingrowth, and one hip showed stable fibrous ingrowth. There was no unstable stem. All acetabular and femoral components were bone-ingrown, and neither pelvic nor femoral osteolysis was identified. The subsequent head penetration, with elimination of the bedding-in wear, resulted in a linear wear rate of 0.032 +/- 0.02 mm per year.

Discussion

Wear of ultra-high molecular weight polyethylene(WHMWPE) prostheses in total joint arthroplasty produces billions of submicron particles annually that may cause a foreign body response leading to extensive bone resorption and gross loosening of the components. Improving the wear resistance of polyethylene, and as a result, reducing the number of particles released to the periarticular tissues, could extend substantially the clinical lifespan of total joint replacements. Effort to improve the wear performance of UHMWPE by method such as high pressure crystallization and fiber reinforcements have not been successful in the past largely because little information on the wear mechanism of UHMWPE in vivo was available [6,10,15]. Implant retrieval studies have shown that this wear occurs by distinct mechanisms involving surface orientation of the material and subsequent rupture of this oriented surface layer during multidirectional motions, which occur at these articulation in vivo [12,13]. This observation led to the development of cross-linked ultrahigh molecular weight polyethylenes (XLP) that are resistant to this type of wear by minimizing surface orientation.

Marathon™ cross linked polyethylene is composed of GUR 1050 (calcium stearate-free) resin consolidated in to cylindrical bars by ram extrusion [11]. Cross linking is achieved by gamma irradiation to 5mrad. Residual free radicals are eliminated by heating the bulk material above the melting point (stabilization). Acetabular components are then machined from this material and placed into a traditional barrier package. Terminal sterilization is with gas plasma.

In hip wear simulator studies, the wear of acetabular components composed of Marathon™ was 85% lower than that of non-irradiated components [11]. The proportional increase in wear resistance was maintained in an abrasive environment and artificial aging.

The reduction in yield strength, ultimate tensile strength and elongation to break are reduced compared to non-irradiated material but very similar to that of components sterilized by traditional method. Because there are no residual free radicals in Marathon™, these material properties are constant over time and not affected by aging (oxidation).

In a recent report [9], with a minimum of 2 years follow up, patients with conventional polyethylene showed a mean linear wear rate of 0.13mm per year and a mean volumetric rate of 87.6mm³ per year. In contrary, the group with Marathon™ cross-linked polyethylene showed a mean linear rate of 0.02mm per year and a mean volumetric rate of 17.0mm³ per year.

Engh et al [5] reported the clinical outcomes (randomized prospective study) after total hip arthroplasty using cross-linked Marathon™ and non-cross-linked Enduron polyethylene liners. At a mean follow-up of 5.7 years, the clinical outcomes among the Marathon and Enduron liners were similar. However, the mean wear rate was 0.01 +/- 0.07 mm/y for the Marathon group, which represents a 95% reduction compared with the mean wear rate of 0.19 +/- 0.12 mm/y for the Enduron group. The results of this study are promising. Clinical results are comparable with traditional poly. The in vivo wear reduction with this crosslinked polyethylene is consistent with the prediction of hip simulator studies. Longer follow-up is needed to determine if the occurrence of osteolysis, nor revision for any reason related to the bearing, are similarly reduced.

References

1. Ayers DC: Polyethylene wear and osteolysis following total knee replacement. Instr Course Lect 1997;46:205-213.

2. Clohisy JC and Harris WH: The Harris-Galante uncemented femoral component in primary total hip replacement at 10 years. J Arthroplasty 1999;14:915-917.

3. Dorr LD, Wan Z: Ten years of experience with porous acetabular components for revision surgery. Clin Orthop Relat Res. 1995;319;191-200.

4. Dorr LD, Lewonowski K, Lucero M, Harris M and Wan Z: Failure mechanisms of anatomic porous replacement I cementless total hip replacement. Clin Orthop 1997;334:157-167.

5. Engh CA Jr, Stepniewski AS, Ginn SD et al: A randomized prospective evaluation of outcomes after total hip arthroplasty using cross-linked marathon and non-cross-linked Enduron polyethylene liners. HYPERLINK "javascript:AL_get(this, 'jour', 'J Arthroplasty.');" J Arthroplasty. 2006 Sep;21(6 Suppl 2):17-25.

6. Ezzet KA: Early failure of Hylamer acetabular inserts due to eccentric wear. J Arthroplasty. 1996; 11:351-3.

7. Fisher J, Leeds, McEwen HML et al: Can polyethylene wear be decreased? 2004 AAOS Meeting, Symposium III.

8. Harris WH: The problem is osteolysis. Clin Orthop 1995;311:46-53.

9. Heisel C, Silver M dela Rosa M and Schmalzried TP: Short term in vivo wear of cross linked polyethylene. J Bone Joint Surg 86-A: 748-751, 2004.

10. Kurtz SM, Muratoglu OK, Evans M and Eddin AA: Advances in the processing, sterilization and crosslinking of ultra-high molecular weight polyethylene for total joint arthroplasty. Biomaterials 1999;20:1659-1688.

11. McKellop H, Shen FW, Lu B, Campbell P and Salovey R: Development of an extremely wear resistant ultra high molecular weight polyethylene for total hip replacements. J Orthop Res 1999;17:157-167.

12. Sakoda H, Voice AM, McEwen HM et al: A comparison of the wear and physical properties of silane cross-linked polyethylene and ultra-high molecular weight polyethylene. J Arthroplasty 2001;16:1018-1023.

13. Schmalzried TP, Kwong LM, Jasty MJ et al: The mechanism of loosening of cemented acetabular components in total hip arthroplasty: Analysis of specimens retrieved at autopsy. Clin Orthop 1992;274:60-78.

14. Tanner MG, Whiteside LA and White SE: Effect of polyethylene quality on wear in total knee arthroplasty. Clin Orthop 1995;317:83-88.

15. Willie BM, Gingell DT, Bloebaum RD and Hoffmann AA: Possible explanation for the white bands artifacts seen in clinically retrieved polyethylene tibial component. J Biomed Mater Res 2000;52:558-866.

16. Wrobleswski BM, Sidney PD, Dowsin D and Collins SN: Prospective clinical and joint simulator studies of a new total joint arthroplasty using alumina ceramic heads and cross-linked polyethylene cups. J Bone Joint Surg Br 1996;78:280-285.

2.2 Comparative Analysis of Ceramic to Ceramic Bearing with Metal to Electron Beam-Irradiated highly cross-linked UHMWPE Bearing

S.-K. Kim, J.-W. Park, J.-H. Wang and J.-G. Kim

Introduction

Ceramics were introduced in total hip arthroplasty to address the problems of friction and wear that were reported with metal on polyethylene articulations. This remarkable sliding characteristics and wettable material could limit wear debries generation and provide longer lifetime of the artificial hip. Extensive clinical study shows that alumina to alumina is the best used in young and active patients, while the classic metal on polyethylene couple remains the gold standard in the remaining population. Compared with metal, ceramic is weak in tension and brittle and fracture is well recognized problem.

Electron beam -irradiated, postirradiation-melted, highly cross-linked polyethylene currently have been increasingly used in hip bearings with increasing wear resistance and oxidative resistance. However, it has been suggested that mechanical property of the cross-linked polyethylene remains poorly understood because thermal processing takes place near the melting transition for ultra high molecular weight polyethylene.

The purpose of this study was to study the clinical results, including observation of osteolysis, penetration of femoral head on the metal to cross-linked ultra high molecular weight polyethylene in a short term follow-up period, thus comparing with ceramic to ceramic couples.

Materials and Method

Total of fifty-two cases of electron-beam irradiated ultra high molecular weight polyethylene liner (Longevity, Zimmer Co, Warsaw, Ind) were examined for this study. Minimum of 2 years of follow -up from early post operative period to maximum follow-up to 3.4 years postoperative radiographs with average 2.6 years were reviewed. Revision arthroplasties were not included in this study and 28mm cobalt chrome (CoCr) femoral heads and uncemented acetabular shell (Zimmer Co) were used in all the examined cases.

We examined 47cases of alumina on alumina total hip arthroplasties which implanted in 44 patients by using Biolox forte (Ceramtec, Plichingen, Germany) with follow-up to 3.5 years. The average age of the patients at the time of operation was 56 years (range, 22 to 75 years) in polyethylene group and 52 years (range, 22 to 62 years) in ceramic group. Ten patients implanted bilaterally on one side metal to polyethylene and on the other side alumina to alumina couple. Clinical and radiological studies included Harris-hip score, dislocation, osteolysis, penetration of head, abnormal sound and related complications.

Results

At maximal 3.6 years follow-up, no hip with both group had been revised any reason. The average postoperative Harris hip score in metal to highly cross-linked ultra high molecular weight polyethylene was 89 (range, 71-100) and 90 (range,75-100) in ceramic to ceramic, thus showed no differences. For the metal to highly cross-linked ultra high molecular weight polyethylene, there was no case of osteolysis and one case of dislocation developed. For ceramic to ceramic, there was no case of osteolysis developed, no dislocation, no abnormal sounds such as squeaking audible.

For the metal to highly cross-linked ultra high molecular weight polyethylene the overall penetration rate was variable with average 0.314+-0.255mm/year (range, 0.091-1.231). For ceramic to ceramic, it was very hard to measure exactly because there was almost no wear and too much radiopaque to measure. There showed average rate of 0.003mm/year (range, 0.001- 0.01). There was no massive wear.

The overall penetration rate for the metal to highly cross-linked ultra high molecular weight polyethylene group was significantly much higher than the overall penetration rate for the ceramic group in a short term follow-up periods. Femoral head penetration was variable during the early postoperative periods of average 2.6 years.

Both magnitude and variability of penetration rate suggested of bedding-in phenomenon which characterizes the creep in ultra high molecular weight polyethylene.

Discussion

This study represents early follow-up observations of wear and development of osteolysis for the electron beam ultra high molecular weight polyethylene with 28mm CoCr femoral heads and ceramic to ceramic couple in uncemented acetabular component in primary THR. In this comparative study, magnitude of wear rate of the highly cross-linked electron-beam irradiated ultra high molecular weight polyethylene was significantly high and variable, compared with ceramic to ceramic and traditional ultra high molecular weight. However, the magnitude of this wear rate is unlikely to account the reduction of material.

As has been reported previously, during early follow-up periods, a large portion of the total femoral head penetration is contributable to the bedding in process. Recently Estok 2nd et al reported that 90 percent of the creep in highly ultra high molecular weight polyethylene had occurred by 2.5 million cycles. Manning et al reported that the total magnitude of penetration during the 1 to 2 years overstate true material loss, whereas the steady-state penetration, after the conclusion of creep and bedding-in process in electron beam-irradiated, melted polyethylene was completed by years. In this study it was concluded that higher magnitude and variability of the wear rate in the early follow-up period was attributed to the bedding-in process in electron beam-irradiated, melted highly cross-linked polyethylene. In the absence of long-term data, it is not evident whether early measures of wear can be used to predict future performance.

Further follow-up is needed to evaluate the effect of bedding-in, the longer-term steady-state wear rate, and the incidence of osteolysis in patients receiving the electron beam ultra high molecular weight polyethylene with 28 CoCr femoral heads.

2.3 Comparison of Uncemented Total Hip Arthroplasty between Metal on Metal and Ceramic on Polyethylene Bearing Surfaces in Young Patients

Y.-H. Kim

Abstract

Reducing wear guarantees the longer survivorship of the implants by reducing the osteolysis and aseptic loosening. Thus, the need for improved bearing surfaces in THA has led to the development and study of alternative bearing materials. We retrospectively reviewed the clinical and radiographic results of the metal-on-metal and ceramic-on-polyethylene articulation by matched pair study. There were 28 hips in the metal-on-metal group and 28 hips in the ceramic-on-polyethylene group. The average periods of follow-up were 111 months in the metal-on-metal group and 106 months in the ceramic-on-polyethylene group. The mean Harris hip score of the final follow-up was 94.5 points in the metal-on-metal group and was 96.1 points in the ceramic-on-polyethylene group. The mean linear and volumetric wear rate of ceramic-on-polyethylene group was 0.08 ± 0.02 mm/yr and 87.42 ± 6.17 mm^3/yr, respectively. Both group showed the excellent clinical and radiographic result with rare radiolucency and osteolysis. But there were three hips showing the unexplained groin pain in the metal-on-metal group. Of these, one hip underwent the revision surgery due to the periacetabular osteolysis which showed the histological findings compatible to the delayed metal hypersensitivity. In conclusion, both the metal-on-metal and ceramic-on-polyethylene articulations are the excellent alternative bearings of the conventional total hip arthroplasty. But, the ceramic-on-polyethylene articulation was the safer option than the metal-on-metal articulation.

Osteolysis resulting from polyethylene wear debris is one of the most common causes of implant failure in young, active individuals who undergo total hip arthroplasty. Reducing wear guarantees the longer survivorship of the implants by reducing the osteolysis and aseptic loosening. Thus, the need for improved bearing surfaces in THA has led to the development and study of alternative bearing materials. These alternative bearing surfaces include metal-on-metal, alumina ceramic-on-alumina ceramic, zirconia-on-polyethylene, alumina ceramic-on-polyethylene or cross-linked polyethylene.

These articulations have great success in reducing wear by disusing the polyethylene or modifying the polyethylene property. But it has been reported that these articulations have various disadvantages becoming new concerns.

Of these new articulations, we have experiences only in metal-on-metal and ceramic-on-polyethylene bearings. The purpose of this retrospective matched pair study was to compare the clinical and radiographic outcomes of the metal-on-metal and ceramic-on-polyethylene bearings in young patients.

Material and Methods

From January 1994 to September 1998, 168 hips (102 patients) underwent total hip arthroplasties with use of metal-on-metal articulations and 84 hips (54 patients) underwent total hip arthroplasties with use of ceramic-on-polyethylene articulations by one surgeon (Y.-H.K.). Of these 252 total hip arthroplasties, 56 hips (43 patients) were enrolled in this study with matched pair variables (28 hips in metal-on-metal and 28 hips in ceramic-on-polyethylene). There were fourteen men and nine women in metal-on-metal group and thirteen men and seven women in ceramic-on-polyethylene group. The average age of the patients at the time of the index operation was thirty-eight years (range, nineteen to fifty years) in metal-on-metal group and forty years (range, twenty-one to fifty years) in ceramic-on-polyethylene group. The average period of the follow-up was 111 months (range, 96 months to 122 months) in metal-on-metal group and 106 months (range, 98 months to 124 months) in ceramic-on-polyethylene group. Other demographic data are listed on Table 1.

	Metal-on-Metal group	Ceramic-on-Polyethylene group
Case	28 hips (23 patients)	28 hips (20 patients)
Age	38.7 (19~50)	40 (21~50)
Sex (M:F)	14:9	13:7
Diagnosis		
Osteonecrosis of the femoral head	21	19
Osteoarthritis	2	1
Old neck fracture	1	
Sequelae of tuberculous hip	2	3
Dysplastic hip	1	2
Rheumatoid arthritis	1	2
Flare index	5.2 (3.8~7.0)	5.4 (3.9~6.9)
Singh index	5.0 (III~VI)	5.1 (III~VI)
Weight	64.9 Kg (45~85)	66.7 Kg (48~82)
Charnley functional class		
A	18	12
B	5	8
C	0	0
Follow-up(month)	111(96~122)	106(98~124)

Table 1:
Demographic data of matched group.

The stem used in the treatment was CLS stem (Sultzer, Bern, Switzerland) made of a titanium alloy with grit-blasted surface. In metal-on-metal group, all patients were treated with the Wagner standard cup (Sultzer, Bern, Switzerland) which has a titanium shell with grit-blasted surface and a 2.4-mm-thick CoCrMo articular surface molded into ultrahigh molecular weight polyethylene (Metasul inlay). The CoCrMo alloy was Protasul-21 WF (Sultzer) which was high-carbon alloys (>0.2% carbon by weight). The polyethylene inlay is inserted in the titanium acetabular shell with a modular snap-fit coupling. The modular femoral head is made of CoCrMo alloy manufactured with extra high precision, only a 28mm size head was used. The femoral head was also high-carbon alloys. In ceramic-on-polyethylene group, all patients were treated with Wagner standard cup (Sultzer, Bern, Switzerland). The polyethylene liner was Sulene™-PE (Sultzer, Bern, Switzerland). The femoral head was third generation alumina head of Biolox® (Ceramtec, Plochingen, Germany) which is composed of high purity alumina more than 99.8% Al_2O_3. The density of Biolox is 3.98 g/cm^3, the bending strength is 580 MPa, the vicker hardness is 2000 HV and the grain size is 1.8 μm.

A posterolateral approach was used for all patients. Femoral stem was tightly inserted with a mallet into the femur after broaching, and an acetabular cup was implanted with tight press-fit after under-reaming by 2mm and fixated with additional 1 or 2 screws. The desired position of the acetabular cup was 35 to 45 degrees of lateral opening and 20 degrees of anteversion. The femoral stem was implanted with 10 degrees of anteversion. Bone graft to the space between the femoral stems and cortices was impacted to facilitated the bone-ongrowth and diminish the potential joint space. The femoral head with 3 type neck length (short, medium, long) was chosen to equalize the limb length and obtain the adequate soft tissue tension. On the day before surgery and for 7 days after it, prophylactic antibiotics were used in all patients. We usually used a first-generation cephalosporin (ceftezole) or a third-generation cephalosporin (ceftriaxone).

Patients were followed clinically, with physical examination, with use of the Harris hip score at six weeks, three, six, and twelve months postoperatively and then once a year. The thigh and groin pain was also evaluated.

The radiographs were analyzed during the follow-up period by two research associates who had not participated in the operation. Radiolucent lines and osteolysis around acetabular and femoral component were measured according to the zones described by DeLee and Charnley [1], and Gruen et al [2] respectively on the AP and lateral radiograph. To be counted, a radiolucent line adjacent to either the acetabular or femoral component needed to occupy at least 50% of the zone.

Measurement of the wear was not successful in metal-on-metal group, for it was not possible to distinguish the edge of the femoral head from the metal articulation surface of the acetabular component on the radiographs. Measurement of the wear in ceramic-on-polyethylene group was performed by the method described by Livermore et al [3]. The fixation status of the femoral component was classified as bone ingrowth, stable fibrous ingrowth, or unstable, according to the method described by Engh et al [4,5]. Definite loosening of the femoral component was defined as progressive axial subsidence of ≥2 mm or a varus or valgus tilting on serial radiographs. A femoral component was considered to be possibly loose when there was a complete radiolucent line surrounding the entire grit-blasted surface on both AP and lateral radiographs. Acetabular loosening was defined radiographically as the presence of a complete radiolucent line measuring >1 mm in all three zones, cup migration of ≥4 mm, or ≥4° of change in cup inclination [6]. Osteolysis was defined, according to the classification described by Zicat et al [7], as a focal area of bone resorption that was ≥2 mm wide at the time of final follow-up and had not been evident on the immediate postoperative radiograph.

During the revision procedures, specimens were retrieved from the periprosthetic tissue. The retrieved tissues were fixed with in neutral buffered formalin and paraffin-embedded sections as well as microbiological cultures were performed. The paraffin sections were stained with hematoxylin and eosin and examined with a light microscope and under polarized light for the presence of metallosis.

Results

Clinical Results

The mean Harris hip score was increased from 53.6 points (range, 21 to 77) preoperatively to 94.5 points (range, 89 to 100) at the final follow-up in the metal-on-metal group and was increased from 48.4 points (range, 26 to 72) preoperatively to 96.1 points (range, 93 to 100) in the ceramic-on-polyethylene group. There was no patient who showed the thigh pain. Groin pain of sudden onset was found in three hips in metal-on-metal group, which had been well-functioning without pain for at least 1 year postoperatively. Of these three hips, one hip had slight degree of pain, while two hips had moderate to severe degree of pain. The one hip with slight degree of pain had the pain appeared at 38 months postoperatively. The pain, however, disappeared after the administration of NSAID (Non-Steroidal Anti-Inflammatory Drug). The other two hips with moderate to severe degree of pain of sudden onset appeared at 25, 74 months postoperatively, but the symptoms never disappeared even after the administration of NSAID. One hip in ceramic-on-polyethylene group showed the groin pain, but this was believed to be caused by heavy work. The chronic reactive protein and erythrocyte sedimentation rate of these patients was in normal range.

Radiographic Results

The incidence of bone formation around the femoral stem per Gruen [2] zone at final follow-up was in Table 2. The fixation status of all the femoral component was classified as bone ingrowth according to the method described by Engh et al [4,5]. No loosening of the femoral stem was observed (Fig.1).

	Metal-on-Metal group (%)	Ceramic-on-Polyethylene group (%)
Zone 1	27 (96.4)	26 (92.8)
Zone 2	25 (89.3)	25 (89.3)
Zone 3	18 (64.8)	16 (57.6)
Zone 4	8 (28.8)	10 (35.7)
Zone 5	11 (39.6)	8 (28.8)
Zone 6	26 (92.8)	26 (92.8)
Zone 7	26 (92.8)	25 (89.3)

Table 2:
Incidence of bone formation around stem per Gruen zone at final follow-up.

The incidence of bone formation around the acetabular cup at final follow-up was 24 hips (85.7%) in zone 1, 25 hips (89.3%) in zone 2, and 19 hips (67.8%) in zone 3 in metal-on-metal group and 23 hips (82.1%) in zone 1, 26 hips (92.8%) in zone 2, and 20 hips (71.4%) in zone 3 in ceramic-on-polyethylene group. Definite acetabular loosening was not observed. In metal-on-metal group, focal osteolysis around the cup at zone 1 was found on the radiograph of one case with the pain appeared at 27 months postoperatively, however, the case is currently under observation until 108 months after operation to see whether the osteolysis progress or not (case 1). The other hip in metal-on-metal group that showed the groin pain at 25 months postoperatively had osteolysis around the cup at zone 2 and proximal femur at zone 7 on the radiograph (Fig. 2). There was progressive huge osteolysis around the cup at zone 2 and around the stem at zone 7 with the increasing size and aseptic loosening of the cup as well on the radiograph taken at 63 months postoperatively (case 2).

The mean linear and volumetric wear rate of ceramic-on-polyethylene group was 0.08 ± 0.02 mm/yr and 87.42 ± 6.17 mm³/yr, respectively.

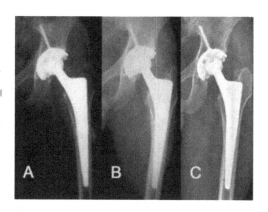

Figure 1:
A) A 38-year male patient underwent the total hip arthroplasty using ceramic-on-polyethylene bearing on the left hip joint due to the osteonecrosis of femoral head.
B) Postoperative 2 year radiograph showed the well-fixed prosthesis without radiolucent line or osteolysis.
C) Postoperative 9 year radiograph at final follow-up showed the bone formation around the prosthesis and calcar rounding. But, there was no radiolucency or osteolysis.

Details on Revision Operations

There was no revision in ceramic-on-polyethylene group. But there was one revision in metal-on-metal group. The reason for revision was the sudden onset of groin pain with the progressive osteolytic lesion and loosening of cup on the radiograph (case 2, Fig. 2). When performing the revision surgery on this patient, we found black tinged metallosis around the hip joint capsule and also at zone 2, where osteolysis had appeared on the radiograph (Fig. 3A). The cavitary defect with black tinged metallosis at zone 2 was curettaged and soft tissue was retrieved for histological analysis. The allogenous morselized bone was grafted to the bony defect and impacted with round acetabular impactor. The acetabular preparation was completed with reverse reaming of the final sized-acetabular reamer. The acetabular cup was press-fitted within the intact acetabular rim and additionally fixed with 2 acetabular screws. During the revision, we exchange metal-on-metal bearing with ceramic-on-polyethylene bearing.

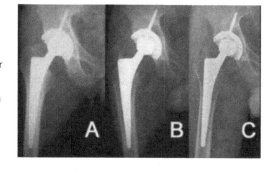

Figure 2:
A) Anteroposterior radiograph of a thirty-nine-year–old man showed a good press fit of acetabular cup at 1 year after operation.
B) Focal pelvic osteolysis in acetabular zone 2 and focal osteolysis in femoral zone 7 appeared at 2 years after the operation with the complaints of groin pain with sudden onset.
C) Progression of the osteolysis with increase of its size resulted in aseptic loosening of the cup at 63 months postoperatively.

Histological Examination

The retrieved tissue at the osteolytic lesion showed multiple perivascular infiltration of lymphocytes and small numbers of macrophages phagocytizing metal debris on one area, but many macrophages containing metal debris were also shown on the other area with rare polymorphonuclear leukocyte, and CD4-positive T-cells, CD8-positive T-cells and CD68 defined macrophages appeared in anti-CD immunostain in the several different regions (Fig. 3B, C and D). We could not observe the polyethylene laden macrophages and microbiological culture was negative.

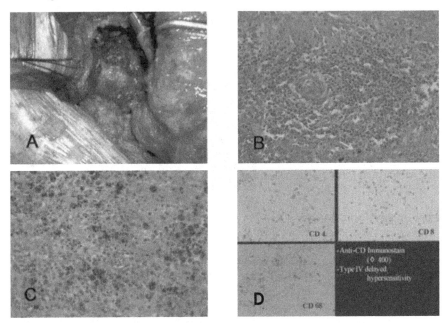

Figure 3:
A) Intraoperative finding of the osteolytic lesion of the hip at revision seen in Fig. 2 showed black tinged metallosis with the excavation of acetabular bone stock.
B) Histological appearance of the retrieved tissue at the osteolytic lesion showed multiple perivascular infiltration of lymphocytes mixed with a small number of macrophages phagocytizing metal debris(arrow) in one area (Hematoxylin and eosin; original magnification, X 400).
C) Many macrophages containing metal debris with rare polymorphonuclear leukocyte were showed in the other area (Hematoxylin and eosin; original magnification, X 200).
D) CD4-positive T-cells, CD8-positive T-cells and CD68 defined macrophages were appeared in the several different regions (Anti-CD immunostain; original magnification, X 400).

Discussion

Of the various bearings of the total hip arthroplasty, we have been choosing only the metal-on-metal and the ceramic-on-polyethylene articulation. The clinical and radiographic results were excellent in both the articulation until the mid-term period. According to our study, we considered the ceramic-on-polyethylene articulation as the safer option as compared with the various other alternative bearings due to the following disadvantages of them.

First, in the metal-on-Cross-linked Ultra-high molecular weight polyethylene (UHMWPE) articulation, the average wear debris particle size is reduced in hip simulator studies of highly cross-linked UHMWPE [8]. Smaller particles are more osteolytic, which raises concern about the potential for these materials to cause early osteolysis despite the reduced overall wear volume [9]. After cross-linking, the mechanical properties of UHMWPE (yield strength, tensile strength, elongation, and fatigue crack propagation resistance) are reduced [10,11]. The reduction in fatigue crack propagation resistance indicates that if a small defect is present in the material, it may propagate more rapidly into a larger crack.

After in vitro femoral head roughening, wear of both conventional and highly cross-linked UHMWPE in increased [12,13]. The susceptibility of highly cross-linked UHMWPE to increased wear with counterface roughening suggests that a more scratch-resistant femoral head may be beneficial in further reducing wear in vivo. Radiographic studies indicate that 50% to 72% less penetration of the femoral head into the acetabular liner occurs with highly cross-linked than conventional UHMWPE [14-16]. These study results demonstrate slightly less wear reduction than the 90% reduction predicted by wear simulator studies.

Second, in the Alumina ceramic-on-alumina ceramic articulation, although the third generation alumina ceramic was introduced, fracture remains a concern. Early ceramics had insufficient purity, low density, and coarsely grained microstructure, which led to poorer mechanical strength of the ceramic [17]. The current or third generation ceramic manufacturing, using hot isostatic pressing, produces a highly pure, fully dense ceramic with small grain size(1.8 µm). Fracture rates of ceramic femoral heads made with third-generation techniques are approximately 0 to 0.004%, or 4 per 100,000 [17]. But, a fracture rate of 1.9% was also reported with use of alumina ceramic femoral heads in the United States [18]. That the ceramic liner chips occurred on insertion is another problem. The problem of insert chipping was shown to be caused by the impaction of a liner not seated completely within the rim of the shell. Finally, the cost of the ceramic-on-ceramic articulation is the most expensive.

Third, in the metal-on-metal articulation, the clinical success of implants combined with the expected low levels of wear on retrieved implants [19] suggests that this articulation can provide a level of durability comparable to that achieved with McKee-Farrar implants. The concern with the metal-on-metal articulating implants has been the theoretic consequences of the metal-ion serum levels of cobalt [20]. Some authors reported early osteolysis probably caused by delayed-type metal hypersensitivity supported by the histological examinations and immunohistochemical study [21-24], which was comparable to our results.

In the ceramic-on-conventional polyethylene articulation, as above mentioned, the current or third generation ceramic manufacturing, using hot isostatic pressing, produces a highly pure, fully dense ceramic with small grain size(1.8 µm). Fracture rates of ceramic femoral heads made with third-generation techniques are dramatically decreased [17]. The conventional UHMWPE sterilized by gamma radiation in air with shelf life less than 3 years showed the consistent average wear below 0.1 mm/yr [25] as our result, which was believed to be the threshold of the osteolysis [26,27]. So we believe that ceramic-on-conventional polyethylene is the one of the safe options of new articulations.

In conclusion, excellent clinical and radiographic results of uncemented total hip arthroplasty with the third generation ceramic-on-polyethylene articulation were obtained in young patients in the mid-term follow-up, especially in terms of no osteolysis, no loosening and very low wear, which means the third generation ceramic-on-polyethylene articulation is the one of the safe options in new articulation systems to reduce wear. However, although the metal-on-metal articulation showed also excellent clinical and radiographic results, early osteolysis probably due to delayed metal hypersensitivity are remained as a concern.

References

1. DeLee JG, Charnley J. Radiological demarcation of cemented sockets in total hip replacement. Clin Orthop Relat Res 1976-121:20-32.
2. Gruen TA, McNeice GM, Amstutz HC. "Modes of failure" of cemented stem-type femoral components: a radiographic analysis of loosening. Clin Orthop Relat Res 1979-141:17-27.
3. Livermore J, Ilstrup D, Morrey B. Effect of femoral head size on wear of the polyethylene acetabular component. J Bone Joint Surg Am 1990;72-4:518-28.
4. Engh CA, Bobyn JD, Glassman AH. Porous-coated hip replacement. The factors governing bone ingrowth, stress shielding, and clinical results. J Bone Joint Surg Br 1987;69-1:45-55.
5. Engh CA, Massin P, Suthers KE. Roentgenographic assessment of the biologic fixation of porous-surfaced femoral components. Clin Orthop Relat Res 1990-257:107-28.
6. Latimer HA, Lachiewicz PF. Porous-coated acetabular components with screw fixation. Five to ten-year results. J Bone Joint Surg Am 1996;78-7:975-81.
7. Zicat B, Engh CA, Gokcen E. Patterns of osteolysis around total hip components inserted with and without cement. J Bone Joint Surg Am 1995;77-3:432-9.
8. Ries MD, Scott ML, Jani S. Relationship between gravimetric wear and particle generation in hip simulators: conventional compared with cross-linked polyethylene. J Bone Joint Surg Am 2001;83-A Suppl 2 Pt 2:116-22.
9. Green TR, Fisher J, Matthews JB, Stone MH, Ingham E. Effect of size and dose on bone resorption activity of macrophages by in vitro clinically relevant ultra high molecular weight polyethylene particles. J Biomed Mater. Res 2000;53-5:490-7.
10. Baker DA, Bellare A, Pruitt L. The effects of degree of crosslinking on the fatigue crack initiation and propagation resistance of orthopedic-grade polyethylene. J Biomed Mater Res A 2003;66-1:146-54.
11. Collier JP, Currier BH, Kennedy FE, Currier JH, Timmins GS, Jackson SK, Brewer RL. Comparison of cross-linked polyethylene materials for orthopaedic applications. Clin Orthop Relat Res 2003-414:289-304.
12. Good V, Ries M, Barrack RL, Widding K, Hunter G, Heuer D. Reduced wear with oxidized zirconium femoral heads. J Bone Joint Surg Am 2003;85-A Suppl 4:105-10.
13. McKellop H, Shen FW, DiMaio W, Lancaster JG. Wear of gamma-crosslinked polyethylene acetabular cups against roughened femoral balls. Clin Orthop Relat Res 1999-369:73-82.
14. Digas G, Karrholm J, Thanner J, Malchau H, Herberts P. Highly cross-linked polyethylene in cemented THA: randomized study of 61 hips. Clin Orthop Relat Res 2003-417:126-38.
15. Heisel C, Silva M, dela Rosa MA, Schmalzried TP. Short-term in vivo wear of cross-linked polyethylene. J Bone Joint Surg Am 2004;86-A-4:748-51.
16. Martell JM, Verner JJ, Incavo SJ. Clinical performance of a highly cross-linked polyethylene at two years in total hip arthroplasty: a randomized prospective trial. J Arthroplasty 2003;18-7 Suppl 1:55-9.
17. Willmann G. Ceramic femoral head retrieval data. Clin Orthop Relat Res 2000-379:22-8.
18. Callaway GH, Flynn W, Ranawat CS, Sculco TP. Fracture of the femoral head after ceramic-on-polyethylene total hip arthroplasty. J Arthroplasty 1995;10-6:855-9.
19. Sieber HP, Rieker CB, Kottig P. Analysis of 118 second-generation metal-on-metal retrieved hip implants. J Bone Joint Surg Br 1999;81-1:46-50.
20. Brodner W, Bitzan P, Meisinger V, Kaider A, Gottsauner-Wolf F, Kotz R. Serum cobalt levels after metal-on-metal total hip arthroplasty. J Bone Joint Surg Am 2003;85-A-11:2168-73.
21. Kim SY, Kyung HS, Ihn JC, Cho MR, Koo KH, Kim CY. Cementless Metasul metal-on-metal total hip arthroplasty in patients less than fifty years old. J Bone Joint Surg Am 2004;86-A-11:2475-81.

22. Korovessis P, Petsinis G, Repanti M, Repantis T. Metallosis after contemporary metal-on-metal total hip arthroplasty. Five to nine-year follow-up. J Bone Joint Surg Am 2006;88-6:1183-91.

23. Park YS, Moon YW, Lim SJ, Yang JM, Ahn G, Choi YL. Early osteolysis following second-generation metal-on-metal hip replacement. J Bone Joint Surg Am 2005;87-7:1515-21.

24. Willert HG, Buchhorn GH, Fayyazi A, Flury R, Windler M, Koster G, Lohmann CH. Metal-on-metal bearings and hypersensitivity in patients with artificial hip joints. A clinical and histomorphological study. J Bone Joint Surg Am 2005;87-1:28-36.

25. Engh CA, Sychterz CJ, Engh CA, Jr. Conventional ultra-high molecular weight polyethylene: a gold standard of sorts. Instr Course Lect 2005;54:183-7.

26. Dowd JE, Sychterz CJ, Young AM, Engh CA. Characterization of long-term femoral-head-penetration rates. Association with and prediction of osteolysis. J Bone Joint Surg Am 2000;82-A-8:1102-7.

27. Wan Z, Dorr LD. Natural history of femoral focal osteolysis with proximal ingrowth smooth stem implant. J Arthroplasty 1996;11-6:718-25.

2.4 Comparison of Polyethylene Wear against Alumina and Zirconia Heads in Cemented Total Hip Arthroplasty

K. Kawanabe, B. Liang, K. Ise and T. Nakamura

Abstract

We compared the polyethylene wear of 22.225-mm alumina heads with zirconia heads in cemented total hip arthroplasty during a mean follow-up period of 5.4 years. Using a computer-aided technique, we measured polyethylene wear radiologically in 46 hips with alumina heads and 58 hips with zirconia heads. The preoperative diagnosis in all cases was osteoarthritis. The mean linear wear rate of polyethylene sockets against zirconia heads were 0.133 mm/y, significantly greater (P < .01) than the wear rates against alumina heads (0.078 mm/y). Age at operation, patient body weight as well as height, thickness of polyethylene, and socket abduction angle did not influence the wear rates. We speculate that the excessive polyethylene wear was caused by phase transformation of zirconia, leading to an increase of surface roughness.

Intruduction

Zirconia ceramics have better fracture toughness, higher flexural strength and lower wear rates against polyethylene in vitro [8]. The superior mechanical properties of zirconia ceramics have allowed for the development of a large variety of head designs, and more than 350 000 zirconia ceramic heads have been used in THA throughout the world [1]. low-temperature aging degradation is caused by tetragonal-to-monoclinic (T-M) phase transformation, and bearing surface deterioration of yttrium-stabilized tetragonal zirconia polycrystal (Y-TZP) has been observed both in vitro [14] and in vivo [3]. However, no previous report has compared the wear of UHMWPE articulated with alumina and zirconia heads of the same sizes. We report on a radiologic review of hip prostheses with 22.225-mm alumina ceramic and zirconia ceramic heads in cemented THA that were followed up for an average period of 5.4 years.

Patients and Methods

Between February 1996 and February 1999, we carried out 118 primary cemented THAs in 103 patients using Kobelco hip prostheses (K-MAX series, Kobe Steel Co Ltd, Kobe, Japan) in which all-polyethylene acetabular components were articulated with 22.225-mm alumina or zirconia heads and titanium alloy femoral stems. The preoperative diagnosis in all cases was osteoarthritis. The acetabular sockets were machined from GUR 402 UHMWPE. The socket was sterilized with 2.5 Mrad of gamma irradiation in air. The femoral stems were made of titanium alloy (Ti-15Mo-5Zr-3Al), and the heads were sterilized using ethylene oxide gas. The acetabular sockets were fixed with bone cement (CMW1), and the femoral stems were also fixed with bone cement (CMW3) applied using a cement gun, the so-called third-generation technique [4].

Between February 1996 and August 1997, alumina heads were applied for 52 hips (46 patients: 5 men and 41 women); between September 1997 and February 1999, zirconia heads were applied for 66 hips (57 patients: 3 men and 54 women). Alumina ceramics containing 0.25 wt% of MgO were used in the alumina heads, and zirconia ceramics of Y-TZP containing 3 mol% of yttrium oxide were used in the zirconia heads. Hips with a minimum follow-up of 5 years were evaluated for polyethylene wear. Clinical outcome was also evaluated using the hip score of the Japan Orthopedic Association (JOA) in which the maximum score of 100 points is divided into scores for pain (40 points), range of motion (20 points), walking ability (20 points), and activities of daily living (20 points) [6].

Radiologic Analysis

All evaluations and measurements of the radiographs were undertaken by the same observer (BL), who also performed all the assessments blindly as to the type of head being studied, to eliminate interobserver error. The analytic methods used in this study, including the digitization of radiographs and the use of software, were the same as those reported previously [15]. For each patient, the immediately postoperative and most recent anterior-posterior radiographs of the pelvis were selected. The radiographs were scanned using a scanner to generate 600–dots per inch TIFF images. Using customized software (Image-Pro Plus version 4.0), the observer digitized 10 points around the periphery of the head on the radiograph and around the periphery of the polyethylene socket at the cement-socket interface. Although head migration may comprise not only true wear but also polyethylene creep deformation, we defined the migration as linear wear in this study. The direction of wear was also defined relative to a vertical line drawn through the center of the head and perpendicular to an interteardrop line [9]. In addition, the linear wear rate and volumetric wear rate were calculated from the linear wear data, as reported previously [11] and [5]. Correlations of polyethylene thickness and wear rates were analyzed.

Statistical Analysis

The data are expressed as mean ± SD and were assessed using one-way factorial analysis of variance and Fisher's protected least significant difference method as a post hoc test. Values of $P < .05$ were considered statistically significant.

Results

At the final follow-up in the alumina group, 2 hips in 2 patients who died and 4 hips in 4 patients who were lost to follow-up could not be examined. On the other hand, in the zirconia group, 2 hips in 2 patients who died and 4 hips in 3 patients who were lost to follow-up could not be studied further. Two hips in 2 patients with zirconia heads had been revised: 1 hip for aseptic loosening of the proximal femoral stem at 50 months after initial THA and the other because of extensive infection from a liver abscess at 59 months after initial THA. Both hips were excluded from the comparison of polyethylene wear because their follow-up periods were shorter than 5 years. The overall follow-up rates in the alumina and zirconia groups were 92% and 94%, respectively.

As a result, we measured radiologic wear in 104 primary cemented THAs in 90 patients; 46 prostheses had alumina heads and 58 had zirconia heads (Table 1).

	Alumina	Zirconia
No. of hips	46	58
No. of patients	40 (6: bilaterally)	50 (8: bilaterally)
Diagnosis	OA	OA
Sex (n)		
Male	5	3
Female	35	48

Table 1:
Patients and Femoral Heads.

There was no significant difference as to mean age at surgery (P = .41), mean patient body weight (P = .69), or mean patient height (P = .87) between the alumina and zirconia groups. There was no significant difference in JOA hip scores between the alumina and zirconia groups either before surgery (P = .32) or at the most recent follow-up (P = .48). The average thickness of polyethylene was 11.2 mm in the alumina group and was 10.8 mm in the zirconia group, with no significant difference (P = .15). The mean socket angle was 44.6° in the alumina group and 45.9° in the zirconia group, also with no significant difference (P = .16) (Table 2).

	Alumina	Zirconia
Follow-up periods (y)	6.7 ± 0.6	5.4 ± 0.8
Age at operation (y)	58.1 ± 9.8	58.3 ± 11.6
Weight (kg)	54.0 ± 7.7	53.4 ± 6.8
Height (m)	1.51 ± 0.07	1.51 ± 0.06
JOA score		
Preoperative	46.8 ± 12.7	44.2 ± 12.7
Last follow-up	89.3 ± 8.2	88.3 ± 7.2
Thickness of socket (mm)	11.2 ± 1.4	10.8 ± 1.2
Socket angle (°)	44.6 ± 4.4	45.9 ± 4.9

Table 2:
Clinical Data at the Last Follow-up (mean ± SD).

The mean rate of linear wear was 0.078 ± 0.044 mm/y for the alumina group (range = 0.02-0.27 mm/y) and was 0.133 ± 0.073 mm/y for the zirconia group (range = 0.01-0.40 mm/y). The mean rate of linear wear in the zirconia group was significantly greater than that in the alumina group (P < .01). The mean volumetric wear rate was 24.2 ± 15.2 mm^3/y in the alumina group (range = 1.7-71.1 mm^3/y) and was 39.8 ± 23.9 mm^3/y in the zirconia group (range = 1.5-146.8 mm^3/y). The mean volumetric wear rate in the zirconia group was also significantly greater than that in the alumina group (P < .01), although there was no significant difference in the direction of wear (P = .42) between the 2 groups (Table 3).

	Alumina	Zirconia
Wear angle (°)	9.0 ± 55.6	2.2 ± 24.4
Linear wear (mm)	0.52 ± 0.27	0.72 ± 0.38**
Linear wear rate (mm/y)	0.078 ± 0.044	0.133 ± 0.073**
Volumetric wear (mm^3)	160.9 ± 96.4	212.0 ± 125.2*
Volumetric wear rate (mm^3/y)	24.1 ± 15.2	39.8 ± 23.9**

*Significantly higher than alumina head, p< .05.
**Significantly higher than alumina head, p< .01.

Table 3:
Wear Data at the Last Follow-up (mean ± SD)).

Discussion

Our results after a minimum follow-up of 5 years showed that both the mean linear and volumetric wear rates were significantly greater in the zirconia group as compared with the alumina group. No previous report has compared UHMWPE wear against alumina and zirconia heads of the same size. Currently, it is still impossible to clarify the mechanism responsible for these differences in polyethylene wear rate when these 2 kinds of ceramic femoral heads; however, it may reflect the differences in physical properties between alumina ceramics and Y-TZP. Yttrium-stabilized tetragonal zirconia polycrystal belongs to a family of stress-toughened materials with a transformation-toughening mechanism that resists crack propagation. Low-temperature aging degradation is caused by T-M phase transformation, and Y-TZP bearing surface deterioration has been observed in vitro [14] and in vivo [3]. There have been few reports about the effects of loading on the T-M phase transformation of Y-TZP. In one study on T-M phase transformation in retrieved Y-TZP heads, the monoclinic phase was approximately 20% at 3 years postoperation and was approximately 30% at 6 years [3]. In another study [2], a strong correlation was observed between increasing transformation to monoclinic phase and decreasing surface hardness. In addition, the surface of retrieved Y-TZP heads showing high phase transformation was found to have become much rougher [2]. Generally, the surface roughness of the head influences the wear rate [13]. Another important difference between alumina ceramics and Y-TZP is thermal conductivity. It has been reported that the thermal conductivity of Y-TZP is more than 15 times lower than that of alumina [10], which might accelerate the T-M phase transformation of Y-TZP heads in vivo [7].

The T-M phase transformation of Y-TZP, mainly propagation of the transformation into the specimen interior, can be suppressed by the addition of a small amount of Al_2O_3 [16]. Recent improvements achieved by the addition of 0.25 wt % of Al_2O_3 have increased the static and dynamic fracture strength of Y-TZP, giving higher resistance to low-temperature aging degradation and phase transformation. In hip simulator wear tests, when articulated with cross-linked polyethylene, the improved Y-TZP heads induced almost no measurable polyethylene wear [12]. The current K-MAX cemented THA with this improved Y-TZP head and cross-linked polyethylene has been used in our hospital since March 2002.

References

1. Cales B (2000) Zirconia as a sliding material. Clin Orthop 379: 94.
2. Catledge SA, Cook M and Vohra YK (2003) Surface crystalline phases and nanoindentation hardness of explanted zirconia femoral heads, J Mater Sci Mater Med 14:863.
3. Haraguchi K, Sugano N.and Nishii T. Miki H, Oka K, Yoshikawa H (2001) Phase transformation of a zirconia ceramic head after total hip arthroplasty, J Bone Joint Surg Br 83: 996.
4. Harris W.H., McCarthy J.C. and O'Neill D.A. (1982) Femoral component loosening using contemporary techniques of femoral cement fixation, J Bone Joint Surg Am 64:1063.
5. Hashimoto Y, Bauer TW, Jiang M, Stulberg BN (1995) Polyethylene wear in total hip arthroplasty: volumetric wear measurement of retrieved acetabular components, Trans Orthop Res Soc 20:116.
6. Imura S. (1995) Evaluation chart of hip joint functions, Nippon Seikeigeka-gakkai Zasshi (J Jpn Orthop Assoc) 69: 864.
7. Kim YH, Kim JS, Cho SH (2001) A comparison of polyethylene wear in hips with cobalt-chrome or zirconia heads. J Bone Joint Surg Br 83: 742.
8. Kumar P, Oka M. and Ikeuchi K. Shimizu K, Yamamuro T, Okumura H, Kotoura Y (1991) Low wear rate of UHMWPE against zirconia ceramic (Y-PSZ) in comparison to alumina ceramic and SUS 316L alloy, J Biomed Mater Res 25: 813.
9. Livermore J, Ilstrup L, Morry B (1990) Effect of femoral head size on wear in wear of the polyethylene acetabular component. J Bone Joint Surg Am 72:518.
10. Lu Z, McKellop H (1997) Frictional heating of bearing materials tested in a hip joint wear simulator. Proc Inst Mech Eng (H) 211:101.
11. Maruyama M, Capello WN, D'Antonio JA, Jaffe WL, Bierbaum BE (2000) Effect of low friction ion treated femoral heads on polyethylene wear rates. Clin Orthop 370:183.
12. Nakamura T, Tanaka K, Tamura J, Kawanabe K, Takigawa Y, Sugano N, Saegusa Y, Takarori Y, Kondo S, Ninomiya S, Mashima N, Matsushita T(2003) Clinical and laboratory wear studies of zirconia-on-UHMWPE combination in cementless THA. Key Eng Mater 240-242:832.
13. Oka M, Kumar P, Ikeuchi K, Yamamuro T, Nakamura T (1992) Low wear rate of UHMWPE against zirconia ceramic (Y-PSZ) Bioceramics 5:373.
14. Tanaka K. Tamura J. and Kawanabe K. Nawa M, Uchida M, Kokubo T, Nakamura T: (2003) Phase stability after aging and its influence on pin-on-disk wear properties of Ce-TZP/Al2O3 nanocomposite and conventional Y-TZP. J Biomed Mater Res 67A:200.
15. Tanaka K, Tamura J, Kawanabe K, Shimizu M, Nakamura T (2003) Effect of alumina femoral heads on polyethylene wear in cemented total hip arthroplasty. Old versus current alumina. J Bone Joint Surg Br 85:655.
16. Tsubakino H and Nozato R (1991) Effect of alumina addition on the tetragonal-to-monoclinic phase transformation in zirconia-3 mol% yttria. J Am Ceram Soc 74: 440.

SESSION 3

Large Diameter Wear Couples

3.1 Wear of large Ceramic Bearings

T. Pandorf

Abstract

Large diameter ceramic bearings are of increasing interest due to the enlarged range of motion, enhanced stability of the artificial hip joint [1], and reduced risk of dislocations. Larger diameter hard on hard bearings may as well change the wear characteristics due to larger wear areas or different lubrication behaviour from changed diameter tolerances as known from Me-Me large bearings. But not only hard-on-hard bearings are of interest. With new low wear highly cross-linked polyethylene, wear behaviour of large ball heads against XPE liners is in focus.

Three different wear studies were conducted:
1. Ce-Ce: Alumina matrix bearings 40 mm and 44 mm with different diameter tolerances were tested according to DIN EN 14242. Roundness of the ball head and insert as well as clearance of the bearing partners have been varied.
2. Ce-XPE: Mean volume change rates have been compared between a 36 mm Biolox® *forte* ceramic ball head and CoCr ball heads. Both heads articulated against a XPE liner.
3. Ce-Ce: 36 mm diameter bearings in microseparation mode with two different ceramic materials were tested, one a pure alumina, the other an alumina matrix composite.

The different wear studies show:
1. Large ceramic bearings have a very low wear rate. The influence of the clearance on the wear rate is negligible.
2. Using a ceramic ball head against a highly crosslinked polyethylene liner reduces the wear rate by 40% compared to metal ball heads.
3. Even in microseparation mode the wear volume is very low compared to other bearing materials. The wear volume is similar to previously performed microseparation wear studies of 28 mm bearings. The wear volume depends on the used combination of the two different bearing materials. The alumina matrix composite (Biolox® *delta*) has 6 fold less wear when compared with the alumina couple.

The superior wear characteristics of large ceramic bearings have been proven in all tribological test setups. The use of ceramics in a hip replacement will significantly reduce the risk of particle induced osteolysis leading to an increased longevity in the human body.

Introduction

The demands on modern total hip replacements (THR) are getting more and more challenging. The patient expects a long durability implying low wear and minimization of osteolysis risk, an optimisation of function (increased range of motion, lower risk of dislocation), and a long term resistance to high loading since the average patient is younger and more active than the historic one leading to higher mean loading acting on the THR.

The use of large diameter THR (> 28 mm) made of modern alumina matrix ceramics fulfils these demands due to their possibility to provide increased range of motion and their higher stability, i.e. a reduced tendency for dislocation. However, the increased wear volume going along with large diameters for specific material combinations [2,3] and investigations on ceramic-ceramic hard bearing couples [4] exhibiting constant wear rates for different diameter sizes require careful wear investigations on the behaviour of large diameter THR before clinical use.

Material and Methods

Study 1 (Performed by Endolab, Rosenheim, Germany):

For each size, three different combinations regarding clearance and sphericity have been chosen: combination 1 contained ball heads and inserts with sphericity and clearance in tolerance (sphericity of the ball heads less than 5 µm, sphericity of the inserts less than 7 µm, clearance of the combination within tolerance (70 µm)). In the following figures 1 and 2, these wear results are represented by the grey columns. Combination 2 contained ball heads with a sphericity of 15 µm (sphericity of the inserts < 7 µm) and a clearance of 240 µm which is the double value of the upper tolerance at the time being. They are represented in the figures by the white columns. Combination 3 consisted of ball heads with a sphericity of 15 µm (sphericity of the inserts < 7 µm) and a clearance at the lower end of the tolerance band (20 µm). These results are represented by black columns. Tables 1 and 2 are providing an overview of the applied combinations and tolerances.

Size 40	Clearance	Sphericity
Combination 1	70 µm	< 5 µm
Combination 2	240 µm	15 µm
Combination 3	20 µm	15 µm

Table 1:
Geometrical parameters for the tribological studies (size 40 mm).

Size 44	Clearance	Sphericity
Combination 1	70 µm	< 5 µm
Combination 2	240 µm	15 µm
Combination 3	20 µm	15 µm

Table 2:
Geometrical parameters for the tribological studies (size 44 mm).

By choosing these combinations, one obtains a reference measurement (combination 1) yielding the possibility to assess the influence of the sphericity on the wear rate with very large clearance (combination 2) and very low clearance (combination 3). Furthermore, the well-known long-term wear behaviour of hard-hard bearings made of Biolox® *forte* which are being used for a long time and are known as exhibiting extremely low wear rates is used as a reference. This wear rate is 0,05 mm³/Mio. cycles and is marked in the figures by a horizontal black line.

Study 2 (performed by J. Fisher, Leeds, UK):

Size 36 mm Biolox® *forte* alumina (Ceramtec AG, Germany) and cobalt chrome (Durasul®, Zimmer, Switzerland) femoral heads were coupled with highly cross-linked polyethylene inserts (Durasul® Alpha, Zimmer, Switzerland) in the ten station Leeds Prosim Physiological Anatomical Hip Joint Simulator. Five sets of components for each material were studied, four were tested in articulating stations to determine creep plus wear and one was loaded with no articulation to determine creep (viscoplastic deformation of the PE).

The test conditions were a physiological walking cycle with a twin peak Paul type loading curve with a peak load of 3kN and a minimum swing phase load of 100N. Two independently controlled motions of +30°/-15° flexion-extension and ±10° internal/external rotation were applied. The simulator was run at 1Hz for 10 million cycles and the lubricant used was new born calf serum diluted to 25%, with 0.1% sodium acid added. The change in volume of the polyethylene inserts was determined geometrically and the mean volume change rates over the periods 0 - 10, 1 - 10 and 2 - 10 million cycles were calculated.

Study 3 (Performed by I. Clarke, Loma Linda Univ. CA, USA):

The 36 mm ceramic balls and cups were made of Biolox® *forte* (pure alumina oxide) and Biolox® *delta* (alumina matrix composite), respectively (see Table 3). They were diametrically matched.

Pairing Definitions	Samples (N)	Ball head material	Insert material
ff	3	Biolox® *forte*	Biolox® *forte*
df	3	Biolox® *delta*	Biolox® *forte*
fd	3	Biolox® *forte*	Biolox® *delta*
dd	3	Biolox® *delta*	Biolox® *delta*

Table 3:
Test matrix for the microseparation test (cup and ball Ø = 36mm).

The cups were mounted anatomically on a orbital hip simulator with 23° biaxial oscillation and customized for micro-separation test mode. The micro-separation was achieved by displacing the cup fixture with a spring force to achieve a potential of 2mm horizontal displacement. Maximum displacement was achieved during the swing phase of normal walking (Paul load curve). Maximum peak load of 2.0kN running at a gait frequency of 1.0Hz. Cup angle was 50° to the horizontal. The lubricant was Alpha-calf fraction (serum) (Hyclone®, Utah, USA) and was diluted with distilled filtered water to create a protein concentration of 10mg/ml (pH 8.0). The serum test volume was 300ml, this was replaced every event and stored frozen for later debris analysis. EDTA was added to reduce calcium films and/or precipitates (20ml of EDTA per litre of serum). Serum evaporation was compensated for by adding distilled filtered water.

Results and Discussion

Study 1:

For both sizes it can be seen that the medium wear rate after 5 Mio. cycles is in the range of 0,05 mm³/Mio. cycles for all three combinations, i. e. in the range of the long-term behaviour of Biolox® *forte*. The difference between the wear rate of reference combination 1 is small compared to those of combinations 2 and 3 for both sizes. However, the wear rate during running-in phase (up to 2 Mio. cycles) is slightly higher for the large diameters 40 mm and 44 mm, but it can be seen that the medium wear rate continuously decreases with increasing number of cycles. This might be due to a smoothing of these combinations with increased wear time. Together with the well-known bio inertness of the ceramic wear particles and the very low wear rates it can be stated that even a comparatively large deviation from ideal sphericity leads not to an increased wear rate compared to hard-hard bearings made of Biolox® *forte*, regardless of the clearance (Fig. 1,2).

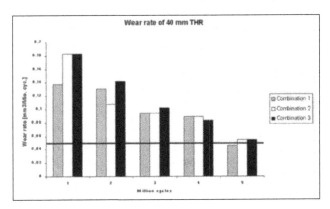

Figure 1:
Wear behaviour of hard-hard bearings made of Biolox® *delta* (40 mm).

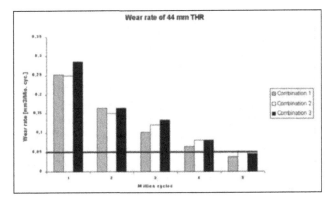

Figure 2:
Wear behaviour of hard-hard bearings made of Biolox® *delta* (44 mm)

Study 2:

The mean steady-state volume change rates after the run in phase are shown in Figure 3. One can see that the cobalt chrome/cross-linked PE bearing combination wears at a mean volume change rate of 8.1 mm³/mio cycles In contrast the rate of volume change of the ceramic/cross-linked PE bearing combination was calculated to be 4.7 mm³/mio. Cycles. This is a 40 % reduction compared to the steady-state wear rate of the cobalt chrome/cross-linked PE bearing combination. Comparing the results over the steady state wear rate for both sets of components, the wear rate of the ceramic/cross-linked PE bearing combination is statistically significantly lower that that of the cobalt chrome/cross-linked PE bearing combination (p < 0.01).

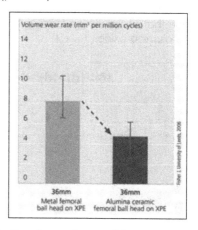

Figure 3:
Mean steady-state volume change rate over 10 million cycles.

The clinical implications of this study relate to the dependency of the wear on the head size for the different material combinations. The long-term wear rate of ceramic hard-hard or ceramic-PE bearings is more or less independent from the diameter [2,5] whereas the wear rate of metal heads increase with increasing diameter, see Figure 4. This means that the actual wear for all diameters is much lower with the ceramic heads due to their superior surface finish, scratch resistance, and wettability. Hence, taking also Into account the excellent biocompatibility of ceramic wear [6] the long-term in-vivo behaviour of ceramic components is even more superior for large diameters compared to metal components.

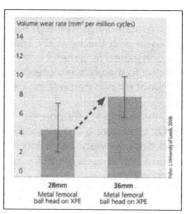

Figure 4:
Increase of wear with increasing metal head size.

Study 3:

The wear rates for all combinations were very low even under severe microseparation test conditions, see figure 4. The ff pairings demonstrated 'average' wear rate of 1.5 mm³/Mc. Clinical wear rates for contemporary alumina THR retrievals range from 0.1 to 3.6 mm³/year [6-8], so clearly the simulator wear rates were in mid-clinical range. The general trend showed that ff pairs had the highest wear rates and dd pairs had the lowest. Overall wear rates were ranked as follows: ff >> (df ~ fd) > dd. Under the microseparation test condition, the 'average' wear rates for the fd and df hybrid pairings were > 3-fold lower than with the historical control (ff). The 'average' for the the dd pairing was 6-fold lower than control and 3-fold lower than the hybrids (fd and df). It is worth mentioning that in the hybrid pairings (df and fd) the wear of the Biolox® *delta* component was higher than that of the Biolox® *forte* component, possibly due to the higher hardness of the alumina oxide.

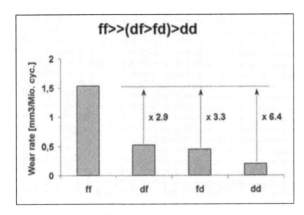

Figure 5:
Wear rate under severe microseparation.

Conclusion

The above discussed results show that large ceramic ball heads have several advantages when compared to metal ball heads. Worth to mention are particularly:

- large ceramic bearings (> 40 mm) are less sensitive to manufacturing tolerances like sphericity and clearance when compared to large metal on metal bearings [see e.g. 10]
- even with the new XPE liners a ceramic head distinctly reduces the wear compared to a metal ball head
- due to the unique material characteristics the Biolox® *delta* material reduces wear rates in ceramic on ceramic bearings even further.

All these findings support the enhanced wear behaviour of large ceramic ball heads, see Figure 6. This is especially valid for the alumina matrix composite Biolox® *delta*. Superior wear behaviour and additional strength are the reasons that this material will be used in the future designs of large diameter ceramic on ceramic bearings.

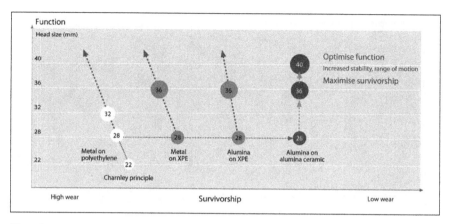

Figure 6:
Tendency of wear rates for different material combinations with increasing head diameter.

References

1. Ceroni Giacometti R, Dalla Pria P. The Development of Large Ceramic Heads to Obtain More Stable THA Wider Range of Motion. A. Toni, G. Willmann (eds.): Bioceramics in Joint Arthroplasty. 6th BIOLOX® Symposium Proceedings. Georg Thieme Verlag, Stuttgart, New York, 2001:11-12.

2. Clarke, I. C., V. Good, L. Anissan, A. Gustafson, Charnley wear model for validation of hip simulator - ball diameter vs. polytetrafluoroethylene and polyethylene wear. Proc. Instn. Mech. Engrs. 211 Part H (1997) 25 – 36.

3. Clarke, I. C., A. G. N. Gustafson, A. Fujisawa, H. Jung; Effect of Femoral-Head Diameter on Polyethylene Wear Rates in Vitro. Seite 301 in: Final Program AAOS New Orleans, LA 1994.

4. Saikko, V. Wear of Alumina on Alumina Total Replacement Hip Joints Studies with a Hip Joint Simulator, 2nd Biolox Symposium.

5. Hendrich C, Goebel S, Roller C, Sauer U, Kirschner S, Schmitz H, Eulert J, Martell JM. In-vivo Wear Rate of Ceramic Heads with Diameters of 28 mm and 32 mm. J.P. Garino, G. Willmann (eds.): Bioceramics in Joint Arthroplasty. 7th BIOLOX® Symposium Proceedings. Georg Thieme Verlag, Stuttgart, New York, 2002: 89-93.

6. Campbell P, Shen Fu-Wen; Mc Kellop H. Biologic and Tribologic Consideration of Alternative Bearing Surfaces. Clin Orthop 2004; 418: 98-111.

7. Böhler M, Mayr G, Goria O, Frank E, Mühlbauer M, Salzer M. Ergebnisse mit der Keramik-Keramik-Gleitpaarung in der Hüftendoprothetik. W. Puhl (ed.): Die Keramikpaarung BIOLOX in der Hüftendoprothetik. 1st BIOLOX® Symposium Proceedings. Georg Thieme Verlag, Stuttgart, New York, 1996: 34-38.

8. Hannouche D, Hamadouche M, Nizard R, Bizot P, Meunier A, Sedel L. Ceramics in Total Hip Replacement. Clin Orthop Rel Res 2005, 430: 62-71.

9. Clarke IC, Manaka M, Shishido T, Oonishi H, Gustafson GA, Boehler M. Tribological and Material Properties for all-Alumina THR - Convergence with Clinical Retrieval Data. H. Zippel, M. Dietrich (eds.): Ceramics in Orthopaedics. 8th BIOLOX® Symposium Proceedings. Steinkopff-Verlag, Darmstadt 2003: 3-17.

10. Dowson D, Hardaker C, Flett M, Isaac GH. A Hip Joint Simulator Study of the Performance of Metal-on-; Metal Joints. Part II: Design. J Arthroplasty 2004;19(9) Suppl 3: 124-130.

3.2 Evolution for Diameters Features and Results

P. Dalla Pria, M. Pressacco, F. Benazzo and S. Fusi

Diameter of the femoral head and joint stability

The success of prosthetic hip surgery, proved by numerous clinical outcomes at an international level, has determined a continuous increase of the number of surgeries. At the same time, the selection of the prosthetic component still remains controversial since it must always be chosen considering the effective benefit for the patient.

The importance of the diameter of the femoral head in relation to the frequency of dislocation in total hip prosthesis has been, for a long time, a topic of extreme interest in the orthopaedic field. In fact, it is well known that dislocation often causes a premature revision of the prosthetic implant [10,11].

Up until today, an appendix extracted from scientific literature regarding this matter, reveals that this topic is still a controversial subject. Woo [23] and Morrey [18] do not point out differences in the frequency of dislocation between femoral heads of 22 mm with respect to those of 32 mm. On the contrary, Pedersen and colleagues [20], in agreement with Kelley et Al. [16] who investigate the same articular diameters but with acetabular component superior to 60 mm, report a statistically significant increase of the frequency of dislocation in heads of 22 mm with respect to those of 28 mm. Similarly, Byström et Al. [8], in a comparative study carried out on 42.987 hip prosthesis on a first implant, illustrate that the revision frequency caused by dislocation of the 28 mm heads was significantly much higher with respect to those caused by the 32 mm heads. Clinical evidence underlines that this is only present in older patients (age > 80 yrs); while in patients with age below 59 years increase of the articular diameter does not necessarily indicate a lower risk of dislocation.

From a study carried out on cadavers of Bartz et al. [1] it has been demonstrated that an increase in the range of motion, determined on four standard femoral diameters (22, 26, 28 e 32 mm), can be reached up to femoral heads equal to 28 mm whereas with larger diameters the increase is of little importance (from 111° to 121°). In disagreement with the results deriving from an in-vitro study of Burroughs et Al. [7] which demonstrate an increase of the value of the range of motion related to the increase of the femoral heads from 28 to 38 mm, with consequent increase of articular stability and a reduction of the risks from impingement.

Some authors also report the sensation of a better personal stability when heads of 36 mm are used with respect to the conventional 28 mm heads [4,22]; therefore, a better sensation of comfort during everyday activities.

It is always not easy to compare this data between them. Apart from the diameter of the head, there are many parameters which can have an effect on the articular stability. Amongst these: the relationship between the diameter of the head and the diameter of the neck, the length of the head, the possible presence of a increase of the rim of the head, the shape of the insert, the surgical approach [18,5,8], the type of impingement (therefore the depth of the acetabular cup), the positioning of the cup and of the stem, the muscular trophism and the behavioural habits of the patient. It should be emphasized that the numerous studies published compare the most common diameters of 22, 28 and 32 mm. With reference to the use of ceramic-ceramic couplings with 36 mm heads, there is very little literature available that demonstrate their clinical importance. This is also due to the fact that dimensional increase of the articular diameter of the prosthesis with respect to the conventional 28 mm heads has been introduced only recently [12].

Large diameter Heads

A perspective comparative study between ceramic-ceramic 28 mm and 36 mm couplings was performed by Zagra and Giacometti Ceroni at the Galeazzi Orthopedic Institute (Milano, Italy) [24].

An acetabular component with a 36 mm liner-head ceramic–ceramic coupling (Delta System, Lima-Lto) has been implanted since 2001. They performed a prospective study to investigate the dislocation rate in the first 2 years after the operation. Two groups of patients have been matched, comparable in diagnosis and age: the first one (370 cases, from March 2001 to March 2004) in which 36 mm heads were implanted, and the second one (223 cases, from January 2001 to March 2004) in which 28 mm heads were used. The surgical technique (postero–lateral approach), the surgeons and the stems (cemented and uncemented) were the same. The number of dislocations was compared in the two groups. There were four dislocations (1.08%) in the first group and 10 (4.48%) in the second. The data confirmed that there was a statistically significant (P = 0.011) decrease of the dislocations in the group of 36 mm heads. Moreover, they evaluated the recurrent dislocations that needed a revision: one in the group of 36 mm head (0.27%) and three in the group of 28 mm (1.34%), confirming the lower rate in the bigger heads.

The use of heads larger than 32 mm seems to reduce the risk of dislocation also in difficult cases. Beaule et al. [2] have successfully used femoral heads with diameter 40 mm and larger to treat recurring dislocations. Good results are reported by Rinaldi et al. [21] in the use of ceramic-ceramic or ceramic-polyethylene 36 mm couplings in revisions and in some cases of bone malformation. Similarly, satisfactory outcomes are reported by Binazzi et al. [6] deriving from the use of 36 mm ceramic-ceramic couplings in the treatment of congenital hip dysplasia.

However, big diameter couplings can also not be as effective as hoped in patients with high risk of dislocation. Lachiewicz and Soileau [17] found no advantages using 36 mm and 40 mm heads in patients age 75 years or older, where preoperative diagnosis was acute femoral neck fracture or non-union, chronic neurological disorder and prior history of alcohol abuse.

The 36 mm coupling can reduce the risks of dislocation but it should not be considered a retentive solution. Even in patients not having a high risk of dislocation positioning should be the most correct as possible. When anteversion is inadequate or when abduction cup angle is over 60° the restraint of the femoral head is dramatically reduced, regardless of the head diameter [9].

Summarizing, large diameter coupling offer a wider ROM and a higher obstacle to the head exit because the dislocation path is longer. These features are not always significant for low/medium demanding patients for whom a well positioned 28 mm coupling is certainly adequate.

The large diameter features can be very important for:
- old people with poor muscular trophism;
- very active and sportive people, regardless the age;
- non-western people, whose usual resting positions (e.g. squatting) require high hip flexion and abduction degrees.

In Asia and Middle East squatting is very popular and hip flexion can achieve 130° [15,19]. The evaluation parameters which are typical for western people should therefore be revised.

In Asian Countries it can be common to choose a cup abduction angle less than 45° and an anteversion higher than 20° to prevent the hip dislocation due to squatting. However, the abduction angle decrease and the anteversion angle increase can cause a supero-anterior impingement when squatting and consequently it can be the cause of the ceramic liner fracture. The use of a 36 mm head or larger could allow for a higher abduction angle and lower anteversion angle.

Stresses in subluxation

When high ROM is required or in case of suboptimal cup positioning a 36 mm coupling can prevent the risk of dislocation; however, the subluxation can occur and the rim of the liner can be highly stressed, especially if made of ceramic material.

We performed a non-linear FEM analysis of a 36 mm ceramic-ceramic coupling in a condition of subluxation in order to know the stress condition of the liner. It is often believed that the thickness of the ceramic is an important factor related to its strength [13,14]. Therefore, we took into consideration two different liners, called 36/44 and 36/48 (manufactured by CeramTec for the Delta System, Lima-Lto), characterized by the outer diameter (respectively 44 and 48 mm) while the inner diameter is 36 mm. This means that the 36/48 liner is two mm thicker than the 36/44 (Fig. 1,2).

We simulated a patient rising from a chair and a subluxation of the head. This situation can occur when the neck impinges against the cup. An angle of 16° between the neck axis and the equatorial plane of the metal shell was chosen (Fig. 3). The joint reaction was applied along the axis of the neck. In fact, this is an approximation because the joint force direction depends on several factors, e.g. the position of the cup and the group of the working muscles but this is not a limit in the study; the aim is to know how the ceramic liner is stressed in a non-spherical contact condition, typical of the subluxation.

We hypothesized a patient weighing 78 kg and according to the in-vivo measurements by Bergmann [3], the applied load for a raising from a chair is approximately 1500 N.

As far as the contact conditions is concerned, we took from the Hertz theory a full elasticity of the head-liner contact, due to the high Young's modulus of Alumina and a friction coefficient of 0,03. For both head and liner a Young's modulus of 380 MPa and a Poisson's modulus of 0,23 were assigned.

The elements in the contact area were suitably increased by the FEM software (I-Deas – UGS, Texas US) because the element dimension has a relevant influence on the stress and contact pressure determination (Fig. 4). After an accurate study, a 0,04 mm element dimension was chosen. This led to a total number of about 120.000 elements and about 200.000 nodes.

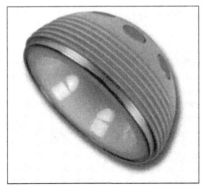

Figure 1:
The PF acetabular cup (Delta System, Lima-Lto).

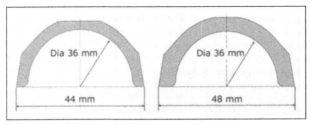

Figure 2:
Comparison between 36/44 (left) and 36/48 (right) ceramic liners. The 36/48 liner is two mm thicker than the 36/44.

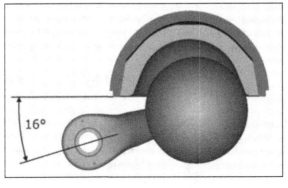

Figure 3:
Simulation of the subluxation. A load of 1520 N is applied.

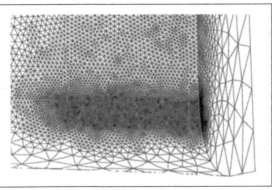

Figure 4:
FEM mesh around the contact area.

Results

The pattern of the stress is shown in Figure 5. Details of the contact pressures and first principal stresses on the contact area are shown in Figures 6 and 7. As forecasted by the Hertz theory, the contact area is elliptical shaped. Contact pressures are equal for both liners. The maximum principal stress for the thicker liner 36/48 is 130 MPa, while for the thinner one 36/44 is 132 MPa. Stresses in both the liners are practically the same, in accordance with the physical laws for the bodies in contact.

Considered that the contact in subluxation is almost punctual, the obtained results can be applied even if the coupling is 28 mm or 32 mm.

Comparing the obtained maximum stress (132 MPa) with the known strength of the BIOLOX® *forte* (560 MPa) and the BIOLOX®*delta* (1250 MPa) we can affirm that accidental subluxations or complete luxations are not critical for the ceramics, neither for BIOLOX® *forte*, nor for BIOLOX® *delta*. Even a single subluxation due to non severe trauma is not dangerous for the Biolox materials.

On the contrary, when subluxation continuously occurs the liner rim can fracture due to fatigue. It means that we have to compare the calculated stress with the fatigue limit stress of the liner material. It is very hard to define the fatigue limit for a ceramic material. Usually, a value equal to 25% of the static strength is chosen. Approximately, we can take 140 MPa for the BIOLOX® *forte* and 310 MPa for the BIOLOX® *delta*. As a consequence, in our conditions a liner made of BIOLOX® *forte* can be stressed close to the fatigue limit, while for the BIOLOX® *delta* the safety factor is still very high (about 2,4).

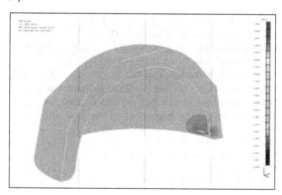

Figure 5:
Overview of the stress distribution (half model).

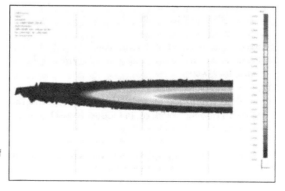

Figure 6:
Detail of the contact pressure (half model). For both the liners the contact pressure is 1,09E3 MPa.

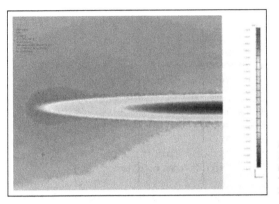

Figure 7:
Detail of the first principal stress (half model). Maximum principal stress for the 36/44 liner is 132 MPa and for the 36/48 liner 130 MPa.

Conclusion

Large diameter heads con offer several advantages in comparison to the traditional 28 mm and 32 mm heads, in terms of lower risk of dislocation and patients' feeling better. In the case of ceramic-ceramic coupling, when high ROM is required because of social habits or sport activities, the use of the more recent Alumina Matrix Composite (AMC) BIOLOX® *delta* is recommended.

Heads of diameter 36 mm, in ceramic or in metal, are also coupled to X-linked UHMWPE liners. The introduction of the X-linked UHMWPE has indeed decreased the concerns related to wear and osteolysis. Although it is our opinion that the problem of wear in the past was more related to the oxidation induced by the Gamma sterilization rather than to the tribological features, a longer longevity can be expected by the use of X-linked polyethylene. One must keep in mind that wear has often been related to thickness. Nowadays it is commonly believed that thickness is no longer a critical factor but it is well known that the fatigue strength of the X-linked polyethylene is lower than the non-reticulated one. Therefore, a correct positioning of the cup is important in order to avoid high stresses on the periphery of the liner, especially when an elevated rim is used [9].

References

1. Bartz RL, Noble PC, Kadakia NR, Tullos HS. (2000) The Effect of Femoral Component Head Size on Posterior Dislocation of the Artificial Hip Joint. J Bone Joint Surg (Am). 82:1300-1307.
2. Beaulé PE, Schmalzried TP, Udomkiet P, Amstutz HC. (2002) Jumbo femoral heads for the treatment of recurrent dislocation following total hip replacement. J Bone Joint Surg (Am). 84:256-263.
3. Bergmann G, ed. (2001) Hip 98-loading of the Hip Joint. : Free University of Berlin.
4. Berizzi A, Tzemtzang M, Aldegheri R. (2006) Head Diameter of 36 mm: New alumina on alumina bearing surfaces. In Proceedings 11th Biolox Symposium. Rome, June 30 – July 1, pp 3-4.
5. Berry DJ, Knock Mv, Schleck CD, Harmsen WS. (2005) Effect of Femoral Head Diameter and Operative Approach on Risk of Dislocation After Primary Total Hip Arthroplasty. J Bone Joint Surg. 87:2456-2463.

6. Binazzi R, Bondi A, Manca L, Marchesini L, Delcogliano M. (2006) Ceramic on ceramic cementless total hip arthroplasty in arthritis following congenital hip disease: an algorithm of the surgical treatment. In Proceedings 11th Biolox Symposium. Rome, June 30 – July 1, pp 237-242.

7. Burroughs BR, Hallstrom B, Golladay GJ, Hoeffel D, Harris WH. (2005) Range of Motion and Stability in Total Hip Arthroplasty With 28-, 32-, 38-, and 44-mm femoral Head Sizes. J Arthroplasty. 20(1):11-19.

8. Byström S, Espehaug B, Furnes O, Havelin L. (2003) Femoral head size is a risk factor for total hip luxation. Acta Orthop Scand. 74(5):514-525.

9. Crowninshield RD, Maloney WJ, Wentz DH, Humphrey SM, Blanchard CR. (2004) Biomechanics of Large Femoral Heads. Clin Orthop Relat Res. 429:102-107.

10. Dorr LD, Wan Z. (1988) Causes of and treatment protocol for instability of total hip replacement. Clin Orthop Relat Res. 355:144-151.

11. Dorr LD, Wolf AW, Chandler R, Conaty JP. (1983) Classification and treatment of dislocations of total hip arthroplasty. Clin Orthop Relat Res. 173:151-158.

12. Giacometti Ceroni R, Dalla Pria P. (2001) The Development of Large Ceramic Head to Obtain More Stable THA with Wider Range of Motion. In Proceedings 6th Biolox Symposium. Stuttgart, March 23-24, pp 11-12.

13. Ha Y-C, Kim S-Y, Kim HJ, Yoo JJ, Koo K-H. (2006) Ceramic Liner Fracture after Cementless Alumina-on-Alumina Total Hip Arthroplasty. Clin Orthop Relat Res. 458:106-110.

14. Hasegawa M, Sudo A, Uchida A. (2006) Alumina ceramic-on-ceramic total hip replacement with a layered acetabular component. J Bone Joint Surg (Br). 88:877-882.

15. Hemmerich A, Brown H, Smith S, Marthandam SS, Wyss UP. (2006) Hip, knee, and ankle kinematics of high range of motion activities of daily living. J Orthop Res. 24:770-781.

16. Kelley SS, Lachiewicz PF, Hickman JM, Paterno SM. (1998) Relationship of Femoral head and Acetabular Size to the Prevalence of Dislocation. Clin Orthop Relat Res. 355:163-170.

17. Lachiewicz PF, Soileau ES. (2006) Dislocation of Primary Total Hip Arthroplasty with 36 and 40-mm Femoral Heads. Clin Orthop Relat Res. 453:153-155.

18. Morrey BF. (1992) Instability after total hip arthroplasty. Orthop Clin North Am. 23:237-248.

19. Mulholland SJ, Wyss UP. (2001) Activities of daily living in non-Western cultures: range of motion requirements for hip and knee joint implants. Int J Rehabil Res. 24:191-198.

20. Pedersen DR, Callaghan JJ, Johnston TL, Fetzer GB, Johnston RC. (2001) Comparison of femoral head penetration rates between cementless acetabular components with 22-mm and 28-mm heads. J Arthroplasty. 16(8):111-115.

21. Rinaldi GP, Bonalumi M, Gaietta D, Capitani D. (2006) 36 mm Ceramic head for "difficult" cases. In Proceedings 11th Biolox Symposium. Rome, June 30 – July 1, pp 17-20.

22. Santori N, Giacomi D, Potestio D, Chilelli F. (2006) Clinical advantages with large diameter heads. In Proceedings 11th Biolox Symposium. Rome, June 30 – July 1, pp 11-16.

23. Woo RY, Morrey BF. (1982) Dislocations after total hip arthroplasty. J Bone Joint Surg (Am). 64(9):1295-1306.

24. Zagra L, Giacometti Ceroni R. (2006) Ceramic-ceramic coupling with big heads: clinical outcome. Eur J Orthop Surg Traumatol. 10-13.

3.3 Design Rationale for Acetabular Cups with alternative Bearings and large Diameter Heads

J. Oehy and M. Shen

Introduction

Total hip arthroplasty (THA) is one of the most successful surgical interventions in medicine with more than 1.3 million THA procedures performed worldwide in 2006. Long-term studies of selected patient cohorts [38,50,53] and hip registries in Sweden and Norway have demonstrated good survivorship rates up to ten years followed by a significant drop during the second decade. To date, younger and more active patients who have longer life expectancies and higher levels of activity are demanding more with respect to durability and functionality of a THA. Hence, development in further improving the THA will be desirable to better suit the needs of current and future THA patients.

Many factors influence the performance of a THA design. For example, the material pairing for articulation has an impact on wear, while the head diameter influences partly the wear performance and partly the stability of the THA. Willert's [55] description of particle disease showed that the foreign-body response to wear particles could progressively deteriorate the bone-prosthesis interface, potentially leading to implant loosening. Thus, a reduction of wear particle generation in THA, via the use of new bearing materials, would be beneficial. Meanwhile, dislocation is a common complication in THA with an occurrence of 2-3% following a primary THA and 10% in revision THA [34]. The expectations regarding a modern, modular THA have changed in recent years. More range of motion while addressing dislocation risks is becoming more important.

The objective of this paper was to review the clinical experience of THA's reported in the literature that could address the following two questions:
Why should alternative bearings be used in THA?
What are the benefits of larger articulation diameters?

Why should alternative bearings be used?

Clinical experience of historical polyethylene

It has been suggested that polyethylene wear and osteolysis associated with historical polyethylene acetabular liners can be caused or increased by third body wear damage to the metallic femoral head, oxidative degradation of gamma sterilization of polyethylene in air, and increased femoral head size. Retrieved polyethylene liners, analysed by Kabo et al [24], demonstrated that surface-replacement components with head diameters ranging from 36 mm to 54 mm had the greatest wear rates of 314 ± 158 mm^3/yr. The average follow-up of those components was 5.7 yr (0.9 to 11.3 yr). Components with smaller head diameters ranging from 22 mm to 32 mm had a noticeably lower average wear rate of 71 ± 47 mm³/yr, with an average follow-up of 10.9 yr (5.1 to 19.5 yr). These smaller components also showed wear rates linearly increased with head diameters. The linear relationship between head size and annual volumetric wear rate associated with the smaller diameter components was similarly reported by others [23]. These findings suggested that limiting the femoral head size to 32 mm was practical to control wear in historical polyethylene liners.

The cascade of wear particle generation, osteolysis, and aseptic loosening can limit the durability of a hip replacement. Numerous publications summarized by Dumbleton et al [14] suggested that the prevalence of osteolysis and loosening rose with increasing wear. A recent study used a pedometer and a step activity monitor to record patient activities and correlated the findings with radiographic analysis of implant wear [46]. The results showed higher in-vivo wear rates associated with higher level of activities. Hence, younger THA patients with historical polyethylene implants, presumably with higher activity levels, might have a lower survivorship compared to older patient group. A survivorship analysis of 5089 Charnley arthroplasties at 20 years [38] showed a 92% survival in patients who underwent THA surgeries at age of 70-80 but a 67% survival in patients at age of 40. Based on these findings, polyethylene wear was clearly a limiting factor in THA's with historical polyethylene liners. Conventional polyethylene THA liners have been in use since the late 80's - 90's with improvements to the historical polyethylene, including packaging in inert environments and improved polyethylene quality. Given the trend of more active, younger patients having THA implants and longer life expectancy in the general population, more wear reduction in the THA designs would be desirable.

Clinical results with new bearing technologies

New bearing materials for THA have been introduced with the aim of reducing wear using two approaches: one is the development of highly crosslinked polyethylene (HXPE) to improve wear resistance and the other is the use of alternative bearing materials to avoid polyethylene altogether. The latter approach has led to the development of ceramic-on-ceramic bearings and metal-on-metal bearings. Extensive in-vitro laboratory studies have evaluated the wear performance of HXPE's [32,36,37], metal-on-metal (MoM) articulation [18,51], and ceramic-on-ceramic (CoC) bearings [6,56] made of alumina or composite ceramics. All these new bearing materials demonstrated noticeably higher wear resistance than the historical polyethylene with both small and larger articulation diameters, i.e., the femoral head size limitation can be reduced by these new bearing materials.

Furthermore, in-vivo wear rates associated with the HXPE, MoM, and CoC bearings have all been demonstrated to be lower than conventional/historical polyethylene-on-metal or conventional/ historical polyethylene-on-ceramic couples [11,20,30,43,47,56]. The in-vivo wear analysis of conventional/historical polyethylene and HXPE typically employs femoral head penetration measurement methods based on x-rays [11,20,30], whereas the analysis of retrieved components is mostly used to provide the in-vivo wear information of hard-on-hard THA [43,47,56]. Because volumetric wear rates are rarely available, Figure 1 shows a comparison of linear wear rates in different bearing material pairings using representative values of 28 mm bearings. All new bearing technologies exhibit clearly improved wear resistance compared to the conventional/historical polyethylene counterpart. Meanwhile, the mid-term clinical results of these new bearing technologies have been quite promising, as summarized in Table 1 (HXPE's), Table 2 (MoM bearings) and Table 3 (CoC bearings). Based on the clinical follow-up data, the MoM and CoC bearings have been suggested as viable solutions for young, high demand and active patients [3,19,25,33,57].

Although the mid-term clinical results of HXPE's listed in Table 1 are promising, it's important to recognize that existing HXPE's are different in many aspects [5,15,26,39], e.g., manufacturing, radiation source, extent of crosslinking, melting or annealing, sterilization method, etc. All these factors may influence clinical outcomes. For example, a recent retrieval analysis of two types of HXPE's, up to 36 months in-vivo, showed noticeable difference in the materials' resistance to oxidative degradation [54]. The difference was attributable to the differences in manufacturing process. The HXPE acetabular liners made from an irradiation crosslinking, melt-annealing, and non-irradiation sterilization method showed no measurable change in its oxidative state up to 36 months, compared to never-implanted controls. Conversely, the HXPE liners made from an irradiation crosslinking, annealing without melt, and irradiation-sterilization method showed increasing oxidation over time in-vivo up to 33 months. To date, these two types of HXPE's have been reported to be more wear resistant than the conventional polyethylene counterparts (Table 1) [11,8]. Longer term follow-ups would be prudent to assure the chemical changes, reflected by the in-vivo oxidation, do not impact the in-vivo THA performance [27].

The existing MoM bearings from different manufacturers are also different in many aspects, e.g., the material's chemistry (carbon content in the base CoCrMo alloy), raw material manufacturing process (wrought versus cast), macro-geometric parameters (diameter and diametral clearance), and micro-geometric parameters (surface topography). Literature of in-vitro and in-vivo studies has reported noticeable differences in the performance of the MoM bearings attributable to the differences in the combination of parameters. The combination of diameter, diametral clearance, and surface topography can influence the resulting lubrication and wear performance of MoM bearings [13]. Additionally, CoCrMo alloys with lower carbon contents have been reported as less wear resistant than CoCrMo alloys with higher carbon contents in several in-vitro studies [51,52]. More recently, higher Co and Cr ion concentrations measured from MoM patients with low carbon CoCrMo alloys, compared to data collected from patients with high carbon CoCrMo alloy MoM bearings [40], appear to corroborate with the in-vitro studies. Hence, careful selections of the combination of parameters will prove to be critical to extend good clinical outcomes in MoM THA's thus far.

Author	HXPE (manufacturer)	Conventional PE Sterilization/ environment	Follow-up (years)	Reduction of head penetration/wear
Digas [11]	Durasul (cemented) (Zimmer)	Gamma / Nitrogen	5	59% linear 3D/ 98% excluding bedding-in
Digas [11]	Longevity (hybrid) (Zimmer)	Gamma / Nitrogen	5	77% linear 3D / 99% excluding bedding-in
Dorr [12]	Durasul (uncemented) (Zimmer)	Gamma / Nitrogen	5	55% linear / 60-75% excluding bedding-in
Bitsch [2]	Marathon (DePuy)	Gamma / Air	5	81% volumetric wear
D'Antonio [8]	Crossfire (Stryker)	Gamma / Nitrogen	5	60% linear/ 72% excluding bedding-in

Table 1:
Clinical outcomes of HXPE THA.

Author	MoM bearing (manufacturer)	No. of cases	Mean follow-up years (range)	Mean age (range)	Revision for any reason	Survival rate
Migaud [33]	Metasul (Zimmer)	39	5.7 (5-7)	39.8 (23-49)	0	100%
Kim [25]	Metasul (Zimmer)	68	7 (5-9)	37 (17-49)	1	not stated
Reitinger [41]	Metasul (Zimmer)	82	8.6 (8-10)	60.1 (46-79)	0	100%
Delaunay [10]	Metasul (Zimmer)	78	8	59.5 (29-73)	1	98.7%
Saito [44]	Metasul (Zimmer)	106	6.4 (5-8)	57.8 (42-79)	1	99.1%
Lombardi [29]	M2a (Biomet)	53	5.7 (5-8)	50 (31-78)	0	100%
Jacobs [22]	Ultima (DePuy)	95	3.9 (3-5.7)	53 (18-75)	1	not stated

Table 2:
Clinical outcomes of MoM bearings.

Author	CoC bearing (manufacturer)	No. of cases	Mean follow-up years (range)	Mean age (range)	Revision for any reason	Survival rate
D'Antonio [9]	Biolox forte (Stryker)	222	5 (0.1-7.2)	53.5 (SD 11.4)	6	97.3%
Yoo [57]	Biolox forte (Aesculap)	93	5.6 (5-6.5)	41 (18-65)	1	not stated
Bizot [3]	Alumina (Ceraver)	57	8 (6-11.5)	46 (21-55)	4	93.7%
Ha [19]	Biolox forte (Aesculap)	74	5.5 (5-6)	37 (19-49)	0	100%
Marcucci [31]	Biolox forte (Zimmer)	162	3.2 (0.3-5.3)	55 (25-74)	1	not stated
Garino [16]	Biolox forte (Wright)	333	1.8 (1.5-3)	52	4	not stated

Table 3:
Clinical outcomes of CoC bearings.

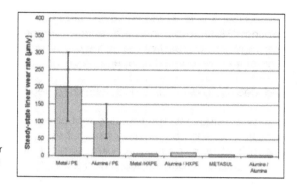

Figure 1:
Comparison of linear in-vivo wear rates of different 28 mm bearings [20,30,43,47,56].

What are the benefits of larger articulation diameters?

Incidence and contributing factors to dislocation

Regarding the contributing causes of THA dislocations, many factors have been reported, including femoral component stem design, acetabular component orientation, surgical approach, soft tissue laxity, femoral head size, and patient factors, whereas the dislocation mechanisms included the levering out of the femoral head due to prosthetic and/or bone impingement and excessive femoral head translation permitted by muscle weakness and soft tissue laxity [7]. Statistically, increased dislocation incidence is observed in females and in elderly [28], and after reoperation procedures [34]. As hip dislocation has a multifactorial etiology, isolating the effect of a single factor has been difficult through clinical studies with limited study population. Crowninshield et al [7] analyzed the hip stability based on biomechanics of large femoral heads and suggested that increased femoral head size could increase hip stability whereas increasing acetabular component abduction greatly diminished the stability advantage of large femoral heads. In a recent study, Berry et al [1] have analyzed dislocation incidence as a function of surgical approach and femoral head size from a large study group. They concluded that a larger femoral head diameter was associated with a lower long-term cumulative risk of dislocation in all three surgical approaches investigated. Figure 2 exhibits the multivariate analysis results of the relative risk of dislocation: 1.7 for 22-mm compared with 32-mm heads and 1.3 for 28-mm compared with 32-mm heads [1]. The cumulative ten-year rate of dislocation was 3.1% following anterolateral approaches, 3.4% following transtrochanteric approaches, and 6.9% following posterolateral approaches.

Different lifestyle and daily living activities

The improvements in hip joint survival rates over the last decades have led to the implantation of THA into younger and more active patients [21]. It is important to recognize that current hip replacements with small articulation diameters do not adequately meet the needs of non-Western cultures or Asian populations, where many activities are performed while squatting, kneeling, or sitting cross-legged. These positions demand a greater range of motion (ROM) than typically required in Western populations [48]. For example, one study reports that 130°-full hip flexion is required to squat and 90°-100° hip flexion is required to sit with legs crossed [35]. The markedly improved wear resistance in HXPE's [36,37] and MoM bearings [18,43], especially with reduced femoral head size limitation on wear, has led to an increased interest in the use of larger size femoral heads to provide a greater ROM, reduce impingement, and improve stability.

Reduced risk to dislocation and decreased healthcare costs

A recent study [45] has reported that approximately two-thirds of dislocations were treated with non-surgical approaches, such as closed reduction, and over one-third of all dislocations required surgical intervention (or open reduction). Both procedures added substantial costs to the treating institution. Closed reduction of dislocation increased medical costs by an average of 27% relative to the cost of a primary THA and surgical intervention (or open reduction), which sometimes followed closed reduction, increased total costs by an average of 148%. Hence, a reduction of dislocation risk apparently can give rise to economic benefits to the healthcare systems. Since smaller head diameters are associated with a higher risk of dislocation [1], the use of larger diameter femoral heads in THA will prove to be beneficial.

The effect of larger head sizes for THA on the type of impingement, ROM, and joint stability has been reported recently in an in-vitro study using an anatomic full-size hip model [4]. The results have shown that femoral heads larger than 32 mm provided greater ROM and virtually eliminated component-to-component impingement. Additionally, the flexion angle before dislocation has been significantly increased and the displacement between the femoral head and acetabulum required to produce dislocation has been increased as well. These findings suggest that larger femoral heads have a potential to provide greater hip ROM and joint stability. Recent clinical studies using large femoral heads in conjunction with alternative bearing technologies have provided consistent results in clinical setting, i.e., a significant reduction of dislocation associated with larger femoral heads: HXPE [17], MoM bearings [49] and CoC bearings [58].

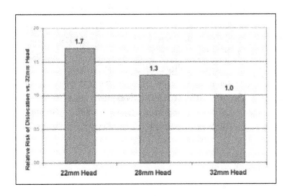

Figure 2:
Relative risk of dislocation for different head diameters [1].

Summary

The improvements in THA performance given rise by alternative bearings such as HXPE, MoM and CoC are significant. They have provided significantly higher wear resistance compared to historical polyethylene and reduced the limitation on femoral head size. The higher wear resistance is beneficial in leading to longer implant durability while meeting increased demands by younger and/or active patients. Furthermore, the ability to use larger femoral heads improves ROM and joint stability, leading to enhanced THA functionality, providing opportunities to perform a wider range of activities of daily living, and to reduce incidence of dislocation. Recent studies using larger femoral heads have demonstrated a significant reduction of dislocation after primary and revision surgeries. To date, modern THA designs in conjunction with alternative bearings and larger femoral heads can offer opportunities not only to improve THA durability and functionality but also to support the efforts to lower healthcare costs.

References

1. Berry DJ, et al (2005) Effect of femoral head diameter and operative approach on risk of dislocation after primary total hip arthroplasty. J Bone Joint Surg (Am) 87-A:2456-2463.
2. Bitsch R, et al (2007) Reduction of osteolysis with crosslinked polyethylene at five years. 74th Annual Meeting AAOS, paper 208.
3. Bizot P, et al (2004) Hybrid alumina total hip arthroplasty using a press-fit metal-backed socket in patients younger than 55 years. A six- to 11-year evaluation. J Bone Joint Surg (Br) 86-B:190-194.
4. Burroughs BR, et al (2005) Range of motion and stability in total hip arthroplasty with 28-, 32-, 38-, and 44-mm femoral head sizes. An in vitro study. J Arthroplasty 20(1):11-19.
5. Collier JP, et al (2003) Comparison of cross-linked polyethylene materials for orthopaedic applications. Clin Orthop Relat Res 414:289-304.
6. Clark IC, et al (2005) Severe simulation test for run-in wear of all-alumina compared to alumina composite THR. In: D'Antonio JA, Dietrich M (eds) Bioceramics and alternative bearings in joint arthroplasty, Darmstadt, Steinkopff, pp 11-20.
7. Crowninshield RD, et al (2004) Biomechanics of large femoral heads. What they do and don't do. Clin Orthop Relat Res 429:102-107.
8. D'Antonio JA, et al (2005) Five-year experience with Crossfire® highly cross-linked polyethylene. Clin Orthop Relat Res 441:143-150.
9. D'Antonio J, et al (2005) Alumina ceramic bearings for total hip arthroplasty. Five-year results of a prospective randomized study. Clin Orthop Relat Res 436:164-171.
10. Delaunay CP (2004) Metal-on-metal bearings in cementless primary total hip arthroplasty. J Arthroplasty 19(8, suppl 3):35–40.
11. Digas G, et al (2007) Five years experience of highly cross-linked polyethylene in cemented and uncemented sockets: Two randomized studies using radiostereometric analysis. 53rd Annual Meeting ORS: poster 392.
12. Dorr LD, et al (2005) Clinical performance of a Durasul highly crosslinked polyethylene acetabular liner for total hip arthroplasty at five years. J Bone Joint Surg (Am) 87-A:1816–1821.
13. Dowson D, et al (2004) A hip joint simulator study of the performance of metal-on-metal joints. J Arthroplasty 19(8, suppl 3):124–130.
14. Dumbleton JH, et al (2002) A literature review of the association between wear rate and osteolysis in total hip arthroplasty. J Arthroplasty 17 (5):649-661.
15. Dumbleton JH, et al (2006) The basis for a second-generation highly crosslinked UHMWPE. Clin Orthop Relat Res 453:265-271.
16. Garino JP (2000) Modern ceramic-on-ceramic total hip systems in the United States. Early results. Clin Orthop Rel Res 379:41-47.
17. Geller JA, et al (2006) Large diameter femoral heads on highly cross-linked polyethylene. Minimum 3-year results. Clin Orthop Relat Res 447:53-59.

18. Goldsmith AAJ, et al (1999) A comparative joint simulator study of the wear of metal-on-metal and alternative materials combinations in hip replacement. Proc Instn Mech Engrs Part H 214:39-47.

19. Ha YC, et al (2007) Cementless alumina-on-alumina total hip arthroplasty in patients younger than 50 years. A 5-year minimum follow-up study. J Arthroplasty 22(2):184-188.

20. Hendrich C, et al (2006) Highly crosslinked ultra molecular weight polyethylene-(UHMWPE-) acetabular liners in combination with 28 mm BIOLOX® heads. In: Benazzo F, Falez F, Dietrich M (eds) Bioceramics and alternative bearings in joint arthroplasty. Darmstadt, Steinkopff, pp 181–184.

21. Herberts P and Malchau H (1997) How outcome studies have changed total hip arthroplasty practices in Sweden. Clin Orthop Rel Res 34:44-60.

22. Jacobs M, et al (2004) Three- to six-year results with the Ultima metal-on-metal hip articulation for primary total hip arthroplasty. J Arthroplasty 19(7):48-53.

23. Jasty M, et al (1997) Wear of polyethylene acetabular components in total hip arthroplasty. An analysis of one hundred and twenty-eight components retrieved at autopsy or revision operations. J Bone Joint Surg (Am) 79-A:349-358.

24. Kabo JM, et al (1993) In vivo wear of polyethylene acetabular components. J Bone Joint Surg (B) 75-B:254-258.

25. Kim SY, et al (2004) Cementless Metasul metal-on-metal total hip arthroplasty in patients less than fifty years old. J Bone Joint Surg (Am) 86-A:2475–2481.

26. Kurtz SM, et al (2006) Anisotropy and oxidative resistance of highly crosslinked UHMWPE after deformation processing by solid-state ram extrusion. Biomaterials 27:24-34.

27. Kurtz SM, et al (2006) Significance of in vivo degradation for polyethylene in total hip arthroplasty. Clin Orthop Rel Res 453:47-57.

28. Levy RN, et al (1995) Outcome and long-term results following total hip replacement in elderly patients. Clin Orthop 316:25-30.

29. Lombardi AV, et al (2004) Mid-term results of a polyethylene-free metal-on-metal articulation. J Arthroplasty 19(7):42-47.

30. Manning DW, et al (2005) In vivo comparative wear study of traditional and highly cross-linked polyethylene in total hip arthroplasty. J Arthroplasty 20(7):880-886.

31. Marcucci M, et al (2006) 28mm head in ceramic/ceramic total hip replacement. In: Benazzo F, Falez F, Dietrich M (eds) Bioceramics and alternative bearings in joint arthroplasty. Darmstadt, Steinkopff, pp 65–71.

32. McKellop H, et al (1999) Development of an extremely wear-resistant ultrahigh molecular weight polyethylene for total hip replacements. J Orthop Res 17(2):157–167.

33. Migaud H, et al (2004) Cementless metal-on-metal hip arthroplasty in patients less than 50 years of age. Comparison with a matched control group using ceramic-on-polyethylene after a minimum 5-year follow-up. J Arthroplasty 19(8, suppl 3):23–28.

34. Morrey BF (1997) Difficult complications after hip joint replacement. Dislocation. Clin Orthop Relat Res 344:179–187.

35. Mulholland SJ, Wyss UP (2001) Activities of daily living in non-western cultures: range of motion requirements for hip and knee joint implants. J Rehabilitation Research 24:191-198.

36. Muratoglu OK, et al (2001) A novel method of crosslinking ultrahigh molecular weight polyethylene to improve wear, reduce oxidation, and retain mechanical properties. J Arthroplasty 16(2):149–160.

37. Muratoglu OK, et al (2001) Larger diameter femoral heads used in conjunction with a highly crosslinked ultrahigh molecular weight polyethylene. J Arthroplasty 16(8, Suppl. 1):24–30.

38. Older J, (2002) Charnley low-friction arthroplasty. A worldwide retrospective review at 15 to 20 years. J Arthroplasty 17(6):675-680.

39. Oonishi H, et al (2006) Wear of highly cross-linked polyethylene acetabular cup in Japan. J Arthroplasty 21(7):944-949.

40. Pfister AJ (2003) Total hip arthroplasty with metal-on-metal bearing surface in younger patients – a one to six-year follow-up. Doctoral thesis, Basel University, Basel, Switzerland.

41. Reitinger A, et al (2003) Clinical eight to ten years results with the cementless Alloclassic/Metasul (2nd generation) hip total endoprosthesis. Orthopädische Praxis 39 (9):544–547.

42. Rieker CB, et al (2001) In-vitro comparison of the two hard-hard articulations for total hip replacements. Proc Instn Mech Engrs Part H 215:153-160.

43. Rieker CB and Koettig P (2002) In vivo tribological performance of 231 metal-on-metal hip articulations. Hip International 12(2):73-76.

44. Saito S, et al (2006) Midterm results of Metasul metal-on-metal total hip arthroplasty. J Arthroplasty 21(8):1105-1110.

45. Sanchez-Sotelo J, et al (2006) Hospital cost of dislocation after primary hip total hip arthroplasty. J Bone Joint Surg (Am) 88-A:290-294.

46. Schmalzried TP, et al (2000) Wear is a function of use, not time. Clin Orthop Relat Res 381:36-46.

47. Semlitsch M, et al (1997) Clinical wear behaviour of ultra-high molecular weight polyethylene cups paired with metal and ceramic ball heads in comparison to metal-on-metal pairings of hip joint replacements. Proc Instn Mech Engrs, 211 (part H):73–87.

48. Singh U and Wason SS (1988) Multiaxial orthotic hip joint for squatting and cross-legged sitting with hip-knee-ankle-foot-orthosis. Prosthetics and Orthotics International 12:101-102.

49. Smith TM, et al (2005) Metal-on-metal total hip arthroplasty with large heads may prevent early dislocation. Clin Orthop Relat Res 441:137-142.

50. Sochart DH (1999) Relationship of acetabular wear to osteolysis and loosening in total hip arthroplasty. Clin Orthop Relat Res 363:135–150.

51. St John KR, et al (1999) Comparison of two cobalt-based alloys for use in metal-on-metal hip prostheses: Evaluation of the wear properties in a simulator. In: Disegi JA, Kennedy RL, Pillar R (eds) Cobalt-base alloys for biomedical applications, ASTM STP 1365:145–155.

52. Tipper JL, et al (1999) Quantitative analysis of the wear and wear debris from low and high carbon content cobalt chrome alloy used in metal on metal hip replacements. J Mat Sci: Materials in Medicine 10:353–362.

53. Urban JA, et al (2001) Ceramic-on-polyethylene bearing surfaces in total hip arthroplasty. Seventeen to twenty-one-year results. J Bone Joint Surg (Am) 83-A:1688–1694.

54. Wannomae KK, et al (2006) In vivo oxidation of retrieved cross-linked ultra-high-molecular-weight polyethylene acetabular components with residual free radicals. J Arthroplasty 21(7):1005-1011.

55. Willert HG (1977) Reactions of the articular capsule to wear products of artificial joint protheses. J Biomed Mater Res 11(2):157–164.

56. Willmann G (2000) Ceramic femoral head retrieval data. Clin Orthop Relat Res 379:22-28.

57. Yoo JJ, et al (2005) Alumina-on-alumina total hip arthroplasty. A five-year minimum follow-up study. J Bone Joint Surg (Am) 87-A:530-535.

58. Zagra L, et al (2004): THA ceramic-ceramic coupling: The evaluation of the dislocation rate with bigger heads. In: Lazennec JY, Dietrich M (eds) Bioceramics in joint arthroplasty, Darmstadt, Steinkopff, pp 163–168.

3.4 Use of Modular Femoral Stem combined with large Diameter Femoral Head in Alumina-on-Alumina Total Hip Arthroplasty

Y.-S. Park, Y.-W. Moon and S.-J. Lim

Abstract

While the clinical use of alumina-on-alumina bearings in total hip arthroplasty has demonstrated excellent clinical results with a low rate of osteolysis, relatively few head and liner options of alumina implants compared with conventional metal-on-polyethylene articulations continue to be one potential disadvantage that may often lead to impingement or dislocation after total hip arthroplasty. We hypothesized that a modular femoral stem that offered a variety of intraoperative adjustment options for producing appropriate femoral offset, length, and version would be favored to optimize stability following alumina-on-alumina total hip arthroplasty. It was also postulated that larger diameter femoral heads that allow for a greater range of motion prior to prosthetic impingement could reduce the risk of dislocation following alumina-on-alumina total hip arthroplasty. When reviewing a consecutive series of 136 alumina-on-alumina total hip arthroplasties performed with use of the S-ROM modular stem combined with 32-mm femoral head at our institution, we have found no ceramic fractures or bearing failures, and only one early postoperative dislocation that resolved with closed reduction was identified during the short follow-up period. Given the extremely low wear rates of alumina-on-alumina bearings even with larger femoral head diameters, our findings may increase potential for use of 32-mm femoral head combined with the S-ROM modular stem in both straightforward and complex total hip arthroplasties that are at high risk for prosthetic impingement or dislocation.

Introduction

Alumina ceramic, now in its third generation, has been markedly improved in terms of its mechanical properties, including purity, grain microstructure, and burst strength, through the evolution of design features and manufacturing processes over the past three decades and through the introduction of proof-testing [1,2]. Recent clinical studies on improved alumina bearings in combination with modern total hip implant designs have shown very low wear rates and substantially improved survivorship rates of the prostheses [3-5]. These favorable results have led to the increased use of an alumina-on-alumina bearing as an alternative to a conventional metal-on-polyethylene articulation, particularly for young, active patients.

Nonetheless, relatively few head and liner options of alumina implants compared with conventional metal-on-polyethylene articulations continue to be one potential disadvantage that may often lead to impingement or dislocation after total hip arthroplasty [6]. Neck-liner impingement may occur more commonly in Asian patients who frequently squat or sit in a cross-legged position.

Evidence of contact between the femoral neck and the acetabular rim has also been recognized as a common occurrence in Western populations following total hip arthroplasty, with impingement seen in more than half (56%) of retrieved polyethylene acetabular liners [7]. Under impingement conditions and over an extended period of time, a polyethylene acetabular liner is more likely to deform rather than fracture, leading to excessive generation of wear particles and consequent osteolysis and aseptic loosening of components. In contrast, the same impingement in a hip with an alumina liner may not be clinically evident until sudden fracture occurs. Therefore, there is a possibility of underestimation of impingement following alumina-on-alumina total hip arthroplasties.

Recently, Hasegawa et al presented a cautionary report that a modular layered acetabular component incorporating a thin alumina insert (Kyocera, Kyoto, Japan) had poor durability because of unexpected mechanical failures including alumina liner fracture and component dissociation [8]. We have also reported that even the third-generation and proof-tested alumina ceramics might fracture (1.7%, 6/357 hips) if used in poorly conceived constructs, such as a stem with a circular neck cross-section combined with a 28-mm-diameter femoral head, resulting in a relatively low head-to-neck ratio [9]. After experiencing this worrisome frequency of alumina ceramic failure probably caused by prosthetic impingement, we have modified our method of the clinical use of an alumina-on-alumina bearing in total hip arthroplasty by incorporating a modular stem combined with a larger diameter femoral head.

We hypothesized that a modular femoral stem that offered a variety of intraoperative adjustment options for producing appropriate femoral offset, length, and version would be favored to optimize stability following alumina-on-alumina total hip arthroplasty. It was also postulated that a larger diameter femoral head that allow for a greater range of motion could reduce the risk of prosthetic impingement or dislocation following an alumina-on-alumina total hip arthroplasty.

Materials and Methods

We retrospectively analyzed a consecutive series of 136 cementless alumina-on-alumina total hip arthroplasties performed with use of a modular stem combined with a larger femoral head. The senior author performed all the total hip arthroplasties through an anterolateral approach. All the patients received the S-ROM femoral component (DePuy, Leeds, United Kingdom) with a 32-mm alumina ceramic femoral head. The S-ROM femoral component is a proximally modular femoral stem, which consists of a polished, distally fluted stem and a circumferentially porous-coated sleeve. The sleeve is tightly fitted to the proximal calcar bone and the mating stem can be placed independently in a position of appropriate femoral offset, length, and version, thereby providing a maximal joint stability. In addition to its advantages in controlling biomechanics of the hip, the S-ROM stem also offers a trapezoidal shape of the neck cross-sectional geometry in an attempt to minimize femoral neck impingement against either the ceramic insert or the outer cup itself. A cementless Duraloc Option acetabular component (DePuy) with an alumina ceramic liner of inner diameter 32-mm was used in all the patients. The titanium-alloy acetabular socket with a porous-coated outer surface was press-fit into a 2-mm under-reamed acetabulum, and, if the socket fixation was not rigid, one or more screws were inserted. All ceramic implants were hot isostatic pressed, laser-marked, and proof-tested third-generation BIOLOX® *forte* alumina (CeramTec, Plochingen, Germany).

At each of the designated follow-up visits, all of these patients were evaluated clinically and radiographically with special attention to noise or squeaking, ceramic chipping or fracture, and dislocation.

Results

All of the patients had no remarkable noise or squeak in his or her hips receiving an alumina-on-alumina total hip arthroplasty. We have also found no chipping or actual fracture of the alumina head or liner during insertion or in vivo use, and only one (0.7%) early postoperative dislocation that resolved with closed reduction was identified during the short follow-up period of 12 months.

Summary and Conclusion

As loading conditions are more complex and variable in vivo, it is difficult to demonstrate the exact mechanism of ceramic failure; however, we believe that the high contact pressure generated by repetitive impingements between the femoral neck and the acetabular liner may be the principal cause of contemporary alumina ceramic failure. Therefore, it is extremely important to make every effort to prevent impingement by meticulous component positioning and, whenever possible, the use of a larger femoral head combined with the optimal design of acetabular liner and femoral neck to realize the potential long-term durability of a total hip arthroplasty with an alumina-on-alumina bearing. Given the extremely low wear rates of alumina-on-alumina bearings even with larger femoral head diameters [10], our findings may increase potential for use of 32-mm femoral head combined with the S-ROM modular stem in both straightforward and complex total hip arthroplasties that are at high risk for prosthetic impingement or dislocation.

References

1. Willmann G. Ceramic femoral head retrieval data. Clin Orthop Relat Res. 2000; 379:22-8.
2. Nizard R, Sedel L, Hannouche D, Hamadouche M, Bizot P. Alumina pairing in total hip replacement. J Bone Joint Surg Br. 2005; 87:755-8.
3. Bizot P, Hannouche D, Nizard R, Witvoet J, Sedel L. Hybrid alumina total hip arthroplasty using a press-fit metal backed socket in patients younger than 55 years: a six- to 11-year evaluation. J Bone Joint Surg Br. 2004; 86:190-4.
4. Yoo JJ, Kim YM, Yoon KS, Koo KH, Song WS, Kim HJ. Alumina-on-alumina total hip arthroplasty. A five-year minimum follow-up study. J Bone Joint Surg Am. 2005; 87:530-5.
5. D'Antonio J, Capello W, Manley M, Naughton M, Sutton K. Alumina ceramic bearings for total hip arthroplasty: five-year results of a prospective randomized study. Clin Orthop Relat Res. 2005; 436:164-71.
6. Barrack RL, Burak C, Skinner HB. Concerns about ceramics in THA. Clin Orthop Relat Res. 2004; 429:73-9.

7. Shon WY, Baldini T, Peterson MG, Wright TM, Salvati EA. Impingement in total hip arthroplasty: a study of retrieved acetabular components. J Arthroplasty. 2005; 20:427-35.
8. Hasegawa M, Sudo A, Uchida A. Alumina ceramic-on-ceramic total hip replacement with a layered acetabular component. J Bone Joint Surg Br.2006; 88:877-82.
9. Park YS, Hwang SK, Choy WK, Kim YS, Moon YW, Lim SJ. Ceramic failure after total hip arthroplasty with an alumina-on-alumina bearing. J Bone Joint Surg Am. 2006; 88:780-7.
10. Fisher J, Jin Z, Tipper J, Stone M, Ingham E. Tribology of alternative bearings. Orthop Relat Res. 2006; 453:25-34.

Ceramic Knee Implants

4.1 Ceramic Femoral Prosthesis in TKA – Present and Future

M.-C. Lee and J.-W. Ahn

Introduction

Total knee arthroplasty is a reliable procedure for the treatment of severely damaged knee joints in patients with osteoarthritis or rheumatoid arthritis. Despite good long-term results, the ultimate failure mode of TKA is osteolysis caused by wear debris from polyethylene. The osteolysis tends to cause aseptic loosening and instability of components, which leads to pain and revision [8,17]. Certainly, in case of elderly patients with lower activity levels, even total knee prostheses with conventional design and materials have achieved excellent long-term results. Over the past 10 years, however, greater demands are recently placed on total knee arthroplasties for younger, more active patients [24]. Therefore, in an attempt to minimize such PE wear, several modifications of the traditional approach to TKR have been introduced. Implant design and surgical instruments are continuously developing, including the use of more conforming articular surfaces [7]. Improvements in manufacturing quality, elimination of sterilization by gamma irradiation in air and cross-linking have reduced the PE wear [16,64]. However, wear and mechanical failures of gamma inert sterilized and highly cross-linked polyethylene have been observed [11,12].

Alternative bearing surfaces have the potential of greatly reducing wear at the articulating surfaces of total knee replacements, thereby minimizing the possibility of periprosthetic osteolysis. While ceramic bearing surfaces have been used extensively in total hip replacement, the data for such biomaterials in total knee is relatively sparse. In this report, we summarize the material properties, applications, clinical experiences, advantages, concerns and future developments of ceramics in TKA.

Material Properties

Ceramics are crystalline solid chemical compounds with a high chemical covalent-ionic bond. This broad definition includes a wide variety of materials, with very few of them finding practical use in the field of orthopedic implants. Special performance is required in physical and mechanical properties to be able to be considered for this use. The material properties that make ceramics a desirable bearing surface are their hardness, wettability and biocompatibility [4,9]. Ceramics are extremely hard making them wear and scratch resistant. These material properties mean less volumetric wear, smaller particle size and decreased cytotoxity when compared with polyethylene [2,62]. Ceramics are wettable because their ionic structure creates a hydrophilic surface and fluid-film lubrication [39]. The ability to be wetted well by a liquid is a prerequisite for low wear rate in tribological system. Ceramics are extremely well wetted by polar liquids, such as for example synovial fluid. It spreads out over the surface rather than beading up as happens with metal. This characteristic should minimize adhesive wear seen with metal on polyethylene because of improved lubrication. Ceramics exist in their highest oxidative state conferring them chemical stability, resistance to corrosion and reliable long-term behavior in vivo [9]. In addition, ceramics are insoluble in water making hydration as a means of degradation impossible [63]. Approximately 10% to 15% of Americans report sensitivity to Ni often with a cross-reactivity with Co [26,36]. All metals in contact with biological systems undergo corrosion and release metal ions [15]. Adverse reaction ranging from mild rashes to severe pain has been linked to allergic responses to these ions, particularly from metals known as sensitizers such as nickel, cobalt and chromium [58]. The use of ceramic bearing surfaces provides one alternative in cases where metal sensitivity is a concern.

Alumina

The two ceramic materials in clinical use today as bearing surfaces are aluminum oxide, called alumina or Al_2O_3 and zirconium oxide, or zirconia, ZrO_2 [18]. Alumina is monophasic polycrystalline, very hard, very stable, and highly oxidized, with a very low coefficient of friction and low bending stress [21,55]. Alumina can not be produced with full theoretical density (no porosity) because the long sintering time results in grain growth. Large grain size translates into a reduction in strength and an increase in fracture. It is known that incorporating materials such as CaO or MgO can prevent the grains from growing during the sintering process and produce materials with higher strength as a result of smaller grain size [56]. Modern manufacturing methods such as hot isostatic pressing (HIP) can practically guarantee the production of ceramic bearings with near-zero internal porosity and with a fine, uniform grain size distributed evenly throughout the material. The strong crystalline structure of alumina is also responsible for an unfavorable material characteristic, which is the brittleness or the low resistance to the propagation of cracks [6]. Alumina exhibits low fracture toughness values [20], which are lower than those of the metals used in orthopedic surgery. This means that the material has no way to deform without breakage.

Zirconia

Zirconia was introduced to overcome the limitations of alumina that are related to the mechanical properties of the material [13]. Zirconia, when properly manufactured, has a higher strength, which should reduce the risk of catastrophic failure. The fracture toughness of ZrO_2 is reported as nearly twice that of Al_2O_3. The strength of Al_2O_3 in bending is greater than 500 MPa, whreas ZrO_2 ranges from 500 to 1000 MPa in bending strength [54]. Zirconia, in contrast to alumina, is an unstable material, existing in three crystalline phases: monoclinic, tetragonal, and cubic. It can undergo transformation from one form (phase) to the next. The tetragonal phase that is the most resistant tends to transform into the monoclinic phase. The addition of stabilizing materials such as yttrium oxide, Y_2O_3, during manufacture can control the phase transformation of zirconia, thereby improving the mechanical properties of the material. Yttrium-stabilized tetragonal zirconia polycrystals (Y-TZP) has the highest mechanical strength of the 3 phases and therefore is used for surgical applications [14]. A serious limitation of Y-TZP relates to its instability; Phase transformation of Y-TZP can occur at a relatively low temperature in the presence of water and pressure [51,52,66].

Alumina Zirconia Composites

This is a high-performance ceramic biocomposite material that combines the excellent material properties of alumina ceramics in terms of chemical stability, hydrothermal stability, biocompatibility and extremely low wear and of zirconia ceramics with its superior mechanical strength and fracture toughness [29,34,35]. Therefore, it provides the opportunity to manufacture small and thin components to ensure the same surgical techniques as well as the same instruments as for the standard metal components. The first example of the future generation of ceramic components to be marketed in the United States is an alumina matrix composite (BIOLOX® delta, CeramTec Medical Products Division, Plochingen, Germany). It consists of zirconia particles dispersed in a dense, fine-grained alumina matrix with further additives such as SrO and Cr_2O_3 to fabricate alumina matrix composite (AMC). Because the material is relatively new, its reliability and advantages are not known.

Surface Modifications of Metals

Alumina and zirconia ceramics are brittle materials and may fracture in vivo. The use of these materials is more limited in total knee than total hip arthroplasty because of the complex geometry and relatively limited thickness of a total knee femoral component [49]. The metal zirconium treated with a 5-µm thick zirconia surface (Oxinium, Smith & Nephew, Mepmphis, TN) is new ceramic technology that provides improvements over CoCr alloy for resistance to roughening, frictional behavior and biocompatibility [10]. Prosthetic components are produced from a wrought zirconium alloy (Zr-2.5%Nb) that is oxidized by thermal diffusion in heated air to create a zirconia surface about 5-µm thick [30]. The oxide is not an externally applied coating, but rather a transformation of the original metal surface into zirconium oxide ceramic. Like titanium, the metallic elements of zirconium and niobium are very biocompatible, with minimum biologic availability and electrocatalytic activity [28]. Nano-hardness testing indicated that the OxZr is more than twice as hard as CoCr on the articular surface [23,33]. Mechanical testing and finite element analysis of OxZr and CoCr femoral components showed equivalent device fatigue strength between the materials, both being in the range of 450 MPa [59]. In contrast to the limitations exhibited by monolithic ceramics such as alumina and zirconia, OxZr does not exhibit brittle fracture during crush test [57]. In vitro knee simulator wear studies have consistently demonstrated less wear with OxZr compared with CoCr articulating on UMHWPE [19]. Collectively, knee simulator tests indicate that OxZr components can reduce wear of the polyethylene counterface by 40%-90% depending on test conditions. Numerous clinical studies are being organized to compare the performance of OxZr and CoCr components since the first surgery in 1997. The first study to be published showed more rapid regaining of functional milestones and no adverse effects had been observed at the 2-year evaluation [30,31]. A much longer time period will be required to measure difference in polyethylene wear and implant survivorship [50].

Applications

Ceramic materials have been used in total hip replacement (THR) for more than 30 years. Ceramics in TKA are not yet popular. There has been limited use of ceramic TKA in Japan for many years. The articulation of hip and knee joint is very different. In hip components, the predominant failure mode is abrasive-adhesive wear because they are more conforming. In knee components, however, the predominant failure mode is fatigue due to cyclic loading of the components because of the different curvatures of the femoral condyles and the top of the tibia plateau. It remains to be seen whether the use of ceramics for knee prostheses can offer real advantages with respect to traditional metal.

Clinical experiences with ceramic prostheses

To our knowledge, the first total knee prostheses employing alumina ceramics were introduced by Oonish in Japan in 1980 [41]. In a first generation, the femoral and tibial components were made of alumina ceramics, combined with a polyethylene insert attached to the tibia component. These components were implanted with or without cement in 137 patients. Relatively large numbers of early radiolucent lines were observed when the cementless fixation was used [42]. The authors reported high rates of loosening, sinking and implant failure in cementless fixation with a follow-up ranging from 20 to 25 years [43]. Thereafter, some refinements of the ceramic TKA designs have been carried out to improve the kinematical properties and the fixation of components with bone. In a second-generation of such prosthesis, developed in 1990, the alumina ceramic tibial component was changed to a titanium alloy tibial component to be fixed with cement, because an alumina tibial tray was thick and brittle and a relatively high occurrence of sinking and radiolucent lines was observed when cementless fixation was used. In a third-generation introduced in 1993, the principles of cement fixation were retained in this design. The femoral components were coated with alumina ceramic beads for enhancing the cement fixation. Second- and third-generation ceramic components were implanted in 534 joints, all using bone cement. In a total of 249 joints after 6 to 14 years of follow-up, no cases of loosening or sinking were observed [47].

Akagi et al. [1] reported 223 TKAs with the Bisurface® ceramic prosthesis. The femoral component and the tibial tray were made of alumina ceramic and titanium alloy, respectively and the prosthesis had a unique ball-and-socket joint to further improve knee flexion. All implants were fixed with bone cement. The survival rate of the implant was 94% after six years of follow-up. No aseptic loosening and no alumina ceramic femoral component breakage occurred. Koshino et al. [27] reported 90 TKAs in severe rheumatoid arthritis using the ceramic Yokohama Medical Ceramic Knee (YMCK). The femoral component of YMCK model was made of alumina ceramic and the tibial component consisted of an UHMWPE firmly fixed on a tibial tray made of alumina ceramic. All implants were fixed with bone cement. They had a survival rate equal to 99.1% at 8 years, without periprosthetic osteolysis. Yasuda et al. [65] performed prospective randomized study of 218 patients undergoing cruciate-retaining TKA with the CoCr alloy prosthesis (Kinemax®, Howmedica) or the LFA-1® (Low Friction Anatomical, Kyocera, Kyoto, Japan) prosthesis composed of alumina ceramic femoral component and a titanium-alloy tibial component with a UHMWPE insert. In each surgery, both components were fixed with cement. In the mid-term follow-up evaluation, the clinical results of the ceramic TKA were equivalent to those of the CoCr alloy TKA.

Zirconia was introduced as a ceramic with higher strength and toughness than alumina ceramic [60]. Thus, a zirconia femoral component can be manufactured with virtually identical dimensions to a CoCr design. In Japan, zirconia ceramic has been used for TKA (KU type, Kyocera Corp, Japan) since 2001 [40]. In the US, Bal et al. [5] reported the clinical results of 39 TKAs with a zirconia ceramic femoral component. The clinical and radiographic results were excellent at 2 year follow-up and none of the femoral components failed catastrophically at this short follow-up. Clinical trials with Y-TZP femoral components are ongoing in the US.

Tribologic properties

In vitro wear studies

Wear properties are different for alumina and zirconia against polyethylene and for either of these materials against themselves. Ueno et al. [61] showed that in a knee simulation study, an alumina ceramic femoral prosthesis generated less polyethylene wear than a CoCr alloy femoral component with exactly the same design and size.

Knee simulation study [60,61] of wear comparisons between zirconia ceramic and CoCr femoal components articulating against UHMWPE showed 4- to 5-fold wear reduction in zirconia ceramic components, depending on the test conditions.

Retrieved implants

Besides in vitro wear studies, detailed observations of wear for retrieved implants are important to examine actual clinical performance of artificial joints. There are few reports to date to investigate the wear patterns of explanted ceramic total knee prostheses.

Oonishi et al. [44] compared the surfaces of retrieved UHMWPE inserts between a combination with alumina and that with CoCr alloy. The UHMWPE surfaces of tibial plates and the surfaces of femoral components were examined using SEM and a metallographic microscope. The wearing patterns of the UHMWPE were different between the two and the surface of the latter combination showed more burnishing and polyethylene-folding phenomenon caused by third-body wear. The alumina surface of femoral condyles showed very slight changes while the CoCr alloy surface had more scratches. Later, they reported the detailed wear pattern and wear volume for a retrieved ceramic prosthesis that was used for a long period (23 years) [45]. The surface roughness (average surface roughness, Ra, and maximum surface roughness, Rmax) was not different between the worn and unworn surfaces. The linear and volumetric wear rate was estimated at 0.037 mm/year and 18.8 mm^3/year, respectively. However, in the retrieved metal/UHMWPE bearing surfaces of similar period [46,47], the surface roughness (Ra, Rmax) was significantly higher for the worn surface than for the unworn surface. The linear wear rate was calculated as 0.08 mm/year. The authors concluded that the low wear rate and the mild wear pattern suggested the possibility of reduced wear of the UHMWPE against the alumina femoral component and the usefulness of the alumina knee prosthesis was recognized even after long clinical use.

Biologic consideration

It takes decades to study the long-term results of newly introduced total knee prostheses. Thus, it is particularly important to examine in vivo polyethylene wear generation in such new prostheses before they come into widespread use. Apart from total hip arthroplasty, it is difficult to determine in vivo polyethylene wear using postoperative radiographs. In this regard, it is useful to measure in vivo polyethylene wear by isolating and analyzing polyethylene wear particles in synovial fluid from well-functioning knee after TKA. Biologic response to ceramic particulate debris should be similar to UHMWPE if the size distribution is similar, because of the inert nature of both materials. It seems likely that the low wear rates of ceramic prostheses will generate a smaller particle size distribution.

Minoda et al. [37] reported that in the comparison of medial pivot knee design, the polyethylene wear particles with an alumina femoral component were fewer in number by almost a factor of 10 and were "rounder", ie, had a smaller aspect ratio (particle shape), than for a CoCr femoral component.

Concerns of ceramic TKA

Fracture

The unexpected failure of ceramic components in vivo is a concern for the surgeon, even though clinical reports of TKA performed with ceramic components have yet to identify catastrophic component breakage as a failure mode [3]. Flaws in the ceramic material, such as microscopic pores, notches, inconsistencies and scratches can be introduced during fabrication or surface machining of the finished bearing [6,20]. With repetitive loading, stress concentration at a material imperfection can result in a crack migration through the material, with catastrophic failures as the ultimate result. In particular, the femoral condyles can be considered as curved cantilevers under bending load. Thus, the application to total knees, and particularly the femoral component, can be more vulnerable to the unexpected fractures [38]. Therefore, in ceramic TKA, every precaution should be taken while implanting the ceramic component without forceful impaction with a hammer, with final seating achieved by reducing the knee in extension [48].

Component Fixation

During about the first decade of application of alumina ceramic in TKA, based on the biocompatibility of the ceramics, a more stable and reliable cementless fixation was expected in ceramic TKA. However, the frequent occurrence of the radiolucent lines and the subsequent loosening of one or both components were observed, mostly ascribed to micromovements due to not sufficiently achieved initial press fit [53]. Experience in early applications of ceramic knee prosthesis implied the need for using cement to fix ceramic components on bone surface. Leyen et al. [32] reported that tensile bond strength of ceramic and bone cement interface in TKA is low compared to titanium and bone cement interface. As the cement-ceramic bond strength is low, satisfactory fixation strength of ceramic TKA may require a design that allows mechanical interlocking. However, such a design may probably promote cement cracking and therefore loosening in the long term [25].

Loss of Option

The most common practical disadvantage associated with the use of ceramic components in TKA is the dramatic loss of options available to the surgeon. As mentioned above, ceramics are brittle and less resistant to the propagation of cracks with low fracture toughness values. This requires more bone resection and thicker component than the corresponding metal prosthesis with limited component options available in order to avoid high tensile stresses and unexpected failures. Major prerequisite for the successful development of ceramic total knee components is the use of existing designs to ensure the same surgical techniques as well as the same instruments as for the standard metal components.

Future

Since the introduction of alumina ceramics in total knee arthroplasty during the late 1970, existing wear data and clinical results to date have been encouraging. However, the benefits of ceramics can not often be accessed because of their brittle character, fixation problem to bone and the difficulty of fabricating them into the necessary prosthetic shapes. To address the brittleness of ceramics, OxZr was introduced. Numerous clinical studies have shown satisfactory short-term clinical results but much longer time period will be required to identify the role of this new ceramic technology. Recently, alumina matrix composite material with higher mechanical strength has been introduced. It may allow us to produce structurally reliable ceramic total knee components without increasing the thickness of the cross-sections and the dimensions of bone resections. Total knee systems with otherwise well proven designs and a long track record of clinical success will identify the precise role of ceramics in total knee replacement surgery. Furthermore it has to be proven that the new ceramic components result in a sufficient quality of life for the young and active patient.

References

1. Akagi M, Nakamura T, Matsusue Y, Ueo T, Nishijyo K, Ohnishi E (2000) The bisurface total knee replacement: a unique design for flexion. J Bone Joint Surg Am 82:1626-1633.
2. Archibeck MJ, Jacobs JJ, Black J (2000) Alternate bearing surfaces in total joint arthroplasty: biologic considerations. Clin Orthop 379:12-21.
3. Bal BS, Oonishi H (2003) Ceramic femoral components in total knee replacement. In: Zippel H, Dietrich M (eds): Bioceramics in Joint Arthroplasty. 8th BIOLOX-Symposium Proceedings. Steinkopff-Verlag, Darmstadt, pp135-136.

4. Bal BS, Garino J, Ries M, Rahaman MN (2006) Ceramic materials in total joint arthroplasty. Semin Arthoplasty 17:94-10.

5. Bal BS, Greenberg DD, Buhrmester L, Aleto TJ (2006) Primary TKA with a zirconia ceramic femoral component. J Knee Surg 19:89-93.

6. Barrack RL, Burak C, Skinner HB (2004) Concerns about ceramics in THA. 429:73-79.

7. Bartel DL, Bicknell VL, Wright TM (1986) The effect of conformity, thickness, and material on stresses in ultrahigh molecular weight components for total joint replacement. J Bone Joint Surg Am 68:1041-1051.

8. Benevenia J, Lee FY, Beuchel F, Parsons JR (1998) Pathologic supracondylar fracture due to osteolytic pseudotumor of knee following cementless total knee replacement. J Biomed Mater Res 43:473-477.

9. Bierbaum B, Nairus J, Kuesis D, Morrison JC, Ward D (2002) Ceramic on ceramic bearings in total hip arthroplasty. Clin Orthop 405:158-163.

10. Bourne R, Barrack R, Rorabeck CH, Salehi A and Good V (2005) Arthroplasty options for the young patient. Clin Orthop 416:191-196.

11. Bradford L, Kurland M, Sankaran H (2004) Early failure due to osteolysis in highly crosslinked ultra-high molecular weight polyethylene: a case report. J Bone Joint Surg Am 86:1051-1056.

12. Bradford-Collons L, Baker DA, Graham J (2004) Wear and surface cracking in early retrieved highly crosslinked Durasul acetabular liners. J Bone Joint Surg Am 86:1271-1282.

13. Cales B (2000) Zirconia as a sliding material: histologic, laboratory, and clinical data. Clin Orthop 379:94-112.

14. Clarke IC, Manaka M, Green DD, Williams P, Pezzotti G, Kim YH, Ries M, Sugano N, Sedel L, Delauney C, Nissan BB, Donalson T, Gustafson GA (2003) Current status of zirconia used in total hip implants. J Bone Joint Surg Am 85 (Suppl 4):73-84.

15. Davidson JA (1993) characteristics of metal and ceramic total hip bearing surfaces and their effect on long-term ultra high molecular weight polyethylene wear. Clin Orthop 294:361-378.

16. Digas G, Karrholm J, Thanner J (2003) Highly cross-linked polyethylene in cemented THA: randomized study of 61 hips. Clin Orthop 417:126-138.

17. Engh GA, Dwyer KA, Hanes CK (1988) Polyethylene wear of metal backed tibial components in total and unicompartmental knee prosthesis. J Bone Joint Surg Br 74:9-17.

18. Fruh HJ, Willman G, Pfaff HG (1997) Wear characteristics of ceramic on ceramic for hip endoprostheses. Biomaterials 18:873-876.

19. Good V, Ries M, Barrack RL, Widding K, Hunter D, Heuer D (2003) Reduced wear with oxidized zirconium femoral heads. J Bone Joint Surg Am 85 (Suppl 4):105-110.

20. Hannouche D, Nich C, Bizot P, Meunier A, Nizard R, Sedel L (2003) Fractures of ceramic bearings. Clin Orthop 417:19-26.

21. Hannouche D, Hamadouche M, Nizard R, Bizot P, Meunier A, Sedel L (2005) Ceramics in total hip replacement. Clin Orthop 430:62-71.

22. Heimke G, Leyen S, Willmann G (2002) Knee arthroplasty: recently developed ceramics offer new solutions. Biomaterials 23:1539-1551.

23. Hunter G, Pawar V, Salehi A, Long M (2004) Abrasive wear of modified CoCr and Ti-6Al-4V surfaces against bone cement. In: Shrivatsva S (ed) Medical Device Materials Park, OH, ASM International pp91-97.

24. Insall JN, Aglietti P, Baldini A, Easley ME (2001) Meniscal-bearing knee replacement. In: Insall JN, Scott WN (eds) Surgery of the Knee, Churchill Livingstone, Philadelphia, pp1717-1738.

25. Janssen D, Stolk J, Verdonschot N (2006) Finite element analysis of the long-term fixation strength of cemented ceramic cups. Proc Inst Mech Eng 220:533-539.

26. Korovessis P, Petsinis G, Repanti M (2006) Metallosis after contemporary metal on metal total hip arthroplasty: five to nine year follow-up. J Bone Joint Surg Am 88: 1183-1191.

27. Koshino T, Okamoto R, Takagi T, Yamamoto K, Saito T (2002) Cemented ceramic YMCK total knee arthroplasty in patients with severe rheumatoid arthritis. J Arthroplasty 17:1009-1015.

28. Kovacs P, Davidson JA (1996) Chemical and electrochemical aspects of the biocompatibility of titanium and its alloys, ASTM STP 1272. American Society for Testing and Materials, West Conshohocken, PA, pp163-178.

29. Kuntz M (2006) Validation of a new high performance alumina matrix composite for use in total joint replacement. Semin Arthoplasty 17:141-145.

30. Laskin RS (2003) An oxidized Zr ceramic surfaced femoral component for total knee arthroplasty. Clin Orthop 416:191-196.

31. Laskin RS (2003) The need for alternative bearings. Orthopedics 26:966-968.

32. Leyen S, Vetter S, Plank H (2004) Analysis and investigation of the adhesive strength of ceramic and bone cement in knee arthroplasty. In: Lazennec JY, Dietrich M (eds): Bioceramics in Joint Arthroplasty. 9th BIOLOX-Symposium Proceedings. Steinkopff-Verlag, Darmstadt, pp57-59.

33. Long M, Rieser L, Hunter G (1998) Nana-hardness measurements of oxidized Zr-2.5 Nb and various orthopaedic materials. Trans Soc Biomaterials 21:528.

34. Merkert P (2003) Next generation ceramic bearings. In: Zippel H, Dietrich M (eds):Bioceramics in Joint Arthroplasty. 8th BIOLOX-Symposium Proceedings. Steinkopff-Verlag, Darmstadt, pp123-125.

35. Merkert P, Kuntz M (2006) Future applications in ceramics. In: Benazzo F, Falez F, Dietrich M (eds): Bioceramics in Joint Arthroplasty. 11th BIOLOX-Symposium Proceedings. Steinkopff-Verlag, Darmstadt, pp283-288.

36. Milosev I, Trebse R, Kovac S (2006) Survivorship and retrieval analysis of Sikomet metal on metal total hip replacements at a mean of seven years. J Bone Joint Surg Am 88: 1173-1182.

37. Minoda Y, Kobayashi A, Iwaki H, Miyaguchi M, Kadoya Y, Ohashi H, Takaoka K (2005) Polyethylene wear particle generation in vivo in an alumina medial pivot total knee prosthesis. Biomaterials 26:6034-6040.

38. Mittelmeier W, Ansorge S, Klub D, Kircher J, Bader R (2006) Ceramic knee endoprostheses: reality or future? In: Benazzo F, Falez F, Dietrich M (eds): Bioceramics in Joint Arthroplasty. 11th BIOLOX-Symposium Proceedings. Steinkopff-Verlag, Darmstadt, pp126-131.

39. Muller MP, Degreif J, Rudig L (2004) Friction of ceramic and metal hip hemi-endoprostheses against cadaveric acetabula. Arch Orthop Trauma Surg 124:681-687.

40. Nakamura T, Oonishi E, Yasuda T, Nakagawa Y (2004) A new knee prosthesis with bisurface femoral component made of zirconia ceramic. Key Eng Mater 254/256:607-609.

41. Oonish H, Hasegawa T (1981) Cementless alumina ceramic total knee prostheses. Orthop Ceramic Implants 1;157-160.

42. Oonishi H, Aono M, Murata N, Kushitani S (1990) Alumina versus polyethylene in total knee arthroplasty. Clin Orthop 282:95-104.

43. Oonishi H, Fujita H, Itoh S, Kim SC, Amino H (2002) Development and improvement of ceramic TKA for 19 years and clinical results. Key Eng Mater 218/220:479-483.

44. Oonishi H, Fujita H, Itoh S, Amino H, Usuji E (2002) Surface analysis on retrieved ceramic total knee prosthesis. Key Eng Mater 218/220:499-502.

45. Oonishi H, Kim SC, Kyomoto M, Masuda S, Asano T, Clark IC (2005) Changes in UHMWPE properties of retrieved ceramic total knee prosthesis in clinical use for 23 years. J Biomed Mater Res Appl Biomater 74B:754-759.

46. Oonishi H, Kim SC, Iwamoto M, Ueno M (2006) PE wear in ceramic/PE bearing surface in total knee arthroplasty: clinical experiences of more than 24 years. In: Benazzo F, Falez F, Dietrich M (eds): Bioceramics in Joint Arthroplasty. 11th BIOLOX-Symposium Proceedings. Steinkopff-Verlag, Darmstadt, pp101-110.

47. Oonishi H, Kim SC, Kyomoto M, Iwamoto M, Masuda S, Ueno M (2006) Ceramic total knee arthroplasty: advanced clinical experiences of 26 years. Semin Arthoplasty 17:134-140.

48. Pria PD, Giorgini L, Kuntz M, Pandorf T (2006) Ceramic knee design. In: Benazzo F, Falez F, Dietrich M (eds): Bioceramics in Joint Arthroplasty. 11ᵗʰ BIOLOX-Symposium Proceedings. Steinkopff-Verlag, Darmstadt, pp115-123.

49. Ries MD (2006) Oxidized zirconium in total joint arthroplasty. Semin Arthoplasty 17:161-164.

50. Ritter MA, Faris GW (2003) Alternative TKR bearing surfaces: the femur? you have got to be kidding. Orthopedics 26:967-980.

51. Sato T, Shimada M (1984) Crystalline phase change in yttria-partially-stabilized zirconia by low temperature annealing. J Amer Ceram Soc 67:212-213.

52. Sato T, Shimada M (1985) Transformation of yttria-doped tetragonal ZrO2 polycrystals by annealing in water. J Amer Ceram Soc 68: 356-359.

53. Schreiner U, Scheller G (2003) Osseointegration of ceramic implants: past, present and future. In: Zippel H, Dietrich M (eds): Bioceramics in Joint Arthroplasty. 8ᵗʰ BIOLOX-Symposium Proceedings. Steinkopff-Verlag, Darmstadt, pp119-122.

54. Sedel L, Nizard R, Bizot P, Meunier A (1998) Perspective on a 20-year experience with ceramic on ceramic articulation in total hip replacement. Semin Arthoplasty 9:123-134

55. Skinner HB (1999) Ceramic bearing surfaces. Clin Orthop 369:83-91.

56. Skinner HB (2006) Ceramics in total joint surgery: the pros and cons. Semin Arthoplasty 17:196-201.

57. Sprague J, Salehi A, Tsai S, Pawar V, Thomas R, Hunter G (2004) Mechanical behavior of zirconia, alumina, and oxidized zirconium modular heads. In: Brown S, Clarke IC, Gustafson A (eds) ISTA 2003, vol 2. International Society for Technology in Arthroplasty, Birmingham, AL, pp31-36.

58. Thomsen M, Thomas P (2006) Hypersensitivity reactions in association to arthroplasty. In: Benazzo F, Falez F, Dietrich M (eds): Bioceramics in Joint Arthroplasty. 11ᵗʰ BIOLOX-Symposium Proceedings. Steinkopff-Verlag, Darmstadt, pp111-113.

59. Tsai S, Sprague J, Hunter G, Thomas R, Salehi A (2001) Mechanical testing and finite element analysis of oxidized zirconium femoral components. Trans Soc Biomaterials 24:163.

60. Tsukamoto R, Chen S, Asano T, Ogino M, Shoji H, Nakamura T, Clarke IC (2006) Improved wear performance with crosslinked UHMWPE and zirconia implants in knee simulation. Acta Orthopaedica 77:505-511.

61. Ueno M, Ikeuchi K, Nakamura T, Akagi M (2003) Comparison of the wear properties of polyethylene plate in total knee prostheses using different femoral component material. Key Eng Mater 240/242:801-804.

62. Walter A (1992) On the material and the tribology of alumina-alumina couplings for hip joint prostheses. Clin Orthop 282:31-46.

63. Willmann G (1998) Ceramics for total hip replacement: what a surgeon should know. Orthopedics 21:173-177.

64. Won CH, Rohatgi S, Kraay MJ (2000) Effect of resin type and manufacturing method on wear of polyethylene tibial components. Clin Orthop 376:161-171.

65. Yasuda K (2004) Long-term clinical results of cruciate-retaining total knee arthroplasty using the alumina ceramic condylar prosthesis. Scientific Exhibit No. SE035. AAOS Meeting, San Francisco.

66. Yoshimura M, Noma T, Kawabata K, Somiya S (1987) Role of H_2O on the degradation process of Y-TZP. J Mater Sci Lett 6:465.

4.2 Finite-Element-Analysis of a Cemented Ceramic Femoral Component in Total Knee Arthroplasty

Ch. Schultze, D. Klüß, A. Lubomierski, K.-P. Schmitz, R. Bader and W. Mittelmeier

Introduction

The femoral components of total knee replacement are generally made of metal and are mainly implanted with bone cement. Common complications in total knee arthroplasty (TKA) include abrasive wear, malpositioning and material fatigue [2]. In comparison to metal, ceramic components provide a better biocompatibility as well as higher scratch and wear resistance. Laboratory tests showed a decrease in the wear debris rate with the bearing couple ceramic-on-polyethylene to more than one third compared to the couple metal-on-polyethylene [1,9]. Another benefit of ceramic implants also exists in the avoidance of allergic reactions in comparison to metal. A disadvantage of ceramic implants is the low fracture toughness respectively the brittle characteristics [19]. Hence the risk of implant damage resulting from stress peaks has to be minimised by an optimal load transmission in the adjacent bone stock. The load transmission also influences the long-time behaviour of the bone cement. Local cement breakage and cement wear debris induce inflammatory reactions, which can finally lead to aseptic loosening [11,4].

The objective of this study was to examine the load situation and the possible mechanisms leading to stress fractures in a newly developed cemented femoral component made of an alumina matrix composite ceramics (BIOLOX® *delta*) with the Finite Element Method (FEM).

Materials and Methods

In the present study the physical model was reduced to the femoral component, the cement layer, the femur and the tibia inlay.

For the three dimensional analysis the CAD-model of an existing femoral component was implemented in the CAD-software CATIA V5 (Dassault Systèmes, SIMULIA, Providence, RI, USA) to generate the cement layer with a thickness of 1.0 mm. The anatomical femoral bone morphology was prepared from computer tomography (CT) data using the software Amira (Mercury Computer Systems). Afterwards the bone resection was simulated according to the surgical manual. All components were assembled in the software Patran (MSC, Santa Ana, CA, USA) and were meshed with 8-node-hexahedron-elements (Fig. 1). Contact was defined between the distal femur and the proximal bone cement layer, between the distal cement layer and the proximal femoral component and between the distal femoral component and the proximal tibia inlay.

A load of 1400 N [8] was transmitted to a rigid surface connected to the proximal end of the femur, while the polyethylene tibia inlay was fixed at the distal surface. Additionally, worst cases like stumbling (8-times body weight), bone defects in the medial distal femoral condyle and malpositioning of the tibia inlay were examined.

Except the femur all materials were assumed as homogenous and isotropic with an linear-elastic behaviour [5,12,17]. For the femur, an elastic ideal-plastic material behaviour according to Zacharias [20] and Rho [14] was defined. All analyses were performed with regard to large deformations using the solver ABAQUS (Dassault Systèmes, SIMULIA, Providence, RI, USA).

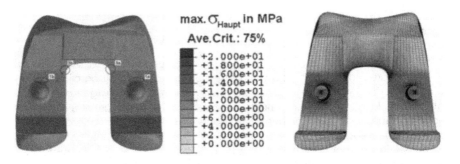

max. σ_{Haupt} in MPa
Ave.Crit.: 75%

+2.000e+01
+1.800e+01
+1.600e+01
+1.400e+01
+1.200e+01
+1.000e+01
+8.000e+00
+6.000e+00
+4.000e+00
+2.000e+00
+0.000e+00

Figure 1:
Zones with high principal stresses at the inner surface of the femoral ceramic component.

Results

At a load of 1400 N, the highest principal stresses were calculated in the zones 3a and 3b (Fig. 1) with values of 37 MPa. Furthermore, high stresses appeared in the zones 1a and 1b. At the worst case during stumbling (8-times body weight) the highest stress was 565 MPa in the zones 3a and 3b. Simulating a femoral bone defect, the stresses adjacent to the defect increased in zone 3a to 39 MPa. With a malpositioned tibia inlay the highest stress occurred in zone 1b.

The increase of the load from 1400 N to 5600 N (8 x BW) during stumbling caused an increase of the maximal stress by a factor of 15. However, all calculated stresses were lower than the ultimate strength [13] of the BIOLOX® *delta* ceramic.

The highest von Mises stress in the tibia inlay was 7 MPa (1400 N) respectively 35 MPa (8 x BW). At the worst case during stumbling the yield point of 18 MPa was exceeded by a factor of 2. In the cement layer the highest von Mises stress appeared in the boundary and amounted 7 MPa (1400 N) respectively 405 MPa (8-times body weight). During stumbling, the compressive strength of 80 MPa [15] was exceeded. The highest von Mises stresses in the femur were between 25 MPa (1400 N) and 245 MPa (8 x BW). The yield point of 100 MPa [20] was exceeded during stumbling.

Discussion

Stress analyses of artificial knee joints via FEM and experimental testing were conducted predominantly at the tibial site so far [3,7]. Ueno et al. [16] accomplished experimental and FE analyses of a zirconia femoral component. Huang et al. [10] report a case in which a metal femoral component broke in zone 1a. Since metal components are subject to ductile fracture in the long term performance while ceramics tend to brittle fracture, the results are not directly comparable. However, in the FE-analyses the same endangered areas (zone 1a) are shown. This also applies for the studies of Cook et al. [6] and Wada et al. [18], who reported fractures of metal femoral components in zone 3a.

Ueno et al. [16] detected the same endangered zones for a ceramic femoral component in an experimental and FE analyses, where the effect of modifications of the material properties on the amount of stresses in the femoral component was investigated. Also, the risk of damage of the femoral component by malpositioning or femoral bone defect was demonstrated, corresponding to the results of the worst case simulation in our present study. Our results show that the femoral component was not exposed to principal stresses beyond the ceramics tensile strength of 1150 MPa [13] in each load case. Of all simulated worst case scenarios, stumbling appeared to cause the highest stresses in the femoral component with values up to 15 times the stress caused during gait.

References

1. Ansorge S, Bader R, Mittelmeier W. Knieendoprothesen aus Keramik - eine Alternative?. Ärztliches Journal Orthopädie 2006; 4: 34-35.
2. Bader R, Mittelmeier W, Steinhauser E. Versagensanalyse von Knieendoprothesen: Grundlagen und methodische Ansätze zur Schadensanalyse. Orthopäde 2006; 35: 896-903.
3. Beilas P, Papaioannou G, Tashman S, Yang KH. A new method to investigate in vivo knee behaviour using a finite element model of the lower limb. J Biomech 2004; 37: 1019-1030.
4. Breusch SJ, Schneider U, Kreutzer J, Ewerbeck V, Lukoschek M. Einfluß der Zementiertechnik auf das Zementierergebnis am koxalen Femurende. Orthopäde 2000; 29: 260-270.
5. CeramTec AG. BIOLOX® delta – Eine neue Keramik für die Orthopädie. Firmeninformationsschrift 10/2004.
6. Cook SD, Thomas KA. Fatigue failure of noncemented porous-coated implants. J Bone Joint Surg 1991; 73-B: 20-24.
7. D'Lima DD, Patil S, Steklov N, Slamin JE, Colwell CW Jr. The Chitranjan Ranawat Award: in vivo knee forces after total knee arthroplasty. Clin Orthop Relat Res 2005; 440: 45-49.
8. D'Lima et al. Tibial forces measured in vivo after total knee arthroplasty. J Arthroplasty 2006; 21 (2): 255-262.
9. Greenwald S, Garino JP. Alternative Bearing Surfaces: The Good, the Bad, and the Ugly. J Bone Joint Surg 2001; 83-A: 68-72.
10. Huang CH, Yang CY, Cheng CK. Fracture of the femoral component associated with polyethylene wear and osteolysis after total knee athroplasty. J Arthroplasty 1999; 14: 375-379.
11. Jacobs JJ, Hallab NJ, Skipor AK, Urban RM. Metal Degradation Products. Clin Orthop Relat Res 2003; 417: 139-147.
12. Klüß et al. Finite-Elemente-Untersuchung zur Impingement-bedingten Schädigung von Implantaten für den Hüftgelenkersatz. Materialprüfung 2007. in print.
13. Rack et al. A new ceramic material for orthopedics. J Biomech 2006; 39: 1371-1382.
14. Rho JY, Hobatho MC, Ashman RB. Relations of mechanical properties to density and CT numbers in human bone. Med Eng Phys 1995; 17: 347-355.
15. Simpson PMS, Dall GF, Breusch SJ, Heisel C. In-vitro-Freisetzung von Antibiotika aus SmartSet HV- und Palacos-R Knochenzement und deren Einfluss auf die mechanischen Eigenschaften. Orthopäde 2005; 34: 1255-1262.

16. Ueno M, Apgar M, Sarin V. Mechanical stress analysis and burst testing of zirconia femoral component for total knee arthroplasty. Key Eng Mat 2002; 218-220: 573-576.

17. Van Lenthe GH, De Waal Malefijt MC, Huiskes R. Stress shielding after total knee replacement may cause bone resorption in the distal femur. J Bone and Joint Surg, 1997; 79: 117-122.

18. Wada M, Imura S, Bo H, Baba H, Miyazaki T. Stress fracture of the femoral component in total knee replacement: a report of 3 cases. Int Orthop 1997; 21: 54-55.

19. Willmann G. Investigation of explanted hip and acetabulum hip prostheses. Biomed Tech 2001; 46: 343-350.

20. Zacharias T. Präoperative biomechanische Berechnung von Femur-Hüftendoprothesen-Systemen zur Ermittlung der individuellen Primärstabilität nach Roboterimplantation. Dissertation, Universität Rostock 2000.

4.3 Advanced Testing of Ceramic Femoral Knee Components

T. Pandorf and M. Kuntz

Abstract

For over 35 years, ceramics in joint replacement are known for their excellent biocompatibility, extremely low wear rates and excellent wettability. Ceramic on ceramic bearings have shown excellent survival rates. Also in hard on soft bearings, i. e. ceramic ball head against (highly crosslinked) polyethylene, a reduction in wear rate compared to metal on (highly crosslinked) polyethylene was shown in-vitro as well as in-vivo.

In knee arthroplasty a ceramic component has several advantages: First of all, there is no ion release implying no risk for potential allergies. Secondly, the extreme hardness of the material leads to a scratch resistance surface and less PE wear over time. In the past, ceramic femoral components in knee applications were limited in the variety of design possibilities due to necessary thickness of the component resulting from the associated fracture risk of ceramics.

By the development of an alumina matrix composite material with increased mechanical properties it is possible to develop a ceramic femoral component which has nearly the same design as a metal component and uses the same surgical approach as well as instruments. This offers the surgeon the opportunity to choose intraoperatively between metal or ceramic femoral components. Extensive in-vitro testing derived from in-vivo loading situations has shown that ceramic femoral components achieve execellent superior mechanical test results. The reliability of the components is build on testing of the design by two burst tests and a fatigue test to evaluate the design of the ceramic component. A proof test which is performed on each individual component before release for sale ensures highest quality of the ceramic knee components.

Introduction

Total Knee Arthroplasty (TKA) is one of the most successful and common effective treatment for degenerative diseases of the knee joint. Despite the positive clinical results, concerns still remain with regard to the material properties and design limitations of the implant systems. This is particularly true if we consider that improvements in surgical techniques are not strictly followed by enhanced performance of the knee prosthesis.

In TKA loosening of components due to UHMWPE wear remains the leading cause for revision surgery. Other possible causes of failure are wrong positioning, inadequate design of the prosthesis, infection and allergy against implant materials [1]. The advantages of ceramics concerning lubrication, friction, and wear properties compared to Cobalt-Chrome alloy (CoCr) vs. Ultra-High Molecular Weight Polyethylene (UHMWPE) surfaces in total joint arthroplasty are well recognized [2-5]. Moreover, ceramics have the additional advantage of being biocompatible in opposite to the well-known difficulties coming along with the metal ion release of metal components [6-9]. Thus, a non-allergic implant potentially could improve functional and long-term results.

However, for many surgeons, these advantages are counterbalanced by fatigue resistance, the fear of ceramic fracture, and the difficult revision surgery when a fracture of ceramic components occurs [10,11].

The use of ceramic materials are not be taken into consideration for knee arthroplasty in the same way as it is acknowledged in total hip arthroplasty (THA). Indeed, while ceramic bearings are nevertheless a suitable alternative to metal in THA, clinical experience with ceramic biomaterials in TKA is still very limited [2,12-15].

Biolox® *delta* is an alumina matrix composite (AMC) featuring better mechanical properties than pure alumina oxide or zirconia oxide (flexural strenght = 1300 MPa, 1100 MPa and 550 MPa for Biolox® *delta*, zirconia oxide, and alumina oxide, respectively).

Consequently, ceramic femoral components for total knee replacement articulating against XPE were designed with shapes and dimensions equivalent to the appropriate metal components.

Mechanical testing of the ceramic femoral component

The mechanical strength of Biolox® *delta* exceeds by far the properties of conventional materials like CoCr, Ti or high purity alumina oxide. Nevertheless, due to the brittle behaviour and the statistical distribution of the mechanical strength which is characterized by Weibull's modulus, it is necessary to ensure a minimum mechanical strength of each produced component. This is accomplished by the "proof test" which means overloading the component up to a load level significantly higher than the in-vivo stresses. Due to the specific design characteristics, the fixation technique and the specific kinematics of the knee joint the femoral component is exposed to a variable load situation and stress distribution. Thus, a sophisticated mechanical test concept is necessary in order to identify critical loading situations and to provide a highly reliable ceramic prosthesis. In the following, the development of the "proof-test" will be described.

The mechanical proof-test was developed by subsequent steps of load/stress analysis and design of an adequate mechanical test equipment. The procedure was organized as follows:

1. Analysis of relevant maximum in-vivo loading conditions
2. Analysis of the "boundary conditions", i.e. the fixation of the ceramic prosthesis on the bone. Identifying worst-case conditions
3. Finite Element analysis: Identifying regions of highest stress concentration at variable external loading
4. Design analysis and accommodation
5. Development of an adequate mechanical test equipment which produces stresses comparable to the in-vivo conditions
6. Performing mechanical tests with ceramic femoral components
7. Life time analysis
8. *Validation* of the test concept: comparison of test results and stress analysis

9. Assign *"safety margin"*, i.e. required overload tolerance of the ceramic component with respect to worst case load in-vivo

10. Establish *"proof test"*, i.e. in-production mechanical testing of each individual component in order to provide safety margin

In the following, the most important features of each item are being discussed:

In-vivo loading conditions: It is distinguished between alternating regular loading with a high cycle number during life time and irregular worst case loading which is assumed to appear rarely during life time. The relevant regular loading is represented by raising from a chair and normal walking. The most critical irregular worst cases are stumbling or impact loading. The load transfer, stress distribution and the anticipated cycle number during life-time are distinguished and taken into account for the development of the test concept. The commonly assumed maximum in-vivo loads are shown in Figure 1.

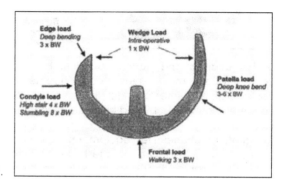

Figure 1:
Assumed maximum in-vivo loads [16].

Boundary conditions: The prosthesis is cemented on the resected femoral bone. Thus, the load transfer from the hard and stiff ceramic component through the cement is essential for the development of the internal stresses. For the assessment of the boundary conditions, all *extreme* situations have been taken into account, i.e. perfect bonding of cement to bone and prosthesis, debonding of the cemented interface and cement damage. The principle is shown in Figure 2.

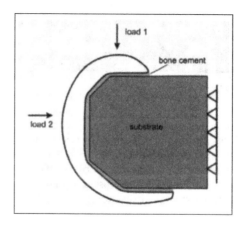

Figure 2:
In-vivo like boundary conditions for the femoral component.

Finite Element Analysis: External loading generates internal stresses inside the component which are typically concentrated to certain positions. The critical positions for all load situations have been quantitatively analysed, see e.g. Figure 3.

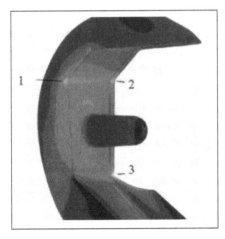

Figure 3:
Example of the stress maxima (1, 2, 3) for one loading situation.

Design analysis and accommodation: From step 3 it is evident that stress concentration is mainly generated by geometric features, e.g. the shape of the corners at the interface to the cement. Significant reduction of stress concentration was achieved by some minor corrections of design details.

Adequate mechanical test equipment: The in-vivo stress distribution is reproduced by mechanical tests. Two main tests are performed by load transfer either from outside (regular load) or inside (wedge load) on the condyles of the prosthesis, see Figure 4.

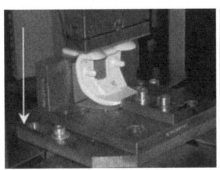 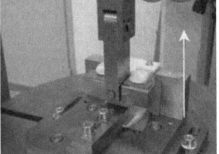

Figure 4:
Regular (left) and wedge (right) test setup.

Mechanical tests: A large number of regular and wedge tests have been performed with ceramic femoral knee components of identical condition as those intended for implantation (incl. grinding and polishing). The equipment has been improved by means of handling and reproducibility. The fracture origin is analysed for each test using high resolution microscopy. The analysis has shown that the components represent regular materials condition.

Validation: The deformation of the ceramic components during the tests was measured by using strain gauges distributed at all of the relevant positions, see Figure 5. It has been shown that the mechanical tests exactly produce the intended stress distribution.

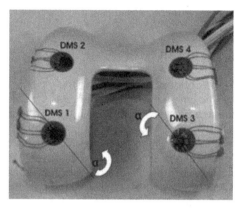

Figure 5:
Regular (left) and wedge (right) test setup.

Life time analysis: Life time relevant tests like wear, static and cyclic loading and exposure to synovia like environment have been performed with ceramic components, see Figure 6, as well as with standardized test specimens. There is only marginal material degradation even after conditions which simulate severe loading for more than 20 years. The high safety margin of the ceramic component is thus maintained during the full anticipated implant duration time.

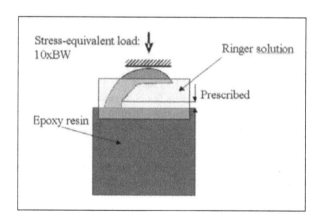

Figure 6:
Setup of the cycling loading test.

Safety margin: The mechanical tests are designed in order to simulate in-vivo loading conditions. Nevertheless, in order to reduce the probability of an unexpected fracture of the implanted component, the acceptance criteria for the test load are chosen significantly higher than the worst case in-vivo load. According to widely accepted rules for components in critical applications the safety margin was chosen to the highest recommended level. Therefore, the tests are performed with 16 x bodyweight for the regular test and 10 x bodyweight for the wedge test.

Proof test: The mechanical tests have been shown to represent reliably all loading conditions which are relevant in-vivo. These tests are accommodated such that they are suitable for *in-production* application. Thus, each individual component is "proof tested" before release to the customer to make sure that all components provide the full safety margin as derived in the sophisticated test concept.

Conclusion

The concept of developing the proof-test values and acceptance criteria from the maximum in-vivo loads ensures together with the Biolox® *delta* material and a suitable and good product design (Multigen Plus system, Lima, Italy) a structurally reliable and useful knee solution. The design is close to that of the appropriate metal knee so that the same surgical approach and instrumentation can be used for both knee solutions. Clinical observations in the framework of a multicenter study in different European countries have been started. Nevertheless, a longer follow-up is needed to validate the performance of ceramic components and to confirm the high safety margin of the ceramic femoral knee component.

References

1. Bader R, Mittelmeier W, Steinhauser E. Failure analysis of total knee replacement: Basics and methodological aspects of the damage analysis. (In press, Orthopäde, 2006).
2. Sonny Bal B, Greenberg DD, Buhrmester L, Aleto TJ. Primary TKA with a Zirconia Ceramic Femoral Component. J Knee Surg 2006;19:89-93.
3. Jacobs JJ, Hallab NJ, Skipor AK, Urban RM. Metal degradation products: a cause for concern in metal-metal bearings? Clin Orthop 2003;417:139-147.
4. Greenwald AS, Garino JP. American Academy of Orthopaedic Surgeons. Committee on Biomedical Engineering; American Academy of Orthopaedic Surgeons. Committee on Hip and Knee Arthritis. Alternative bearing surfaces: the good, the bad, and the ugly. J Bone Joint Surg Am 2001;83 Suppl 2 Pt 2:68-72.
5. Oonishi H, Tsuji E, Mizukoshi T et al. Wear of polyethylene and alumina in clinical cases of alumina total knee prostheses. Bioceramics 1991;3:137-145.
6. Baur W, Hönle W, Schuh A. Histopathologic changes in tissue surrounding revised metal-metal-bearings. BIOmaterialien 2004; 5(2): 86.
7. Bos I, Willmann G. Morphologic characteristics of periprosthetic tissues from hip prostheses with ceramic-ceramic couples. Acta Orthop Scand 2001; 72(4): 335-342.
8. Campbell P, Shen Fu-Wen; Mc Kellop H. Biologic and Tribologic Consideration of Alternative Bearing Surfaces. Clin Orthop 2004; 418: 98-111.
9. Fisher J, Galvin A, Tipper J, Stewart T, Stone M, Ingham E. Comparison of the Functional Biological Activity and Osteolytic Potential of Ceramic on Ceramic and Cross Linked Polyethylene Bearings in the Hip. J.A. D'Antonio, M. Dietrich (eds.): Bioceramics and Alternative Bearings in Joint Arthroplasty. 10th BIOLOX® Symposium Proceedings. Steinkopff Verlag, Darmstadt 2005: 21-24.
10. Abernethy PJ, Robinson CM, Fowler RM. Fracture of the metal tibial tray after kinematic total knee replacement. A common cause of early aseptic failure. J Bone Joint Surg Br 1996;78(2):220-225.

11. Wright J, Ewald FC, Walker PS, Thomas WH, Poss R, Sledge CB. Total knee arthroplasty with the kinematic prosthesis. Results after five to nine years: a follow-up note. J bone Joint Surg Am 1990;72:1003-1009.

12. Oonishi H, Aono M, Murata N, Kushitani S. Alumina versus polyethylene in total knee arthroplasty. Clin Orthop 1992;282:95-104.

13. Yasuda K, Miyagi N, Kaneda K. Low friction total knee arthroplasty with the alumina ceramic condylar prosthesis. Bull Hosp Jt Dis 1993;53:15-21.

14. Oonishi H, Fujita H, Itoh S, Kin S, Amino H. Development and improvement of ceramic TKP for 19 years and clinical results. Key Eng Mat 2002;14:479-482.

15. Oonishi H, Kim SC, Kyomoto M, Masuda S, Asano T, Clarke IC. Change in UHMWPE properties of retrieved ceramic total knee prosthesis in clinical use for 23 years. J Biomed Mater Res B Appl Biomater 2005;74:754-759.

16. Wimmer, M. Internal Paper, 2005.

4.4 Reasons using a Ceramic Femoral Component and First Clinical Experience

F. Benazzo, P. Dalla Pria, W. Mittelmeier, D. Tigani, C. Zorzi, D. Ganzer, C.H. Lohmann, E.G. Cimbrelo, C.R. Merchan, E.M. Saura, A.U. Lizaur, J.F. Couceiro and S. Burelli

Introduction

Metal sensitivity can be considered an emerging issue in TKA (Hallab, 2001). Wear of the polyethylene liner has been addressed with better design of the components, improvement of the material itself and improved surgical techniques (Gioe, 2004; Fehring, 2004, Tsukamoto, 2006). However, for the increasing number of young active people candidate for a variety of reasons to surgery, the issue of wear still remain of paramount importance.

Considerable advancement in both fields have been made with the introduction of femoral components made of oxidized zirconium (Oxinium®) (Ezzet, 2004), while Titanium prosthesis addresses more specifically the problem of allergy.

Ceramic is an unique material combining different features, such as strength and hardness, negligible wear, biocompatibility with no ions release neither intolerance issues, high lubrication and wettability (White, 1994). It has a long and proven history in THR, while in Japan it has been in use since almost two decades in TKA (Oonishi, 2005).

The purpose of this investigation, involving an international group of surgeons, is to verify the feasibility of the use on a larger scale of a femoral component of a well known and time-proven prosthesis (Multigen Plus, Lima Lto Spa, Italy), made of Biolox® delta ceramic (CeramTec AG, Germany) in order to assess the efficacy, functional and radiological performance of this Delta Ceramic Multigen Plus and to detect any infrequent complications or problems after long term and wide-spread use.

Materials and Methods

The expected total number of patients, that are going to be enrolled, according to the inclusion and exclusion criteria, is 200. Patients are submitted to a total knee arthroplasty (TKA) with a Biolox® delta femoral component, Ti6Al4V alloy tibial plate and an UMWPHE liner EtO sterilized (Multigen Plus System, Lima-Lto Spa, Italy) and are fixed with a high quality high viscosity cement. The Biolox® delta femoral component is manufactured by CeramTec AG for Lima-Lto Spa.

All surgical procedures are performed by only one surgeon for each centre and all of them are trained and experienced in performing the same surgical procedure with the similar CoCrMo Multigen Plus femoral component.

Intraoperative evaluation includes data concerning time of surgery (from cut to closure), type of anaesthesia, antibiotic and anticoagulation prophylaxis, blood loss, and bone stock quality.

Patients are evaluated preoperatively, immediately postoperatively and 3 months, 1 year, 2 year, 5 years after surgery. Clinical performance is assessed with the Hospital for Special Surgery (HSS) Score (Ranawat, 1973), including the evaluation of the range of motion.

Patients physical functional outcome and quality of life are evaluated using standard self-administered questionnaires, respectively by Western Ontario and MacMaster (WOMAC) Universities Osteoarthritis Index Score and SF-36 Score.

Radiographic analysis requires full-length, anteroposterior, lateral and patella (Merchant view) x-rays in order to determine preoperatively joint configuration (axes, joint space narrowing, osteophytes, calcifications or ossifications) and the degree of deformity and postoperatively to assess alignment, component position and femoral flexion angle, tibial angle and total valgus angle. The radiographic examination also includes the presence and the location of any periprosthetic radiolucent lines. Radiological evaluation is performed by an independent qualified examiner, according to the Knee Society evaluation and scoring system (Ewald, 1989).

Ethics Committees approval was obtained for this study at each of the participating centres and written informed consent is be obtained from all enrolled patients.

Surgical technique

The surgical approach is the standard medial parapatellar with posterior cruciate ligament retaining, without patella replacement and without the use of navigation system.

Particular attention is given to the femoral preparation: bone cuts are accurately checked in order to avoid any stress raising point during the insertion of the femoral component, and to obtain an uniform cement layer. For the same reason the holes for the two pegs are enlarged with a specially designed punch.

The femoral component is driven in place with a holder, and the cement squeezed out putting the leg in extension with the trial liner in.

The post-operative does not present any particular issue.

Results

Since the beginning of the study in October 2006, the study is presently in the enrolment phase. This starting group of enrolled patients, currently 36, includes 80% of female and 20% of male with a mean age of 67 years (range 54 - 75). The mean body mass index (BMI) is 28 kg/m^2 (range 20,83 - 33). The prevalent preoperative diagnosis in the enrolled patients is osteoarthritis. Up to this initial phase of the clinical trial, no complications have been detected.

Discussion

Issues:

The prevalence of metal sensitivity among the general population is approximately 10% to 15%, with nickel sensitivity having the highest prevalence and a common cross-reactivity between nickel and cobalt (Hallab, 2001). Immunological metallic-specific responses are cited as possible causes for osteolysis, postoperative complications and early implant loosening and may suggest an involvement in a poor implant performance or in implants failure (Hallab, 2005, Gawkrodger, 2003).

More than 30 years of clinical experience (Sedel, 2004) and in-vitro/in-vivo research have demonstrated a high biocompatibility of Biolox ceramic materials, consisting of ultra pure aluminium oxide ceramics. Testing for hypersensitivity has been conducted in vivo by epicutaneous tests and in vitro by lymphocyte transformation testing (LTT) showing no allergic reactions and demonstrating that Biolox® delta is a bio-inert material.

Furthermore, in vitro tests have been performed to investigate the potential chrome release. There is uncertainty over the possible biological effects and implications caused by the long term loading of the human body with metallic wear particles and metal ions. Whether released metal ions have a tumour-causing effect is still not absolutely certain (Visuri 1996, Witzleb 2006). Anyway, results of analysis performed on Biolox® delta revealed a clear evidence of no indication of ions release in a toxically relevant concentration.

In conclusion, Biolox® delta reveals a high biocompatibility.

Benefits of delta Ceramic includes the potential to achieve low wear, while avoiding the problems of brittleness which plagues other ceramics.

The Implant has the advantage of combining a well established and proven design with the potential benefits of the delta ceramic material. In addition the technique of implantation is familiar to any arthroplasty surgeon.

Patients will be assessed both clinically and radiologically at 3-6 –12 months and then annually. At each visit both clinical assessment with established scoring systems and x-rays will be made in order to establish clinical outcome data, surgical accuracy and implant longevity.

References

1. Ranawat CS, Shine JJ. Duo-condylar total knee arthroplasty. Clin Orthop Relat Res. 1973 Jul-Aug;(94):185-95.
2. Ewald FC. The Knee Society total knee arthroplasty roentgenographic evaluation and scoring system. Clin Orthop Relat Res. 1989 Nov;(248):9-12.
3. Hallab N, Merritt K, Jacobs JJ. Metal sensitivity in patients with orthopaedic implants. J Bone Joint Surg Am. 2001 Mar;83-A(3):428-36.
4. Hallab NJ, Anderson S, Stafford T, Glant T, Jacobs JJ. Lymphocyte responses in patients with total hip arthroplasty. J Orthop Res. 2005 Mar;23(2):384-91.
5. Gawkrodger DJ. Metal sensitivities and orthopaedic implants revisited: the potential for metal allergy with the new metal-on-metal joint prostheses. Br J Dermatol. 2003 Jun; 148(6):1089-93.

6. Sedel L. Thirty Years Experience with all Ceramic Bearings. Proceedings 5th International Biolox Symposium 2000, Thieme Verlag.

7. Visuri T, Pukkala E, Paavolainen P, Pulkkinen P, Riska EB.Cancer risk after metal on metal and polyethylene on metal total hip arthroplasty. Clin Orthop Relat Res. 1996 Aug;(329 Suppl):S280-9.

8. Witzleb WC, Ziegler J, Krummenauer F, Neumeister V, Guenther KP. Exposure to chromium, cobalt and molybdenum from metal-on-metal total hip replacement and hip resurfacing arthroplasty. Acta Orthop. 2006 Oct;77(5):697-705.

9. Ezzet KA, Hermida JC, Colwell CW Jr, D'Lima DD. Oxidized zirconium femoral components reduce polyethylene wear in a knee wear simulator. Clin Orthop Relat Res 2004; 428:120–124.

10. Gioe TJ, Killeen KK, Grimm K, et al. Why are total knee replacements revised? Analysis of early revision in a community knee implant registry. Clin Orthop Relat Res 2004; 428:100–106.

11. Fehring TK, Murphy JA, Hayes TD, et al. Factors Influencing wear and osteolysis in press-fit condylar modular total knee replacements. Clin Orthop Relat Res 2004; 428:40–50.

12. White SE, Whiteside LA, McCarthy DS, Anthony M, Poggie RA Simulated knee wear with cobalt chromium and oxidized zirconium knee femoral components Clin Orthop Relat Res. 1994 Dec;(309):176-84.

13. Oonishi H, Kim SC, Kyomoto M, Masuda S, Asano T, Clarke IC. Change in UHMWPE properties of retrieved ceramic total knee prosthesis in clinical use for 23 years. J Biomed Mater Res B Appl Biomater. 2005 Aug;74(2):754-9.

14. Tsukamoto R, Chen S, Asano T, Ogino M, Shoji H, Nakamura T, Clarke IC. Improved wear performance with crosslinked UHMWPE and zirconia implants in knee simulation. Acta Orthop. 2006 Jun;77(3):505-11.

4.5 Comparison of In-Vivo Wear between Polyethylene Inserts articulating against Ceramic and Cobalt-Chrome Femoral Components in Total Knee Prostheses

H. Oonishi, S.-C. Kim, H. Oonishi, M. Kyomoto, M. Iwamoto and M. Ueno

Abstract

In the late 1970s, the use of a combination of alumina ceramics and ultra-high molecular weight polyethylene (UHMWPE) was started for total knee prostheses (TKPs) to reduce UHMWPE wear and suppress bone resorption, based on good clinical results in total hip prostheses. In this study, to examine the *in vivo* efficacy of alumina ceramic bearing surface of TKP, we compared retrieved alumina ceramic TKPs with cobalt-chrome (Co-Cr) alloy TKPs by surface observation and linear wear measurement. In the scanning electron microscopic observations, many scratches due to clinical use were observed only on the retrieved Co-Cr alloy femoral component. The damage in the form of scratches on the articulating surface was linear and produced by rubbing of microscopic asperities against the Co-Cr alloy surface. The linear wear rate of the retrieved Co-Cr alloy TKPs was 0.027–0.358 mm/year. In contrast, the wear of the retrieved alumina ceramic TKPs was stably low and linear; the linear wear rate was estimated to be 0.026 mm/year. The lower wear rate and milder nature of wear observed in TKP with UHMWPE insert and alumina ceramic femoral component combination suggest the possibility of retention of high performance of this TKP even during prolonged clinical use.

Introduction

Total knee prostheses (TKPs) are being widely used because they are successful and effective in the treatment of degenerative knee joint diseases. However, the wear debris from the ultra-high molecular weight polyethylene (UHMWPE) insert in TKP induces aseptic loosening of the TKP remains a majority of the revisions as well as total hip prostheses (THPs) [1,2]. In order to reduce polyethylene wear, clinical application of highly pure alumina ceramics in THPs was initiated in Europe and Japan in the 1970s. In 1971, Boutin et al. first reported the clinical results of alumina-on-alumina ceramics in THPs in France [3,4]. In 1977, the clinical results of THPs obtained by Shikita and Oonishi et al. in Japan indicated that the wear of UHMWPE cups was lower in combination with an alumina ceramic head than in combination with a metallic head [5,6]. Consequently, based on the good clinical results with these THPs, Oonishi et al. started using a combination of alumina ceramics and UHMWPE in TKPs in the late 1970s [7].

Subsequently, some refinements of the ceramic TKP designs have been carried out to date to improve the kinematical properties and the fixation of TKP with the living bone (Fig. 1). The first generation TKP used from 1981 to 1985 consisted of an alumina ceramic femoral component, an alumina ceramic tibial component,

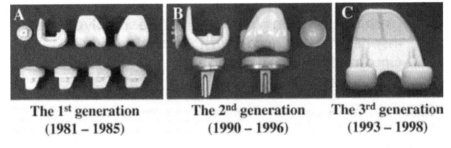

The 1st generation   The 2nd generation   The 3rd generation
(1981 – 1985)   (1990 – 1996)   (1993 – 1998)

Figure 1:
Refinements of the ceramic total knee prosthesis designs.

and an UHMWPE insert. Polycrystalline alumina of 99.5% or higher purity was used as an alumina ceramic raw material. The stem of alumina ceramic was positioned at the center of the tibial component so that the load was transmitted from the stem to the cortical bone in the posterior portion of the tibia. Small and shallow groves were observed on the portion of the bone that was in contact with the femoral and tibial components. Both femoral and tibial components can be used as cemented and cementless fixation. With regard to the first generation TKPs, 137 joints have been followed-up for 20 to 25 years after implantation. The rates of loosening, sinking, and revisions were very high with cementless fixation but very low with cemented fixation [8–10]. The second generation TKPs used from 1990 to 1996 comprised an alumina ceramic femoral component, a titanium alloy tibial component, and an UHMWPE insert. The alumina ceramic tibial component in the first generation TKP was replaced with the titanium alloy tibial component that was required to be fixed with bone cement; this was because the alumina ceramic tibial component was thick and brittle and a relatively high incidence of sinking and occurrence of radiolucent lines was observed on the components in the case of cementless fixation. In the third generation TKPs used from 1993 to 1998, a porous coating of ceramic beads was applied on the surface of the femoral component in order to improve the fixation between bone cement and the ceramic femoral component. Subsequently, there has been a remarkable progression in ceramic applications in the field of total knee arthroplasty. We have developed a new high-strength alumina ceramic by improving both raw material quality and production process, through the application of hot isostatic pressing treatment. This alumina ceramic has been used for fabricating the femoral component of the TKPs since 1997. Due to the high mechanical strength of this ceramic [11], the limitations regarding TKP designs were reduced. Moreover, the thickness of the alumina femoral component is equal to that of the metallic one. Since 2001, a tetragonal zirconia polycrystal (TZP) ceramic as a multiphase material has been used for TKP (KU type; Kyocera Corp., Kyoto, Japan) largely due to its higher strength than that of alumina ceramic (Fig. 2) [12–14]. We have previously reported the clinical results of the second and third generation ceramic TKPs (total 534 joints, 1990–2005). All the components were implanted using bone cement. After 6–14 years of follow-up of 249 joints, no case of loosening or sinking was observed [15]. Radiolucent lines were observed at the rate of 4.3% and 2.1% at the medial and lateral tibial areas, respectively (Fig. 3). Osteolysis had not occurred in any of the followed-up cases. Since good clinical results were obtained with the ceramic femoral component and UHMWPE tibial insert, their basic structures have been retained

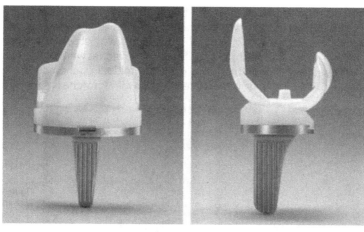

Figure 2:
Zirconia ceramic total knee prosthesis (KU type).

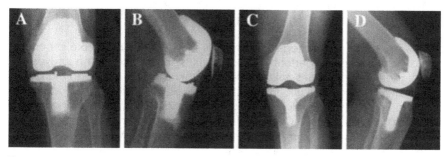

Figure 3:
Radiographs of the patient implanted with the second generation TKP after 14 years of implantation (A: anteroposterior, B: lateral) and the third generation TKP (C: anteroposterior, D: lateral) after 6 years of implantation.

in our current TKPs, which have the potential of extremely low clinical wear rate that in turn will reduce the risk of osteolysis.

In our previous studies, we compared the surfaces of retrieved UHMWPE inserts articulated against an alumina ceramic femoral component with those articulated against a cobalt-chrome (Co-Cr) alloy femoral component that were used for short term [16]. The former was the first generation TKP (KOM type, Kyocera Corp.). In the postmortem retrieval analysis, no loosening was observed after 6 years of implantation. The latter TKP (PCA type; Howmedica Corp., Rutherford, NJ, USA) that was retrieved due to late infection after 3 years of implantation also showed no loosening. The UHMWPE insert surfaces in the alumina ceramic TKP were found to have gentle sloping machine marks on non-load-bearing areas, while machine marks on load-bearing areas, i.e., worn areas, completely disappeared after 6 years of implantation (Fig. 4, A). Overall observation revealed that almost all the surfaces were smooth and burnished without scratches or pits. The UHMWPE folding phenomenon that is thought to be caused by third-body wear, which occurs as a result of interposition of UHMWPE wear particles between the components, was also observed at certain sites but to a small extent. It was suspected that a part of the tip of this folded UHMWPE was torn into debris when a force was transmitted onto the tip from the femoral component. In the case of the Co-Cr alloy TKP, burnishing was observed at sites where the machine marks had disappeared, and small scratches were observed at these sites after 3 years of implantation (Fig. 4, B). The folding phenomenon was frequently observed, and the folding area intermingled with scratches at many sites.

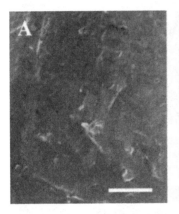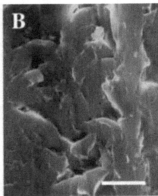

Figure 4:
SEM images of worn areas of retrieved UHMWPE insert surfaces.
A: Alumina ceramic TKP (KOM type), B: Co-Cr alloy TKP (PCA type). Bar; 10 μm.

The *in vivo* surface damage and wear of the UHMWPE inserts are important indicators of the clinical performance of the TKPs. This is because the survivorship rate of the TKPs alone does not completely capture the clinical performance of the UHMWPE insert in a TKP. In this study, we observed the worn surface of retrieved TKPs that were implanted for long term and evaluated their *in vivo* wear. The results of TKPs with Co-Cr alloy/UHMWPE bearing surface were compared with those of TKPs with alumina ceramic/UHMWPE bearing surface in order to examine the efficacy of ceramic bearing surface of TKP.

Materials and Methods

Retrieved TKP

Six retrieved UHMWPE inserts that were being clinically used for 6–23 years were studied. Of these, 3 inserts were articulated against the ceramic femoral components. The remaining inserts were articulated against the Co-Cr femoral component. The clinical data are summarized in Table 1. In the first case, the retrieved Co-Cr TKP (PCA type, Howmedica Corp.; Case 1) was implanted in a female patient in October 1987 and retrieved in July 2004 because of the loosening of the femoral and tibial components with metallosis. In the second case (Case 2), the retrieved TKP (I/B I type; Zimmer Inc., Warsaw, IN, USA) was implanted in a female patient with osteoarthritis of the knee in April 1983 and retrieved in June 2004 because of the loosening of the tibial component. In the third case, the retrieved Co-Cr TKP (I/B I type; Case 3) was implanted in September 1981 and retrieved in September 2004 because of the loosening of the femoral and tibial components. These retrieved Co-Cr TKPs comprised Co-Cr alloy femoral components and UHMWPE inserts that were gamma sterilized in air. In the fourth case, the retrieved alumina ceramic TKP (KU3 type, Kyocera Corp.;

Case 4) was implanted in a female patient with osteoarthritis of the knee in January 1999 and retrieved in March 2005 because of infection at the surgical site. In the fifth case, the retrieved alumina ceramic TKP (N-KOM type, Kyocera Corp.; Case 5) was implanted in a female patient with rheumatoid arthritis (mutilans type) in January 1994 and retrieved in November 2004 because of the loosening of the tibial component. In the last case, the retrieved alumina ceramic TKP (KOM type, Kyocera Corp.; Case 6) [17] was implanted in a female patient with osteoarthritis of the knee in 1979 and retrieved in January 2002 because of painless subsidence of the tibial component due to osteoporosis. This KOM-type implant was used in a clinical trial of the first generation TKPs. These retrieved ceramic TKPs comprised alumina ceramic femoral components and ethylene oxide gas-sterilized UHMWPE inserts.

Case No.	TKP system	Femoral component	Original disease	Reason for revision	Clinical Use (year)	Comments
1	PCA	Co-Cr	RA	Loosening of femoral and tibial-component	16.8	Facture of insert
2	I/B I	Co-Cr	OA	Loosening of tibial-component	21.2	Delamination
3	I/B I	Co-Cr	OA	Loosening of femoral and tibial-component	23.0	–
4	KU 3	Alumina	OA	Infection	6.2	–
5	N-KOM	Alumina	A (mutilance)	Loosening of tibial-component	10.8	–
6	KOM	Alumina	OA	Sinking of tibial-component	23.0	–

Table 1:
Clinical data of the retrieved TKPs.

Methods

The worn surfaces of the retrieved femoral components and UHMWPE inserts were observed under an optical microscope (VHX-200 optical microscope; Keyence Corp., Osaka, Japan) and a scanning electron microscope (SEM) (S-3400N scanning electron microscope; Hitachi Ltd., Tokyo, Japan); the latter was used at an acceleration voltage of 15 kV.

The surface roughness was measured by a surface roughness tester (Surfcom 570A; Tokyo Seimitsu Corp., Tokyo, Japan). Each measurement consisted of 3 parallel traces along the medial-lateral direction at 0.8-mm intervals for the unworn and worn surfaces of the retrieved femoral components. In order to evaluate the surface conditions, the surface features of the bearing surfaces of the retrieved femoral components were observed with a confocal laser scanning microscope (LSM) (OLS1200; Olympus Corp., Tokyo, Japan).

The shapes of the medial and lateral areas of the UHMWPE inserts in the Co-Cr alloy TKPs were determined by a shape tracer (Contourecord 1600, Tokyo Seimitsu Corp.). The linear wear was calculated by comparing the current shapes of the retrieved components with their estimated original shapes; the estimations were derived from the marginal (i.e., unworn) shapes of the inserts because the data of their actual original shapes could not be obtained. On the other hand, the shapes of the UHMWPE inserts in the alumina ceramic TKPs were determined by a three-dimensional coordinate measurement instrument (BHN-305; Mitsutoyo Corp., Kawasaki, Japan). We measured the shapes of 2 articulating areas at 1-mm intervals anteroposteriorly and at 3-mm intervals lateromedially. We calculated the linear wear by comparing the measurement result with the original shape of the insert that was determined from the product's plan.

Results and Discussion

Osteolysis caused by wear debris from UHMWPE inserts is a serious problem with TKP [1,2]. The material used for fabricating the femoral component is an important factor with regard to the wear of the UHMWPE insert in TKPs. To evaluate the *in vivo* wear, we performed a retrieval analysis to compare the different types of TKPs: TKPs having combinations of the UHMWPE insert with the Co-Cr alloy and alumina ceramic femoral components.

Figure 5 shows the optical microscopic images of the surfaces of the Co-Cr alloy femoral component. Low-magnification (10x) optical microscopic observations of the worn areas of both the Co-Cr alloy femoral component condyles (excluding Figure 5, E) revealed frosting, which might be caused by many scratches. Fig. 6 shows the SEM images of typical worn surfaces of the retrieved femoral components and UHMWPE inserts. As shown in Figure 6, A, many scratches parallel to the anterior-posterior direction were clearly observed in these areas. Scratches were also observed on the surface of the UHMWPE insert (Figure 6, B). On the other hand, under SEM, several small pits that measured a few micrometers were observed on the worn areas of the alumina ceramic femoral components and UHMWPE insert surfaces (Figure 6, C). The pits observed in the areas that were not in contact with the UHMWPE insert were believed to have been formed during the manufacturing process. Even high-magnification (350x) observations demonstrated the absence of wear-induced scratches or pits. The surface of the UHMWPE insert was smooth (Figure 6, D). The wear in the UHMWPE insert in the alumina ceramic TKP was not as severe as that observed in the inserts with Co-Cr alloy femoral components in previous and this study [16]. In the retrieved alumina ceramic TKPs, almost all the surfaces were smooth and burnished without any scratches or pits (Figure 6, D). The UHMWPE folding phenomenon that is believed to be caused by third-body wear, which occurs as a result of interposition of UHMWPE wear particles between the components, was also observed in certain areas but to a small extent. It was suspected that a part of the tip of this folded UHMWPE disintegrated to form debris when a force was transmitted onto the tip from the femoral component. In the case of the Co-Cr alloy TKP, burnishing was observed in areas corresponding to the disappeared machine marks; additionally, small scratches were observed (Figure 6, B). The folding phenomenon was frequently observed, and the folded area intermingled with the scratches at many sites.

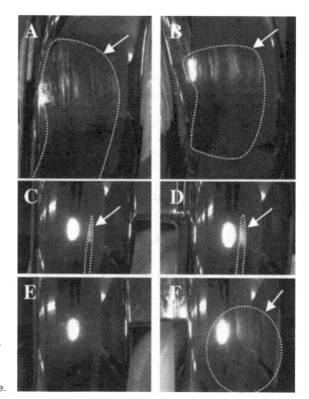

Figure 5:
Optical microscopic images of the surfaces of the Co-Cr alloy femoral component. A: Medial, B: lateral in Case 1, C: medial, D: lateral in Case 2, E: medial and F: lateral in Case 3. Arrows indicate frosting area of surface.

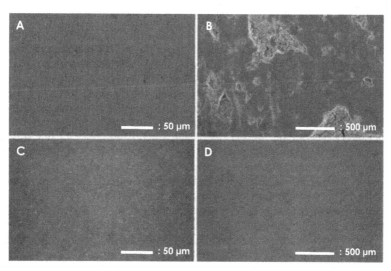

Figure 6:
SEM images of typical worn surface of the retrieved femoral components and UHMWPE inserts. A: Co-Cr alloy (350x), B: UHMWPE (35x) of the retrieved Co-Cr alloy TKP (Case 3), C: alumina ceramic (350x), D: UHMWPE (35x) of the retrieved alumina ceramic TKP (Case 6).

The damage in the form of scratches on the UHMWPE insert surface might be produced due to the rubbing of microscopic asperities against the surface of the femoral component. The Co-Cr alloy femoral component surface (hardness H_v = 285–340), which is not harder than the alumina ceramic femoral component surface (H_v = 1900), is sensitive to third-body wear [11]. Many scratches formed during the clinical use were observed only on the retrieved Co-Cr femoral component. In contrast, the ceramic femoral components substantially maintained their virginal surface qualities, as reported in previous studies [9,17]. The average surface roughness R_a and the maximum surface roughness R_{max} of the unworn and worn surfaces of the retrieved Co-Cr alloy and alumina ceramic femoral components are shown in Table 2. It was found that the R_a and R_{max} of the worn surface of the Co-Cr alloy femoral component were significantly higher than those of the unworn surface. In contrast, the R_a and R_{max} of the worn surface of the alumina ceramic femoral component were not very different from

Case No.	R_a (μm)		R_{max} (μm)	
	Unworn	Worn	Unworn	Worn
1	0.02 (0.00)*	0.03 (0.01)	0.19 (0.02)	0.30 (0.14)
2	0.03 (0.01)	0.05 (0.01)	0.34 (0.20)	0.37 (0.08)
3	0.04 (0.00)	0.04 (0.01)	0.32 (0.03)	0.44 (0.15)
4	0.01 (0.01)	0.01 (0.00)	0.10 (0.03)	0.11 (0.01)
5	0.02 (0.00)	0.02 (0.01)	0.18 (0.02)	0.15 (0.01)
6	0.02 (0.00)	0.02 (0.01)	0.28 (0.11)	0.22 (0.03)

*The standard deviation is in parentheses.

Table 2:
Surface roughness of the unworn and worn surfaces of the retrieved Co-Cr alloy and alumina ceramic femoral components.

those of the unworn surface. Figure 7 shows the A: LSM images, B: 3D images from LSM image, and C: the condition of the Co-Cr alloy and alumina ceramic bearing surfaces of the retrieved TKPs. When third-body wear occurs during the clinical use of a TKP, a hollow may form on the ceramic surface but protrusions may occur on the Co-Cr alloy surface (Figure 7, B, C). (A hollow on the alumina ceramic surface was a grain boundary with a rich glass compound, probably occurred by etching with a body fluid during the clinical use.) Therefore, the ceramic femoral component has a great advantage in terms of the wear of the UHMWPE insert because even under third-body wear conditions, the wear of the insert with the alumina ceramic bearing surface was considerably less than that of the insert with the Co-Cr alloy bearing surface [18,19].

Figure 8 shows the linear wear of the retrieved UHMWPE inserts used in combination with the Co-Cr alloy or alumina ceramic femoral component. The linear wear was calculated as an average of the maximum linear wear in each medial and lateral worn area. In the Co-Cr alloy femoral component, the linear wear values varied for each insert. For example, in Case 1, extreme damage to the medial area of the insert was caused by the penetration of the UHMWPE insert; as a result, the linear wear was greater than 6 mm. Based on these results, the linear wear rate was calculated as 0.027–0.358 mm/year. In contrast, the wear of the alumina ceramic TKPs was stably low and linear; the linear wear rate

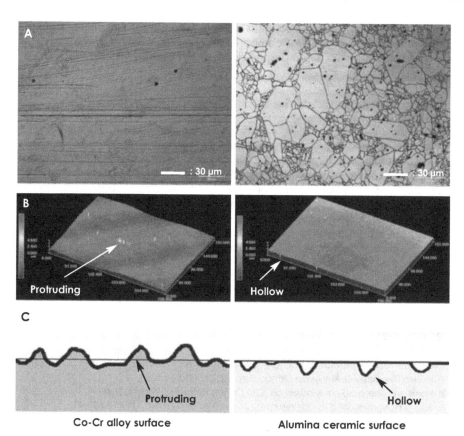

Figure 7:
A: LSM images, B: 3D images from LSM image, and C: the condition of the Co-Cr alloy (Case 3) and alumina ceramic (Case 6) bearing surfaces of the retrieved TKPs with clinical use for 23 years.

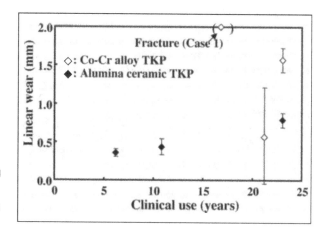

Figure 8:
Linear wear of the retrieved UHMWPE inserts used in the Co-Cr alloy or alumina ceramic TKP. Bar: Standard deviation.

was estimated to be 0.026 mm/year. In addition to surface damage in the form of scratches, the Co-Cr alloy TKP showed a higher wear rate than the alumina ceramic TKP. The lower wear rate and milder nature of wear observed in the latter suggest the possibility of reduced wear of the UHMWPE inserts articulated against the alumina ceramic femoral component. Thus, the alumina ceramic TKP is expected to retain its high performance even when clinically used for a prolonged duration.

Conclusion

Detailed observations of wear of retrieved implants are important to examine the actual clinical performance of artificial joints. In this study, we investigated the surface damage and wear of retrieved Co-Cr alloy and alumina ceramic TKPs that were implanted for long term. The results of TKPs with Co-Cr alloy/UHMWPE bearing surface were compared with those of TKPs with alumina ceramic/UHMWPE bearing surface. The Co-Cr alloy TKPs showed higher wear rate with surface damage due to scratches than the alumina ceramic TKPs. The lower wear rate and milder nature of wear observed in the latter suggest the possibility of reduced wear of the UHMWPE insert articulated against the alumina ceramic femoral component. Thus, the alumina ceramic TKP is expected to retain high performance even during prolonged clinical use.

References

1. Naudie DD, Ammeen DJ, Engh GA, et al. Wear and osteolysis around total kneearthroplasty. J Am Acad Orthop Surg 2007;15(1):53-64.
2. Harris WH. The problem is osteolysis. Clin Orthop Relat Res 1995;(311):46-53.
3. Boutin P. Alumina and its use in surgery of the hip. Presse Med 1971;79:639-40.
4. Boutin P, Christel P, Dorlot JM, et al. The use of dense alumina-alumina ceramic combination in total hip replacement. J Biomed Mater Res 1988;22:1203-32.
5. Shikita T, Oonishi H, Hashimoto Y, et al. Wear resistance of irradiated UHMW polyethylenes to Al_2O_3 ceramics in total hip prostheses. Transactions of the 3rd Annual Meeting of the Society for Biomaterials 3:118, 1977.
6. Oonishi H, Wakitani S, Murata N, et al. Clinical experience with ceramics in total hip replacement. Clin Orthop Relat Res. 2000;(379):77-84.
7. Oonishi H, Hasegawa T. Cementless alumina ceramic total knee prosthesis. Orthopedic Ceramic Implants 1 1981;157-160.
8. Oonishi H, Tsuji E, Mizukoshi T, et al. Wear of polyethylene and alumina in clinical cases of alumina total knee prostheses. Bioceramics 1991;3:137-145.
9. Oonishi H, Fujita H, Itoh S, et al. Surface analysis on retrieved ceramic total knee prosthesis. Key Eng Mater 2002;218-220:499-502.
10. Oonishi H, Fujita H, Itoh S, et al. Development and improvement of ceramic TKP for 19 years and clinical results. Key Eng Mater 2002;218-220:479-482.
11. Nakanishi T, Shikata K, Wang Y, et al. The characteristics of the new material for artificial joints. Key Eng Mater 2006;309-311:1235-1238.
12. Akagi M, Nakamura T, Matsusue Y, et al. The bisurface total knee replacement: a unique design for flexion. J Bone Joint Surg Am 2000;82(11):1626-1633.
13. Akagi M, Ueo T, Takagi H, et al. A mechanical comparison of 2 posterior-stabilizing designs: Insall/Burstein 2 knee and Bisurface knee. J Arthroplasty 2002;17(5):627-634.
14. Akagi M, Kaneda E, Nakamura T, et al. Functional analysis of the effect of the posterior stabilising cam in two total knee replacements. A comparison of the Insall/Burstein and Bisurface prostheses. J Bone Joint Surg Br 2002;84(4):561-565.

15. Oonishi H, Kim SC, Ueno M. PE wear in ceramic/PE bearing surface in TKA: 24 year clinical experience. Presented at the 17th Annual Symposium of the International Society for Technology in Arthroplasty, Rome, Italy, September 2004.

16. Oonishi H, Kim SC, Kyomoto M, et al. PE wear in ceramic/PE bearing surface in total knee arthroplasty: Clinical experiences of more than 24 years. In: Benazzo F, Falez F and Dietrich M, editors. Bioceramics and Alternative Bearings in Joint Arthroplasty, 2006.

17. Oonishi H, Kim SC, Kyomoto M, et al. Change in UHMWPE Properties of Retrieved Ceramic Total Knee Prosthesis in Clinical Use for 23 Years. J Biomed Mater Res Appl Biomater 2005;74B:754-759.

18. Minakawa H, Stone MH, Wroblewski BM, et al. Quantification of third-body damage and its effect on UHMWPE wear with different types of femoral head. J Bone Joint Surg Br 80(5):894-899, 1998.

19. Davidson JA, Poggie RA, Mishra AK. Abrasive wear of ceramic, metal, and UHMWPE bearing surfaces from third-body bone, PMMA bone cement, and titanium debris. Biomed Mater Eng 1994;4(3):213-29.

SESSION 5A

Hard on Hard Bearings

5A.1 Toughening vs. Environmental Aging in BIOLOX® *delta*: A micromechanics study

G. Pezzotti

Abstract

A BIOLOX® *delta* femoral head has been evaluated with respect to its surface micromechanical behavior and its environmental aging response upon increasing elongation time in a hot water vapor environment. A microscopic evaluation of surface phenomena was obtained according to confocal Raman microprobe spectroscopy. The confocal configuration of the optical probe allowed spectroscopic assessments in the very neighborhood of the material surface. After extreme exposure time in moist environment, a portion of zirconia dispersoids transformed from the tetragonal to the monoclinic polymorph on the surface of the sample. A pyramidal diamond indentation technique was applied in order to analyze crack initiation. A significant influence of the transformation to the crack tip opening was observed. However, it should be noted that such an effect is likely to occur only after extremely long exposure in hot vapor environment.

Introduction

Recent trends in biomedical materials research have been aimed to prolong the lifetime of hip prostheses to much greater than ten years, through the development of advanced composite materials such as alumina-zirconia composites [1-3]. These materials have been found to possess superior mechanical properties in addition to full biocompatibility. Proof tests using joint simulators, as well as wear and mechanical testing have been used to investigate the long-term mechanical reliability and biocompatibility of hip prostheses built with advanced biomaterials [4-7].

Among advanced bioceramics, BIOLOX® *delta*, a zirconia-reinforced alumina-matrix composite, has played a pioneering role in the field and is a primary candidate for expanding the medical use of ceramic-on-ceramic joint implants, opening the possibility to long-term wear resistance and superior lifetimes for artificial hip joints. One main characteristic of this material is its high toughness, as compared to monolithic ceramics. The main source of toughening is likely related to the presence in the ceramic microstructure of ≈ 18.0 vol. % zirconia dispersoids, which may eventually undergo a tetragonal-to-monoclinic phase transformation (simply referred to as t → m transformation, henceforth). The toughening behavior of BIOLOX® *delta* is, as we shall show in the remainder of this paper, quite complex and may require further studies for its actual performance. The general notion in transformation toughening is that, in the case of crack initiation and successive propagation in the presence of a transforming zirconia phase, a local (equilibrium) compressive stress field may develop in a characteristic process zone surrounding the crack tip. Such a stress field overlaps the tensile crack-tip stress field and partly impedes crack propagation (i.e., leading to the observed toughening effect). However, this process may also affect the environmental aging behavior of the material surface in biological environment, eventually changing the surface properties.

In this paper, we describe a micromechanical evaluation of the toughening behavior of BIOLOX® delta as received from the manufacturer and after long-term exposure under hot vapor pressure. The impact of phase transformation on the material toughness is quantitatively assessed and evidence provided of the effect of a residual stress field, stored in the tetragonal phase, on the kinetic of t → m phase transformation.

Material and Methods

A commercially available ceramic femoral head (BIOLOX® delta, manu-factured by CeramTec) was tested, which consisted of Al_2O_3 (80.5 vol.%), ZrO_2 (18.0 vol.%) and mixed oxides (1.5 vol. % CrO_2, Y_2O_3 and SrO). The femoral head was kept for increasing times (i.e., ranging between 0 and 300 h) into an autoclave operating at 121° C under a vapor pressure of 1 bar (accelerating test) in order to simulate the effect of environmental aging in human body. After exposure to moist environment, the surface of the femoral head was scanned with a Raman spectroscope (triple monochromator; T-64000, ISA Jovin-Ivon/Horiba Group, Tokyo, Japan) equipped with a charge-coupled detector (high-resolution CCD camera). Raman experiments were performed in a confocal configuration with the laser light from the probe-head focused to a microscopic spot on the sample surface by an optical microscope objective. According to confocal probe calibrations, a pinhole aperture of 100 μm enabled us to obtain an optical (lateral) resolution of about 1 μm and probe sub-surface depth ≈ 6 ?m for both tetragonal and monoclinic zirconia polymorphs. A slightly larger penetration depth (≈ 8 μm) was recorded for the same confocal configuration for the Cr^{3+} fluorescence bands of alumina.

Indentation prints with a pyramidal indenter have been introduced in the material surface before and after exposure to moist environment. Indentation cracks, which propagated from the corners of the indent, were observed by a field-emission-gun scanning electron microscope (FEG-SEM; JSM-6500F, JEOL, Ltd., Tokyo, Japan) and quantitatively analyzed with respect to their crack opening displacement (COD) and crack-tip stress field.

Results and Discussion

Figure 1 shows the dependence of the average monoclinic fraction in the composite, V_m, as a function of aging time in climate test chamber. It has been shown in previous studies [8,9] that a partly transformed zirconia structure can be clearly patterned from the concurrent presence in the Raman spectrum of distinct bands belonging either to the monoclinic or to the tetragonal polymorph. Monoclinic fraction can be calculated according to the relative intensity of selected monoclinic and tetragonal bands [10]. Besides an initial fraction of monoclinic polymorph was already present in the as received femoral head (i.e., about 17 vol. % of the initial 18 vol. % zirconia content, namely ≈ 3 % of the cumulative material volume), the monoclinic volume fraction was observed to

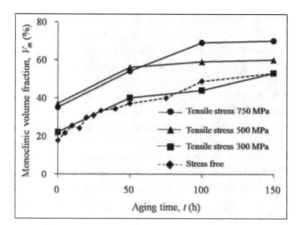

Figure 1:
Plots of monoclinic volume fractions as a function of aging time under different stress conditions (stress here refers to the residual stress stored in the tetragonal phase). The fractions refer to fractions of the zirconia content in the composite.

increase upon increasing aging time in a climate test chamber operating under a vapor pressure of 1 bar at 121° C. The monoclinic content increased with relatively high rate at the initial stage of aging (e.g., the initial 30 h), while a tendency to saturation was observed after relatively long elapsing times. After saturation, the amount of t → m transformation driven by environmentally assisted processes was ≈ 75 vol. % of the initial 18 vol. % zirconia content, namely ≈ 14 % of the cumulative material volume.

It should be noted that analysis of t → m transformation via surface sensitive Raman spectroscopy in general leads to a higher apparent monoclinic content than the depth sensitive conventional X-ray diffraction. The reason is that phase transformation starts from the surface and the monoclinic content decreases with depth within a few microns.

The impact of environmentally driven phase transformation on the material (surface) toughness was evaluated by recording COD profiles from indentation cracks introduced in the material surface either before or after environmental aging test. It has been shown [11] that indentation cracks can be considered as equilibrium cracks, which are thus stably arrested at their threshold stress intensity value for propagation, K_{IC}. Such a toughness value, which refers to quite short cracks and thus involves a minimum contribution from rising R-curve, can be retrieved from the slope of a plot of COD vs. the parameter $8b^{1/2} F(a, x)/\pi E'$. Where E' is the plane strain elastic modulus, and x, a, and b are an abscissa along the crack path (behind the crack tip and with origin at the tip), the distance between the crack tip and the geometrical center of the indentation print, and the half diagonal of the indentation print, respectively. The function $F(a, x)$ represents a weight function given by Fett [12]. Figure 2 shows FEG-SEM images of the indentation crack path in a zone of high COD values (A) and in the neighborhood of the crack tip (B). In both cases, observation is made in the as received material. In Figure 3, two COD plots are shown for typical indentation cracks introduced on the surface of the composite in the as received state and after 300 h aging in moist atmosphere.

From the slopes of the plots, an apparent reduction in surface toughness of the material surface is noticed after the extreme 300 h ageing in autoclave. The amount of monoclinic polymorph was mapped with the Raman microprobe in the neighborhood of the two cracks whose COD are shown in Figure 3. These Raman maps are shown in (Figure 4 A, B) for the as received material and for the

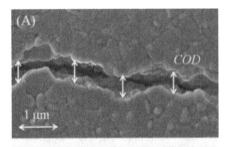

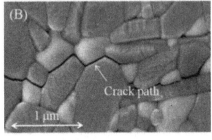

Figure 2:
A) FEG-SEM image of crack path in the an as received material (after thermal etching) taken in an area of relatively large COD; B) crack path in the neighborhood of the crack tip in the as received material.

material exposed for 300 h in autoclave. From a comparison between the above two figures, it can be seen that a clear transformation zone is observed in the as received sample, while in the aged sample the crack runs in a fully transformed area. By considering the surface toughness data in Figure 3, it can be concluded that a significant toughening effect from the formation of a process zone (constrained and subject to compression by the surrounding non-transformed volume of material) can be available only when transformation occurs concurrently to crack propagation.

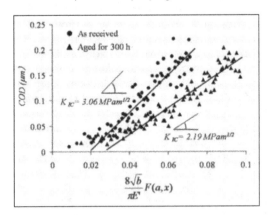

Figure 3:
Plots of COD for the as received and 300 h autoclaved material. The slopes of the plots correspond to the surface material toughness.

However, as these effects are only present after the ageing very close to the surface, it is evident that the macroscopic bulk fracture toughness of the material is not significantly affected by the ageing as it was shown using standard evaluation of fracture toughness.

In order to examine the effect of a surface impingement on the kinetic of phase transformation, we printed a Vickers indentation on the surface of the as received BIOLOX® *delta* material. Then, aging in autoclave was performed

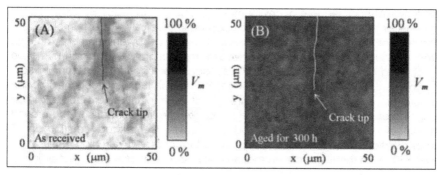

Figure 4 A, B:
Maps of monoclinic volume fraction obtained in the neighborhood of the tip of indentation cracks propagated in the as received sample (A) and in a sample (B) aged 300 h in moist atmosphere.

according to the same schedule as shown above. The results of this experiment are shown in (Figure 5 A, B and C) for the as received material, and after auto-clave exposures of 50 h and 150 h, respectively. As a general trend, it was observed that zones nearby the indent aged faster than the virgin material. It is known [13] that in areas immediately outside the indentation print a tensile stress field is developed. Here, we monitored the kinetic of phase transformation in such tensile stressed zones and obtained for them plots of monoclinic fraction as a function of tensile stress in the tetragonal phase. The stress magnitude was measured from a selected tetragonal band of the zirconia Raman spectrum, as described elsewhere [14,15]. Such plots are shown in Figure 1 for different stress magnitudes. It is known that a tensile stress field in the tetragonal phase provides a driving force for the formation of monoclinic polymorph. In the present composite material, we found no significant alteration of phase transformation kinetic for tensile stresses up to a magnitude of about 300 MPa, while higher tensile stresses significantly accelerated transformation.

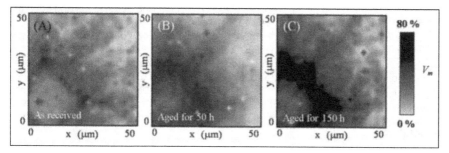

Figure 5 A-C:
Map of monoclinic volume fraction around an edge of indentation print in the as received sample (A), in a sample (B) aged 50 h, and in a sample (C) aged 150 h.

Conclusion

In this study, we have applied combined techniques of micromechanics and confocal Raman microspectroscopy to the characterization of the surface of a BIOLOX® *delta* femoral head. We showed that t → m phase transformation occurs in the femoral head because of environmentally assisted processes. However, it is fair to consider that the testing procedure adopted in this study was extremely severe and not comparable to relevant conditions in human body environment. The high crack-tip toughness level in the as received material, enhanced by a transformation toughening effect, was reduced at the surface after long-term exposure in moist environment. Such a surface effect does not impair the bulk toughness of the femoral head and, thus, the overall strength of the implants. Microscopic Raman mapping at crack paths enabled one to visualize the transformation zone around the tip of an equilibrium crack and to visualize the related contribution of transformation to toughening. We also found that only at a very high tensile stress level > 300 MPa the t → m transformation is significantly accelerated. According to current understanding such extreme conditions can not emerge in-vivo even under worst-case assumptions like third body wear or impingement.

References

1. S. Deville, J. Chevalier, C. H. Dauvergne, G. Fantozzi, J. F. Bartolome, J. S. Moya, and R. Torrecillas, "Microstructural investigation of the aging behavior of (3Y-TZP)-Al $_2$O$_3$ composites," J. Am. Ceram. Soc., 88, 1273-1280 (2005).
2. G. Gregori, W. Burger, and V. Sergo, "Piezo-spectroscopic analysis of the residual stresses in zirconia-toughened alumina ceramics: the influence of the tetragonal-to- monoclinic transformation," Mater. Sci. Eng., 271, 401-406 (1999).
3. P. Merkert, "Next generation ceramic bearings", In: 8th BIOLOX® Symposium, 123-125(2003).
4. T. D. Stewart, J. L. Tipper, G. Insley, R. M. Streicher, E. Ingham, and J. Fisher, "Long-term wear of ceramic matrix composite materials for hip prostheses under severe swing phase microseparation," J. Biomed. Mater. Res. Part B, 66-B, 567-573 (2003).
5. J. L. Masonis, R. B. Bourne, M. D. Ries, R. W. McCalden, A. Salehi, and D. C. Kelman, "Zirconia femoral head fracture," J. Arthroplasty, 19, 898-905 (2004).
6. G. Maccauro, C. Piconi, W. Burger, L. Pilloni, E. De Santis, and I. D. Learmonth, "Fracture of a Y-TZP ceramic femoral head," J. Bone Joint Surg. Br., 86-B, 1192-1196 (2004).
7. J. E. Nevelos, E. Ingham, C. Doyle, A. B. Nevelos, and J. Fisher, "The influence of acetabular cup angle on the wear of "BIOLOX Forte" alumina ceramic bearing couples in a hip joint simulator," J. Mater. Sci., 13, 141-144 (2001).
8. G. Pezzotti, and A. A. Porporati, "Raman spectroscopic analysis of phase transformation and stress patterns in zirconia hip joints," J. Biomed. Optics, 9, 372-384 (2004).
9. G. Pezzotti, "Stress microscopy and confocal Raman imaging of load-bearing surface in artificial hip joints," Expert Rev. Med. Devices, 4, 165-189 (2007).
10. G. Katagiri, H. Ishida, A. Ishitani and T. Masaki, "Direct Determination by a Raman Microprobe of the Transformation Zone Size in Y$_2$O$_3$ Containing Tetragonal ZrO$_2$ Polycrystals," Advances in Ceramics, Vol. 24: Science and Technology of Zirconia III, 537-544 (1988).
11. J. Seidel and J. Rödel, "Measurement of Crack Tip Toughness in Alumina as a function of Grain size," J. Am. Ceram. Soc., 80, 433-438 (1997).
12. T. Fett, "Computation of the Crack Opening Displacements for Vickers Indentation Cracks," Rept. No. FZKA 6757, Forschungszentrum Karlsruhe, Karlsruhe, Germany, (2002).
13. E. H. Yoffe, "Elastic Stress Fields Caused by Indenting Brittle Materials," Philos. Mag. A., 46, 617-628 (1982).
14. V. Sergo and D. M. Clarke, "Deformation bands in Ceria-Stabilized Tetragonal Zirconia/ Alumina: II, Stress-Induced Aging at Room Temperature," J. Am. Ceram. Soc., 78, 641-44 (1995).
15. G. Pezzotti, "Raman piezo-spectroscopic analysis of natural and synthetic biomaterials," Anal. Bioanal. Chem., 381, 577-590 (2005).

5A.2 Clinical Experience with Ceramic on Ceramic in the USA

J. P. Garino

Abstract

Ceramic on Ceramic total hip arthroplasty (THR)has had a very long history as a low wear bearing material. With initial problems related to primarily fixation. That problem seemed to be solved with the advent of reliable cementless components, and the uncoupling of bearing and fixation functions. In the United States, 11 years have now passed since the first Food and Drug Administration (FDA) approved studies began, and four years have elapsed since the FDA approved the first Ceramic-Ceramic hip replacements for general use. Although the results of these multiple studies have continued to demonstrate the superior wear bearings of ceramics, the advent of highly cross-linked polyethylene, the relative lack of liner and ball head options, the occasional fracture, and now the report of an occasional squeaking hip have impeded more robust acceptance of these advanced bearing devices.

Introduction

The use of Ceramic-Ceramic THR began in 1970 at a time when Alumina ceramics were recognized as an ideal bearing surface [1]. Success of the Charnley THR with a polyethylene bearing coupled with fixation issues for the ceramic-ceramic THR devices of the 1970's and 1980's prevented these hip replacements from higher levels of popularity. However, the limitations of the polyethylene bearings became more appreciated in the 1990's, and the search for a better bearing material brought manufacturers and surgeons back to a now 3rd generation of medical grade ceramics. The new strategy of applying these materials was to separate the fixation and bearing aspects of THR. Thus the use of successful stems with a standardized taper, as well as a cementless hemispherical shell with porous coating and a modified interior taper design were developed to take advantage of this low wear material. This was critical as the indications for hip replacements were rapidly expanding into the younger and younger age groups. With the initial success of these hips in Europe, several manufactures embarked on Investigational Device Exemptions (IDE), which were FDA approved scientific studies designed to collect clinical data with the prospect of receiving full FDA approval for sale. After additional unexpected delays due to increased validation requirements by the FDA of ceramic manufacturers, Stryker Orthopedics and Wright Medical Technology were given approval to begin generalized sales of ceramic-ceramic THR in the Winter of 2003.

Data From IDE's

Murphy reported the results of the Wright Medical Technology IDE in 2006 [2]. 709 THR's were performed in 1484 patients. All were ceramic on ceramic using historical controls. These patients included all of the continued access patients in addition to the original 350 patients which were the core group followed by the FDA. The 8-year survival rate for any implant related complication was 97%, while that of the acetabular component was 99.9. There were 4 fractures of ceramic bearings, but these failures compare favorably with polyethylene bearings where the revision rate can be up to 5/1000 hips [3]. With a reoperation of only two hips for instability, Murphy makes the point clear that the relative lack of lipped liners and smaller selection of ball head lengths, that these devices are a safe alternative for the young patient.

D'Antonio has published the IDE data from the Stryker series on a number of occasions [4]. In this particular series, known as the ABC series, two groups of devices were utilized. In the first series, 514 hips were enrolled in a randomized prospective series where 1/3 of the patients received a metal-poly bearing and 2/3 received a ceramic-ceramic bearing. The same femoral component, Omnitfit, was used in all patients. Upon the conclusion of the close of this IDE about 2 years after it had begun, a fourth arm of the study utilizing the newly designed trident cup was opened to several of the investigators. At a minimum of 6 years for the ABC system 284 hips demonstrated no difference in function and patient satisfaction between the ceramic and standard bearing devices. However, there were significantly more revisions in the polyethylene controls (7.5% versus 2.3%). There was significantly more radiolucencies and osteolysis in the poly group as well. There were no reported fractures.

More recent presentations of ceramic- bearings at the 2007 AAOS included an update of the D'antonio data above. In this presentation, the prospective series of 1382 patients had no ceramic fractures. In addition only 4 fractures were reported following the implantation of some 50,000 total hips with ceramic on ceramic bearings. There were no head fractures [5].

Conclusions

Ceramic-Ceramic THR continue to function well in the United States as a low-wear couple for active patients. Because of the lack of approval of stronger and harder 4th generation ceramic materials that would allow for larger ball heads to be used in smaller cups and which would further reduce fractures, the ceramic-ceramic THR has lost some of its appeal. Orthopedic companies do not face the same regulatory hurdles with metal on metal or cross-linked polyethylene, and these alternatives are being pushed a bit harder. But these alternatives have their problems as well including poly fractures and metal allergy. Nonetheless, in spite of the excellent clinical data gathered at an intermediate time frame, the relative lack of flexibility and fear of fracture (and the subsequent legal issues) have stunted the growth of ceramic bearings in the US. When one considers the risk of revision of a THR over the life of a young patient, the use of Ceramic-ceramic bearings are the wear couple that will most likely produce the lowest revision risk of any couple currently available. The already very low fracture rate will be further reduced with the generalized availability of 4th generation ceramics.

References

1. Sedel, L.; Nizard, R.; Bizot, P.; and Meunier, A.: Perspective on a 20-year experience with ceramic-on-ceramic articulation in total hip replacement. Semin Arthroplasty, 9(2): 123-134, 1998.
2. Murphy; SB; Ecker, T; Tannast,M; Bierbaum,B; Garino,J; Howe, J; Hume, E; Jones, R; Keggi, K; Kress, K; Phillips, D; Zann, R: Experience in the United States with Alumina Ceramic-Ceramic Total Hip Arthroplasty. Semin Arthroplasty, 17:120-4, 2006.
3. Heck, DA; Partridge, CM; Rueben, JD, et al: Prosthetic component failures in THR. J Arthroplasty: 10:575-580, 1995.
4. D'antonio, J; Capello, W; Beirbaum, B: Manley, M; Naughton, MB: Ceramic-Ceramic bearings for total hip Arthroplasty: 5-9 year follow-up. Semin Arthroplasty, 17: 146-52, 2006.
5. D'Antonio, J: Ceramic Fractures: Past and Present. Open meeting of the Hip Society, San Diego, February 17, 2007.

5A.3 Why use an all Ceramic Tripolar THR ?
– clinical and experimental data

J.-Y. Lazennec, H. Sari Ali, M. Gorin, B. Roger, A. Baudoin and A. Rangel

A tripolar all ceramic joint is an emerging technology that reduces the risk of dislocation and subluxation in T.H.R. Muscular insufficiency, caricatural lower limbs discrepancies or neurological problems are classical causes for T.H.P. dislocations or subluxations [10,11]. Instability may also be linked to 2 specific mechanisms, lever-out (with impingement) and shear-out (without impingement).

Microseparation and edge loading of femoral ball head on the insert are relevant issues for hard on hard bearing surfaces, either ceramic on ceramic or metal on metal [9,4]. The aim of the system is the reduction of lever-arm dislocation rate occurring during impingement and the optimisation of the "head-insert" relocation phenomenons during T.H.P. function. Based on long-term experience with "classical" PE double mobility systems, the all tripolar ceramic THP offers new solutions without any change regarding the components implantation on the acetabular and femoral sites and the standard THP adjustment. The concept is only an optimization of the joint function for macro and microstability in substitution to classical alumina femoral head. Using two bearing ceramic delta surfaces, the additional intermediate component (bipolar head) acts as a self "adjusting cup", dealing with the variations of pelvic orientation and acetabulum anteversion [8] and the side effects of femoro-tibial rotational variations (Fig. 1).

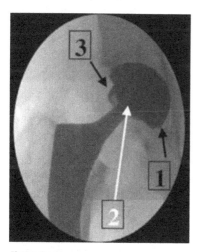 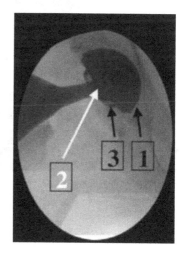

Figure 1:
1 : Standard titanium metal back with ceramic insert
2 : Standard delta ceramic femoral head
3 : Delta ceramic intermediate self-adjusting component

More than 1000 implantations are available to verify the results of the preclinical research studies regarding the adaptation of the intermediate component according to pelvic position and lower limb function.

Preclinical studies

Biomechanical test

The orientation of the cup in terms of anteversion and inclination appreciably influences the range of motion of the joint and its dislocation resistance [8].

The use of the 3D▲ tripolar joint seems an interesting alternative for difficult or unexpected situations of cup adjustment and cases of hip instability.

The position of the rotation center in the cup-ball head system influences joint stability. It has been shown that a few millimetres inset of the rotation centre significantly increases the peak resisting moment against dislocation [6]. This benefit in terms of stability has a significant disadvantage due to the decrease of range of motion (ROM) with classical ball-insert systems.

The 3D▲ tripolar joint allows the location of the centre of rotation much deeper inside the insert without significant negative impact on the ROM [1].

A comparison of the mechanism of dislocation between a standard system (32mm ball head/ceramic insert) and the 3D▲ System (two ceramic on ceramic bearing surfaces with a 32mm self adjusting cup) has been made for impingement situations. The dislocation stability parameter was the torque during subluxation (resisting moment) against levering the head out of the cup [3].

With the Standard system the dislocation appears if there is contact between the neck and the insert because of the moment applied. This dislocation by impingement is in direct relation with the range of motion (Fig. 2).

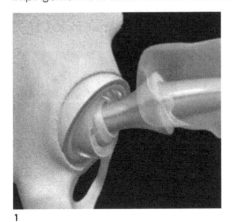

1

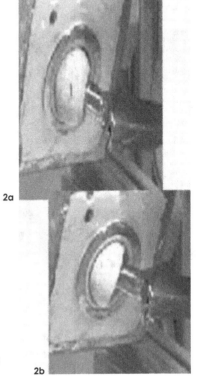

2a

2b

Figure 2:
Sitting position, right hip, postero lateral view
1: classical 32 mm ceramic head.
2a, b: tripolar all alumina delta joint.
For the same sitting position with equivalent internal rotation and hip flexion, the remaining coverage of the tripolar is higher, due to the adaptation of the intermediate component and the inset of the rotation centers.

With the 3D▲ system the mechanism is different and shows different steps:
   During a first step, a rotation of the ball head alone is observed. In a second step the rotation of the bipolar head occurs in the opposite direction because of contact forces. Finally, rotation of the ball head and the bipolar head will appear together [2]. The relative motion of the intermediate component is closely related to the eccentricity between the intermediate component and the femoral head centres.

b Tribological tests

   Micro-separation is more appropriate for the evaluation of ceramic bearings, as clinical wear rates, wear mechanism and wear debris are reproduced.
The aim of tribological tests was to assess the wear characteristics under standard and swing phase micro-separation between 200 and 500 µm for a total of 5 million cycles using the Leeds II Physiological Anatomical hip joint simulator [8].
   In a previous study conventional Biolox Delta components were tested under microseparation conditions in the same simulator with reported wear rates of 0.32 mm^3/million cycles during bedding-in (0-1 million cycles), reducing to a steady state wear rate of 0.12 mm^3/million cycles (1-5 million cycles) [8].
   Furthermore, a stripe of wear appeared on the standard Biolox Delta heads, which increased the surface roughness Ra from <0.005 µm to between 0.02 µm and 0.13 µm.

In the testing of the tripolar joint, there was no visual macroscopic evidence of wear.
   The wear was less than 0.01 mm^3/ million cycles, the detection limit for wear measurement. The 3D▲ tripolar joint showed reduced frictional torque due to articulation at the smaller diameter 22 mm inner femoral head.
   No stripe wear was observed; the surface roughness of the ball heads and the outer and inner surfaces of the bipolar head were smoother at the end of the test indicating that they had undergone a polishing effect.
   There was no change in the surface roughness of the inserts. There was no statistical significant difference in the post-test surface measurements between the standard and micro-separation test conditions for any of the components.
The design of the 3D▲ tripolar joint with the mobile ceramic head prevented edge loading of the head on the edge of the cup, so significantly reduced wear under these severe, but clinically relevant microseperation conditions [5].

Regarding the PE ring, dislocation tests have been performed to evaluate its resistance to secure the ball head inside of the intermediate component. Results are comparable to similar PE rings that have been used for more than 18 years for classical double-mobility hip joint. The wear volume of the PE rings could not be accurately quantified as it was within the systematic error of the soak control ring. The backside of the PE rings showed no damage, with only a light polishing effect being observed in places [6].

Clinical data

   Precise information regarding early clinical results have been obtained from 482 cases prospectively evaluated. No specific learning curve was necessary: the surgeons did not change their implantation procedures for metal back and acetabular insert placements nor for femoral adjustment. The only originality of the system is the interposition of a "double femoral ball head" on the femoral taper. The 22 mm head positioning on the taper is easy as the intermediate cup is secured in a second step using the PE ring [7].

The indications have been focused on risky cases for instability, stiff coxarthrosis, osteonecrosis, revisions, oblique pelvis or significant rotational troubles, neurological troubles and some difficult patients (alcoholic and psychiatric).

Clinical evolution has been comparable to that of standard THP regarding Harris hip score. No dislocation and no fracture have been observed in this series. We experienced a pelvic fracture in a psychiatric patient who intended to self dislocate his tripolar THP during a maniac crisis; the double mobility joint worked and resisted dislocation until an anterior pelvic fracture occurred.

In a few cases, the patients described some loud noise coming from the hip area, analogous to what has been described for classical PE double mobility systems; this noise has been related to the sudden relocation of the intermediate component according to the experience with the double mobility PE joints. This phenomenon disappeared with time without any complications; it has been suggested that the progressive stiffening of the soft tissues and the muscles could be an explanation. Those transitory noisy hips have been observed in suboptimal adjustment of the implants and shortening with excessive pistonning and lack of offset .The phenomenon is completely different from squeaking regarding the sound characteristics and the mechanical aspects.

A specific radiological protocol allows to observe the adaptation of the intermediate component in standing, and sitting positions.

The mobility of the intermediate component is coherent with the previous modelisation studies and with the experimental data. No intermediate component verticalisation has been observed. An increased horizontalisation of the intermediate component has been observed in some cases as an adaptation to excessive frontal inclination of the metal back-insert component. In 11% of the cases, the exact position of the intermediate component could not be analyzed due to the superposition of the metal back. In the other cases the intermediate component is still working after 2 years; the mechanical behaviour remains the same as defined during the experimental studies (Fig. 3).

In some patients with significant anomalies of the lower limb rotational anatomy, the tripolar system has been a "salvage procedure" to solve complex instability situations (Fig. 4a, b).

Nevertheless, the 3D▲ joint cannot compensate suboptimal THP implantations such as excessive shear-out laxity due to shortening of the head-neck length or lack of femoral offset [10,11].

Conclusions

The ceramic tripolar joint is a new solution against THR instability and microseparation consequences such as stripe wear. Functional and radiological results confirm the preclinical studies.

2 year follow-up clinical results are available to assess the decrease of dislocation rates with the all ceramic tripolar system.

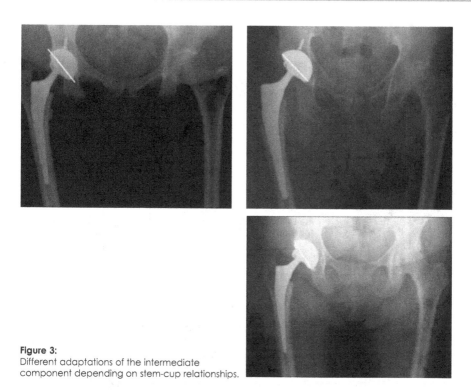

Figure 3:
Different adaptations of the intermediate
component depending on stem-cup relationships.

**Upper view of lower limbs
using the EOS® reconstruction
system (pre-op).**

Figure 4a:
Recurrent anterior subluxation after a cemented monobloc THP (posterior approach).
Tridimensional analysis using the EOS® radiographic system. The lenght of the right limb is increased
after the THP. No excessive acetabular or femoral anteversion. The adaptation has been hip flexion
in standing position, internal rotation of the whole right lower limb inducing a false knee valgus and
patella subluxation. Note the rotational position of the pelvis (right anterior iliac position).

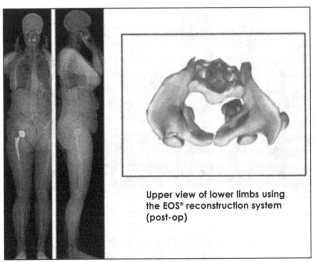

**Upper view of lower limbs using
the EOS® reconstruction system
(post-op)**

Figure 4b:
The solution has been revision of the monobloc femoral stem for shortening of the femur. To solve the instability problem and to optimize the adjustment facing the rotationnal problems, a tripolar hip joint has been used. The acetabular cup has been exchanged for a cementless component, without any modification of the implantation adjustment.
The «false» valgus knee has disappeared and the rotation problem of the pelvis has been solved as well as the patellar syndrom.

References

1. Bader R ,Datzman Th , Steihauser E ,Mittelmeier W , Lazennec J-Y. Biomechanical study of resistance to dislocation of the ceramic - ceramic delta tripolar joint Biomaterialen 2004.
2. Chen Q., Lazennec J. Y., Guyen O., Kinbrum A, Berry D. J., An K. N. Validation of a Motion Analysis System for Measuring the Relative Motion of the Intermediate Component of a Tripolar Total Hip Arthroplasty Prosthesis Med Eng Phys. 2005 Jul;27(6):505-12.
3. Chen Q, Lazennec JY, Prabhakar PP, Berry DJ, An KN. Motion of the intermediate component of an eccentric tripolar T.H.P. Annual Meeting of the Orthopaedic Research Society 2005 poster 1181.
4. Ishida, T; Clarke, IC; Shirasu,, H; Shishido, T; Yamamoto, K; Lazennec, J-Y. Detailed wear mapping of retrieved second-generation metal on metal THR Annual Meeting of the Orthopaedic Research Society 2007 Poster No: 1656.
5. Jennings, L M; Fisher, J; Stewart, T D; Masson, B; Lazennec J-Y. Wear and friction characteristics of the tripolat all ceramic hip prosthesis Annual Meeting of the Orthopaedic Research Society 2006 poster 498.
6. Lazennec J.-Y., Jennings L. M., Fisher J. Masson B. Two Ceramic Bearing Surfaces with a Self Adjusting cup: A New Application of Delta Ceramics to reduce the Risk of Dislocation and Subluxation Bioceramics and alternative bearings in joint arthroplasty Springer Ed 2005.
7. Lazennec JY, Sari Ali E, Rousseau MA, Hansen S. All ceramic tripolar Total Hip Arthroplasty: experimental data and clinical results Bioceramics and alternative bearings in joint arthroplasty 11th BIOLOX Symposium Bioceramics in Joint Arthroplasty, Springer Ed 2006.
8. Lazennec JY, Riwan A,. Gravez F, Rousseau MA., Mora N, Gorin M,. Lasne A, Catonne Y, Saillant G. Hip spine relationships: application to total hip arthrosplasty Hip International/ Vol. 17 , 2 (suppl 5) 2007 pp S91-S104.
9. Stewart T. D., Tipper J. L., Insley G., Streicher R. M., Ingham E., Fisher J., Long-Term Wear of Ceramic Matrix Composite Materials for Hip Prostheses Under Severe Swing Phase Microseparation". JBMR 66B (2003); 562-573.
10. Toni A., Sudanese A., Ceramic on ceramic: long term clinical experience Bioceramics in joint arthroplasty Thieme Ed 2001.
11. Von Knoch M., Berry D. J., Harmsen W. S., Morrey B. F., Late dislocation after total hip arthroplasty. Journal of Bone & Joint Surgery - American Volume. 84-A(11):1949-53, 2002.

5A.4 Lessons from 1st generation Ceramic on Ceramic THA

Y.-J. Cho

Abstract

The alumina head on alumina cup combination was first implanted by Boutin in 1970 with Mittelmeier following with Autophor design in 1972. Such ceramic on ceramic bearing articulation have been used over 30 years and is being used more widely now. The clinical performance of these first generation alumina on alumina THA revealed very variable results between excellent to very poor. The unfavorable results of 1st generation alumina on alumina THA is not due to wear and wear related problems like as in metal–polyethylene THA but mainly due to mechanical failure. This high rate of mechanical failure was due to poor implant design and surgical technique, and most of ceramic articulation performed well and did not contribute to the unsatisfactory results. Some survived 1st generation ceramic THA without loosening shows excellent results without osteolysis. The reported wear rate of ceramic on ceramic combination is very low and is about one fortieth to eighties of wear rate of conventional metal-polyethylene. But some retrieved ceramic heads and sockets shows severe wear comparable to the conventional metal-polyethylene combination. These unexpectedly excessive wear is usually shown in the joints with high inclination of ceramic cup. Osteolysis which is the most common serious problems of metal-polyethylene articulation is extremely rare or minimal in ceramic on ceramic articulation. Even though early clinical use of 1st generation ceramic on ceramic combination was disappointing because of component loosening and fracture, previous data of 1st generation alumina ceramic bearings demonstrates much more wear resistance. These clinical proofs can give us belief that modern alumina ceramics which have a much lower porosity, lower grain size, and higher purity can provide more safe and durable joints.

5A.5 Nine-Year Experience with a Contemporary Alumina-on-alumina THA Implant

H.-J. Kim and J.-J. Yoo

Introduction

There are three options to solve the problems associated with the conventional polyethylene, the wear and subsequent osteolysis. These included ceramic-on-ceramic bearing, metal-on-metal bearing and cross-linked polyethylene. We chose ceramic-on-ceramic bearing based on our experience with the old generation alumina-on-alumina articulation.

We also experienced poor clinical results with the old generation alumina implant. However, the main cause of the poor clinical results was the fixation failure. Long-term survived cases showed no measurable wear, and radiolucency around the implants was usually linear, not cavitary (Fig. 1). We expected good results with contemporary alumina ceramic bearing because many improvements have been made in the manufacture and to the design of ceramic implants [10].

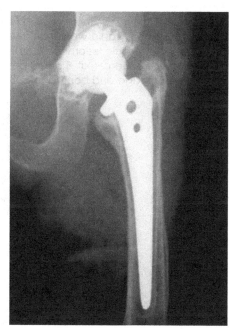

Figure 1:
Radiograph taken at 16 years postoperatively shows radiolucent area around alumina-on-alumina bearing implants. The radiolucent area is linear along the implant margin.

Since November 1997, we have performed total hip arthroplasty (THA) using an implant with alumina-on-alumina bearing surface for relatively young patients. In this manuscript, we described our experience with special regard to wear and ceramic failure. We also described the significance of metal transfer to ceramic head.

Patients and Methods

From November 1997, about 1200 cases of primary THA were performed using an alumina-on-alumina bearing implant, PLASMACUP® SC - BiCONTACT® hip system (AESCULAP AG & Co., Tuttlingen, Germany). The implant was used in all patients younger than 65 years unless a specially designed implant was necessary because of the skeletal condition. The most common cause of THA was osteonecrosis of the femoral head.

THA was performed usually through a posterolateral approach, but sometimes through a direct lateral approach and a lateral approach with a trochanteric osteotomy. Patients were usually allowed to walk with supports after five days and full weight-bearing was permitted after ten weeks.

Clinical and radiographic evaluations were performed at six weeks, three months, six months, and one year, and subsequently annually or biannually. Serial radiographs were examined for component stability, ceramic wear and periprosthetic osteolysis [5,6].

Results

In all cases, implants were stably fixed. Revision surgery was performed in two cases in which ceramic failure occurred. Femoral fracture during insertion of the femoral stem was the most frequent complication, but all fractures healed with or without wiring. Otherwise, there were no serious complications remarkable.

In no case, measurable wear was detected. However, in one case, cavitary periprosthetic osteolytic lesions were detected around the acetabular cup and in the greater trochanter at 8 years postoperatively (Fig. 2). The lesions were treated by curettage and bone graft. During the operation, black discoloration

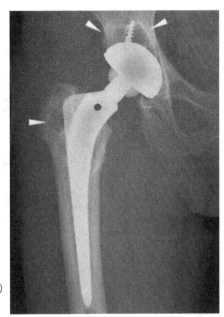

Figure 2:
Radigraph taken at 8 years postoperatively shows geographic osteolytic lesions (arrow head) around the acetabular cup and in greater trochanter.

was observed on the alumina bearing surfaces. Energy dispersive x-ray spectrophotometric analysis confirmed that the black discoloration was a titanium metal stain. Histological examination and elementary mapping analysis with an electron probe micro analyzer confirmed numerous macrophages and abundant alumina particles in the tissue taken from the osteolytic lesions [8]. The mechanism of the ceramic particle production was not clear, but increased wear by the transferred metallic debris via an abrasive or a third body wear mechanism seemed to be the most probable mechanism. In other cases, no osteolysis was detected.

Alumina failure occurred in two cases. In one case, fracture of the alumina femoral head and alumina insert occurred by a major motor vehicle accident causing a large amount of axial force to the femur at four years and two months postoperatively (Fig. 3) [16]. In the other case, peripheral chip fracture of the acetabular insert was detected at 14 months postoperatively (Fig. 4) [15]. There was no history of significant trauma, but the hip joint was unstable preoperatively due to inadequate hip muscle tone following a spinal cord injury. The joint was constantly unstable after arthroplasty and recurrent subluxation caused the chip fracture.

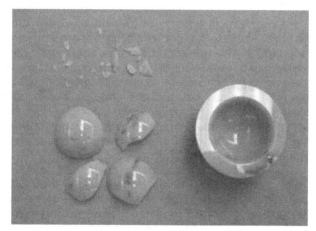

Figure 3:
Photograph shows fractured alumina head and acetabular insert retrieved from a 36-year-old male patient at 4 years and 2 months postoperatively.

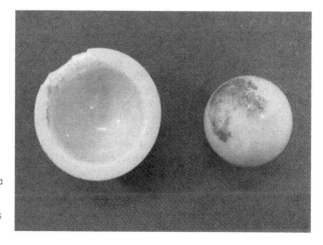

Figure 4:
Photograph shows a black stained alumina head and a fractured alumina insert retrieved from a 25-year-old female patient at 17 months postoperatively.

It was found that metal transfer from the metal shell to the ceramic head occurred when a ceramic head was impinged on a metal shell during intraoperative reduction of the ceramic head [14]. The metal transfer was identified in cases of difficult reduction because of soft tissue tension, but it was confirmed to occur by a light scraping [1]. In a revision surgery case, ceramic bearing surface was found damaged by the transferred metal debris through an abrasive or a third body wear mechanism [14].

Six patients felt noise that seemed to originate from the bearing surface. In all cases, no abnormal findings were detected on plain radiographs and the noise was not disturbing activity. All cases are under simple observation without special examinations.

Discussion

Our experience with the contemporary alumina-on-alumina bearing surface was very satisfactory. Wear was detected in no case, and periprosthetic osteolysis was detected in only one case. These results contradict the results of other studies of conventional metal-on-polyethylene bearing surfaces [7,11].

The mechanical strength of alumina has been substantially improved, but ceramic fractures of contemporary alumina-on-alumina articulation were reported [2]. We experienced two cases of ceramic failure. The failure occurred because of a severe trauma in one case and because of recurrent subluxation in the other case. Fortunately, no ceramic failure occurred during ordinary activity. The most probable cause of the osteolysis in one case of this study was the alumina particles. Transferred metal particles seemed to produce alumina particles by an abrasive or a third body wear mechanism. It is necessary to avoid scraping a ceramic component on metal components or instruments during the operation.

Noise is a recently recognized problem associated with ceramic-on-ceramic bearing surface [3,4,9,12,13]. The etiology of the noise remains elusive at the present time. We found that several patients was feeling noise from the joint, but did not perform special studies to find out the cause of the noise. In no case, the noise was disturbing daily activity.

References

1. Chang CB, Yoo JJ, Song WS, Kim DJ, Koo K-H, Kim HJ (in press) Transfer of metallic debris from the metal surface of an acetabular cup to artificial femoral heads by scraping: comparison between alumina and cobalt-chrome heads (in press) J Biomed Mater Res B.
2. Ha YC, Koo KH, Jeong ST, JJ Yoo, Kim YM, Kim HJ (2006) Cementless alumina-on-alumina total hip arthroplasty in patients younger than 50 years: a 5-year minimum follow-up study. J Arthroplasty 22:184-188.
3. Hozak WJ, Restrepo C, Parvizi J, Purtill JJ, Sharkey PF, Rothman RH (2007) Noisy ceramic hip: is component malpositioning the problem? AAOS Annual Meeting Proceedings 8:374-375.
4. Jarrett CA, Ranawat AS, Bruzzone M, Rodriguez JA, Ranawat CS (2007) The squeaking hip: an under-reported phenomenon of ceramic-on-ceramic total hip arthroplasty. AAOS Annual Meeting Procedings 8:375.

5. Joshi RP, Eftekhar NS, McMahon DJ, Nercessian OA (1998) Osteolysis after Charnley primary low-friction arthroplasty: a comparison of two matched paired groups. J Bone Joint Surg [Br] 80:585-590.

6. Maloney WJ, Jasty M, Harris WH, Galante JO, Callaghan JJ (1990) Endosteal erosion in association with stable uncemented femoral components. J Bone Joint Surg [Am] 72:1025-1034.

7. Maloney WJ, Woolson ST (1996) Increasing incidence of femoral osteolysis in association with uncemented Harris-Galante total hip arthroplasty: a follow-up report. J Arthroplasty 11:130-134.

8. Nam KW, Yoo JJ, Kim YL, Kim Y-M, Lee MH, Kim HJ (in press) Alumina-debris induced osteolysis after metal transfer in contemporary alumina-on-alumina total hip arthroplasty: a case report. J Bone Joint Surg [Am]

9. O'Toole GC, Walter WL, Zicat BA, Walter WK (2006) Squeaking in ceramic-on-ceramic hips: incidence, causes and solutions. AAOS Annual Meeting Procedings 7:483.

10. Skinner HB (1999) Ceramic bearing surfaces. Clin Orthop 369:83-91.

11. Smith E, Harris WH (1995) Increasing prevalence of femoral lysis in cementless total hip arthroplasty. J Arthroplasty 10:407-412.

12. Toni A, Traina F, Stea S, Sudanese A, Visentin M, Bordini B (2006) Early diagnosis of ceramic liner fracture: guidelines based on a 12-year clinical experience with 3710 modern ceramic prostheses. AAOS Annual Meeting Procedings 7:534.

13. Walter WL, Kurtz SM, Hozack WJ, Garino JP, Tuke MA, Parvizi J, Kirsh G, Ellis AM (2007) Retrieval analysis of squeaking alumina ceramic-on-ceramic bearings. AAOS Annual Meeting Procedings 8:374.

14. Yoo JJ, Kim HJ, Kim Y-M (2004) Damage of an alumina-on-alumina bearing surface from a difficult reduction of a total hip arthroplasty. J Bone Joint Surg [Am] 86:376-378.

15. Yoo JJ, Kim Y-M, Yoon KS, Koo K-H, Kim JW, Nam KW, Kim HJ (2006) Contemporary alumina-on-alumina total hip arthroplasty performed in patients younger than forty years: a 5-year minimum follow-up study. J Biomed Mater Res B 78:70-75.

16. Yoo JJ, Kim Y-M, Yoon KS, Koo K-H, Song WS, Kim HJ (2005) Alumina-on-alumina total hip arthroplasty: a five-year minimum follow-up study. J Bone Joint Surg [Am] 87:530-535.

5A.6 Ceramic on Ceramic Bearing in Coren® Hip System

J.-M. Lee

Introduction

The main goal of THA is for the patient to have almost the same functional hip joint as the normal joint, and use the implant as long as possible at the same time. Allowed hip joint ROM (range of motion) may be one of the most important deciding factors for maintaining normal daily activity. However, preexisting total hip arthroplasty systems allow range of joint motion far less than that permitted by the normal hip joint. If one tries to flex the hip joint beyond what is allowed by conventional hip systems, an impingement, even dislocation and loosening may occur.

There have been numerous attempts to improve hip joint range of motion of THA patients but there has only been limited success. Widely used popular metal on polyethylene bearings have exhibited such problems; however, recently similar problems have been often encountered with ceramic on ceramic bearings. In other word, a fracture or chipping which is the biggest concern in ceramic on ceramic bearings may occur, and the impingement may affect a long-term result.

The first Korean designed and manufactured total hip system (Coren® hip system) has developed, making an improvement to avoid such problems, and the concept of impingement and characteristics of design will be hereby addressed.

Flexion is usually allowed up to 135 degrees in the normal hip joint. It is well understood that the diameter of normal femoral head ranges between 45 and 50 mm, and the head neck ratio plays an essential role in deciding hip joint range of motion. However, if femoral heads of metal on polyethylene were manufactured closed to the size of normal femoral head, substantial wear and problems caused by coefficient of friction would be inevitable; therefore the size of 22 mm, not even 28 mm, of femoral heads were limitedly used; and 32 mm was rarely used for its complication. In addition, to overcome the metal's characteristically repeated load, there has been a limitation in reducing the dimension of the neck even it is closely related to larger joint ROM. If forced to reduce the dimension further, the neck area would induce the stress fracture. Therefore, adjusting the head neck ratio has clear limitation in improving hip ROM, and many hip systems yield the maximum hip joint flexion only in the range of 115 to 120 degrees.

Impingement usually occurs even before reaching hip flexion degrees of 110 - 120, and dislocation becomes unavoidable beyond this range. During revision, it is not infrequent to encounter indentations in either anterior or posterior aspect of the acetabular cup. Such finding is attributed to recurrent impingement of the polyethylene liner in either the anterior or the posterior of the acetabular cup during the repeated motions of hip flexion. Indentations caused by such impingement may be easily found in polyethylene liners but in case of ceramic liners, it seems to be impossible to see such indentation. Chip off or the ceramic liner fracture and repeated friction between the stem and the liner may induce failure of the stem.

Anatomical position of the acetabular cup lies 45 degrees in abduction and 10 to 15 degrees in anteversion. Also the femoral stem should be positioned at 5 to 10 degrees in anteversion. Even before reaching the hip flexion degrees of 110 – 120, the anterior becomes impinged and the femoral head becomes slightly dislodged from the cup; furthermore, beyond this point, a posterior dislocation of the femoral head ensues. Hence, numbers of surgeons tend to add more anteversion to the cup to prevent a posterior hip dislocation. Although this may produce less anterior impingement, between the phases of mid-stance and push off during a gait, posterior impingement may occur with prolonged extension of the hip joint. Therefore, excessive anteversion of the cup may induce an anterior hip dislocation.

In conclusion, there is a clear limitation in reducing impingement solely by adjusting an amount of cup anteversion. This raises an important message particularly for Asians, people whom the excessive amount of hip flexion is required during daily activity. Although Harris-Galante II cup has been reported with relatively good results in America, it has been producing poor results for Korean (domestic) population. Such results may be attributed to poor locking mechanism of the cup and recurrent impingement of the polyethylene liner; which then leads to considerable liner dissociation or wear of the implant. Korean population uses much more ROM compared to other nations which increases the chance of impingements, and that caused a difference as a result. Based on several shortcomings, an improvement in hip joint ROM should be made for possibly having better results for both Asian and American populations. (Based on several shortcomings, the result affected by the joint motion of range has bigger meanings in Asian countries, and also has important effect in Western countries.)

Aluminum oxide and zirconium oxide are the ceramic materials widely used in artificial joints. Ceramic material was first introduced in 1970s as a bearing in Mittelmeier total hip arthroplasty system. Characteristically, the ceramics exhibit bioinertness, high degree of hardness, and high wettability, which make them biocompatible. Oxide powders are treated through hot isostatic pressure (HIP) process and this process is known to be a fair technology. Despite all the advantages of using ceramics including low wear rate and low friction coefficient, one drawback that refrain some surgeons from using the ceramic material is the possibility of ceramic fracture. The reported fracture rate ranges from 0.02 - 0.09%, especially Biolox Forte® has as low as 0.004% of reported fracture rate. In preexisting THA systems, an issue of impingement has not been a serious concern among surgeons. However, occurrences of dislocation, loosening, and liner dissociation are considered to be largely related to impingement.

Fortunately, recently popularized bearings such as metal on cross linked polyethylene, metal on metal and ceramic on ceramic have overcame the wear issue, and currently, the bigger sized heads (32 mm, 36 mm) are introduced in the market. Increasing the head size produces an increased ROM, but further also increases the friction torque. Therefore, it is advisable to decrease the surface of the neck area while simultaneously increasing the head size.

The Coren® Hip system is the first Korean designed and manufactured cementless total hip arthroplasty system; its first clinical application was in 2003, and has become widely available in the market since 2006. The femoral stem has a tapered wedge design with three vertical ribs at proximal, and is composed of titanium alloy with corundum blasted surface. The acetabular cup is in a hemispherical configuration with two specially designed screw holes. The surface is a fine titanium plasma spray. The preferred surface bearing is ceramic on ceramic, and the surface area of the neck was maintained at the largest in its initial design, and the area of impingement was carved out in order to reduce the impingement and, at the same time, maximizing the hip joint ROM (Fig. 1). Although assuming that creating an anterior-posterior cut edge is simple in many commercially available total hip systems, may be thought to increase flexion motion, however, its effect was found to be negligible.

In Coren® Hip System, the flexion goal was achieved by mainly carving out upon 45 degrees of both anteromedial and posteromedial corners of the stem. Through this design strategy, 127 degrees, 130 degrees, and 137 degrees of hip joint flexion could be achieved using the size of 28 mm, 32 mm, and 36 mm femoral head, respectively. This may be translated into approximately 10-degree improvement in hip flexion in each head size as compared with other preexisting hip systems. Up to the size of 50 mm acetabular cup is used with 28 mm femoral head, and from the size of 52 mm acetabular cup is used with 32 mm, but soon will be changed to 36 mm (Fig. 2, 3).

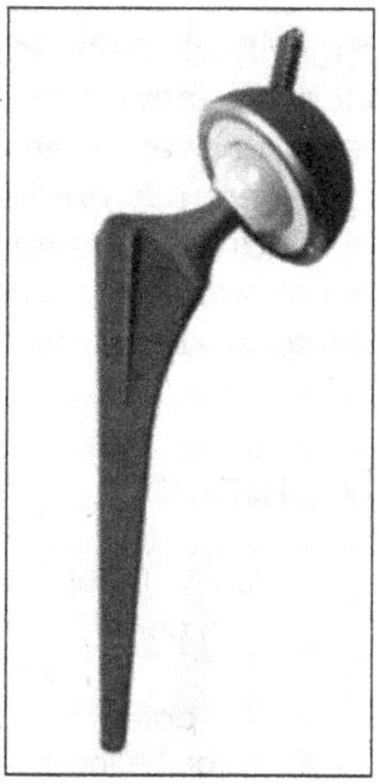

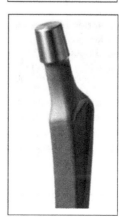

Figure 1:
The Coren® hip system is comprised of a tapered wedge stem, with a design modification in the neck area of the stem, standard ceramic on ceramic articular surface bearing and an acetabular cup.

Figure 2:
A design modification was made in the neck area of the Coren® stem to maximize the range of hip joint motion.

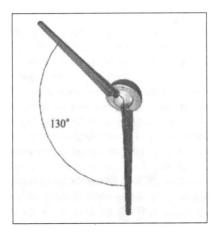

Figure 3:
Using a 32mm femoral head, in an actual
implanted position of prostheses, up to 130
degrees of hip joint flexion can be achieved.

Conclusion

Impingement occurring in THA has been an important deciding factor for the longevity of the implant when using polyethylene on metal bearings; nevertheless since the introduction of ceramic on ceramic bearings, such importance has became even more aware. The first Korean designed and manufactured total hip system (Coren® Hip System) has not only increased the size of head but also significantly modified the neck structure for increased ROM. Considering mentioned facts, Coren® Hip System is expected to be ideal in accomplishing natural and improved hip joint motion as a result.

References

1. D'Antonio J, Capello W, Manley M, Bierbaum B (2002) New experience with alumina-on-alumina ceramic bearings for total hip arthroplasty. J Arthroplasty 17:390-7.
2. Nevelos J, Ingham E, Doyle C, Streicher R, Nevelos A, Walter W, Fisher J (2000) Microseparation of the centers of alumina-alumina artificial hip joints during simulator testing produces clinically relevant wear rates and patterns. J Arthroplasty. 15:793-5.
3. Robert LB, Corey B, Harry BS (2004) Concerns about Ceramics in THA. Clin Orthop Relat Res, 429:73-9.
4. Skinner HB (1999) Ceramic bearing surface. Clin Orthop 369: 83-91.
5. Walter A (1992) On the material and the tribology of alumina-alumina couplings for hip joint prosthesis. Clin Orthop and Rel Res 282.

Hard on Hard Bearings

5B.1 Metallosis in Metal-on-Metal PPF Total Hip Arthroplasties

R. Legenstein, W. Huber and P. Boesch

Abstract

Metallosis in total hip arthroplasty (THA) is a not commonly reported complication. We followed 173 consecutive patients, who had received primary, single and non-cemented proximal press fit (PFF) THA with metal-on-metal bearings made of low carbon content in 1995. Follow-up results are available for a total of 161 (93.1%) patients. The mean age of the patients was 63.3 years (31 to 76). The mean duration of follow-up was 94.5 months (range, 57 to 112). The median Harris hip score at follow-up was 95 points.

36 (20.8%) metallosis cases were observed. 18 cases because of metallosis were revised. Dislocation in metallosis cases occurred in 25%. Revisions were obtained because of 2 femur fractures (1 with metallosis) and 5 infections. The results with metal-on-metal bearings were not satisfactory. Toxic metal concentrations in joint effusions were found. We do not implant or recommend metal-on-metal bearings in total hip arthroplasty anymore.

Introduction

The concept of metal-on-metal bearing systems for total hip arthroplasty (THA) was established in the late 1960s1. In the late 1980s, improved surface finishes were introduced to reduce prosthetic wear and hence to avoid periprostetic osteolytic reactions [2]. A large number of clinical studies described the successful use of metal-on-metal in THAs, which were found to be reliable and to provide an excellent outcome [2-4]. Further studies were highlighting the remarkably low wear rates of metal-on-metal bearings [11,12]. Also in vitro studies have shown that the metal-on-metal combination has excellent wear resistance [5]. Some cases of metallosis have been reported following the use of second generation metal-on-metal THAs6]. Some studies on modern metal pairings are concerned with the histopathologic respons of the periprosthetic tissue and the joints capsule to metal wear debris; but opinions varied widely and the reasons for metallosis are at least unknown [7,8].

Since 1990 we implanted the non-cemented Proximal Press Fit total hip arthroplasty System (PPF, STRATEC, Switzerland) with ceramic-on-polyethylene or metal-on-polyethylene articulation at the hospital in Wiener Neustadt. In June 1994 metal-on-metal bearings were introduced for the PPF System. Metal-on-metal bearing partners were consecutive implanted in all patients with an age below seventy years because we observed in serial radiographs radiolucencies and were first seen within 12 months, but were of no clinical relevance. Periprosthetic radiolucencies around cups and stems occurred because of polyethylene debris-induced granulomas. But the PPF system yields satisfactory medium-term results patients with ceramic-on-polyethylene articulation in 1995 and revealed a clinical survival rate of 95% after 10 years. From 1990 to 1991 we implanted 176 non-cemented PPF total hip arthroplasties with ceramic-on-polyethylene articulation in 170 patients. Of these, 119 patients (122 THA) were followed after 104 to 129 months. Only four cups had been revised for aseptic loosening, but no stem. Two infections and two dislocations occurred. The median postoperative Harris hip score was 91.

The purpose of our study was to analyze metallosis cases of PPF metal-on-metal bearings in the first consecutive year of implantation because periprosthetic osteolysis, dislocations and inexplicable pain of patients occurred. Clinical and radiological signs were observed for identification of metallosis. Histopathological evaluation was done in all revision cases and chemoanalytical metal evaluation was performed in three cases.

Material and Methods

Patients

In 1995, 173 patients received primary, single and non-cemented PPF THAs with metal-on-metal articulation with low carbon content. There were 102 women and 71 men. The average age at the time of surgery was 63.3 years (range, 31 to 76 years). The mean duration of follow-up was 94.5 months (range, 57 to 112 months).

Indications for the 173 (100%) operated hips were primary osteoarthritis (112, 64.7%), congenital hip dislocation (42, 24.3%), osteonecrosis of the femoral head (15, 8.7%), femur neck fractures (1, 0.6%), posttraumatic osteoarthritis (1, 0.6%), osteoarthritis secondary to pyogenic arthritis (1, 0.6%) and rheumatoid arthritis (1, 0.6%).

Follow-up results are available for a total of 161 (93.1%) patients. 11 patients were deceased. 24 patients were revised. 5 patients refused follow-up but granted us good clinical condition via telephone. 11 patients could not be reached, although at least 2 annual results were available from previous follow-ups and only 2 patients had no follow-up since surgery. Before the patient's discharge, an anteroposterior and an axial radiograph of the operated hip were obtained. Clinical and radiographic follow-up was carried out prospectively, initially after 6, 12 and 24 months and then at least every 2 years. Patients who did not attend for routine monitoring were called in again in the year of 2004.

Radiological evaluation

Radiological evaluation was made by a senior orthopaedic surgeon on anterior-posterior and lateral roentgenograms of the hip. Radiolucent areas around the femoral stem were measured using the Gruen [21] zones 1-7 and around the screw socket were measured using the DeLee [22] zones I-III. All radiological changes of the thickness of the periprosthetic femoral and acetabular bone (hypertrophy, atrophy, radiolucency and osteolysis) in any of the above described zones were divided in mild (< 1 mm), moderate (< 2 mm), progressive (> 2-4 mm) and osteolytic (> 4 mm). Postoperative heterotopic ossification were classified according to Brooker [10] (0-IV).

Materials

The non-cemented PPF total hip arthroplasty (PANTITAN (-1995) - STRATEC (1995-2001) - BIOMET (2001-)), manufactured from the titanium forged alloy Ti-Al$_6$-V$_4$, consists of a conical screw socket and a stem with rectangular cross-section, tapering in distal direction. In order to prevent premature distal press-fit, the stem is slightly tapered on the medial side in distal direction, relative to the rasp. The articulating metal head, with a diameter of 28 mm, and the corresponding metal were made of a low carbide alloy with low carbon content (0.00-0.08%). The insert, a construction of the ultra-high-molecular-weight-polyethylene and metal, is pressed inside the cup after its stable implantation. The polyethylene was sterilised with use of gamma irradiation in air.

Surgical technique

The surgeries were performed under spinal or general anesthesia through a modified anterolateral Watson-Jones approach with a horizontal incisicion superior from the trochanter major, a minimal ventral tenotomy of the gluteus medius with refixation after implantation and a ventral capsulectomy. Full weight-bearing was permitted immediately after stable implantation. As a rule two crutches were recommended for six weeks postoperatively. Patients were assessed clinically before the operation, postoperatively at intervals of six months, one year, and then every two years. The patients assigned their degree of pain subjectively to one of four categories: none, mild, moderate or severe. As thrombosis prophylaxis patients received subcutaneous injection of low molecular heparin until five weeks postoperatively. On the day of surgery the patient's received antibiotic prophylaxis, three times a day two grams of a second generation cephalosporin intravenously. Patients were given 50 mg Indomethacin against heterotopic ossification twice a day for at least ten days postoperatively.

Results

Clinical results
Harris Hip score [24]

The median preoperative Harris hip score was 33. At the final follow-up examination the median Harris hip score was 95.

Tönnis score [23]

The postoperative functional outcome score evaluated according to the five parameters of Tönnis showed in the range of motion 78% grade 0, in 12% grade 1, in 8% grade 2 and in 3% grade 3. The Trendelenburg sign occurred in 81% as grade 0, in as 13% grade 1, in 4% as grade 2 and in 1% as grade 3. Pain was observed in 90% as grade 0, in 6% grade as 1, and in 4% as grade 2. The ability to walk was in 86% grade 0, in 11% grade 1, and in 4% grade 2. The patient's subjective evaluation of the operations result was as follows: 93% grade 0, in 6% grade 1, and in 1% grade 2. The functional Tönnis score at the final follow-up examination was in 85% very good, in 11% good and in 4% moderate.

Pain

18 cases (10.4%) had clinical or radiological metalosis signs as follows: 1 patient (0.6%) had periprosthetic osteolysis and pain, 11 patients (6.4%) had osteolysis without pain and 6 patients (3.6%) had pain without osteolysis in the radiographs. Pain caused by metalosis occurred typically inguinal and at an average time of thirty months postoperatively (range, 5 to 85). Pain in the area of the major trochanter and gluteal were concomitant at initial walking. During follow-up

examination most patients' claim on inguinal pain being forced by extended leg lifting. The ability to use stairs only with mild inguinal pain was interpreted by patients mostly as muscle disorder.

Dislocation

Dislocation was observed in one patient without metallosis signs and a cup inclination angle of 53° after 37 months; a revision surgery because of an infection 6 months postoperatively was performed. 10 cases at an average time of 44 months with an average cup inclination of 48°. Out of 36 metallosis cases 7 dislocations were recorded. One of these cases had an extreme cup inclination angle of 70° an a L1 head with an extended neck which can either force dislocation and could have induced metallosis after ten dislocations but revision surgery was refused (see Fig. 5).

Chemical Analysis (Table 1)

In three patients A-C metal concentrations of the joint effusion could be analysed. The serum concentration of one patient was also evaluated. Normal values of the serum/plasma are: Co 0.1-0.5 µg/kg, Cr 0.05-0.1 µg/kg and Mo 0.3-1.2 µg/kg or Co -2 µg/l, Cr -5 µg/l.

Case	Co		Cr		Mo	
A (effusion)	335	µg/kg	635	µg/kg	45	µg/kg
B (effusion)	30	µg/kg	32	µg/kg	3.1	µg/kg
C (effusion)	67410	µg/l	46095	µg/l		
C (serum)	7.5	µg/l	5.25	µg/l		
normal values	0.1-0.5	µg/kg	0.05-0.1	µg/kg	0.3-1.2	µg/kg
	-2	µg/l	-5	µg/l.		

Table 1:
In three patients A-C metal concentrations of the joint effusion could be analysed.
The serum concentration of patient C was also evaluated.

Case A: Dislocation occurred in a forty four year old female patient eighty seven months postoperatively. Radiographs showed local osteolysis in the stem Zones 1 and 7 [21] and massive atrophy in the cup zones 1-3 [22]. The HHS at this time was 93. The cup inclination was 48°. Because of painless head and inlay changing were performed during revision surgery after 102 months. Infection lab and Gram`s method were negative. The mean metal concentrations in the effusion after two measurements were: Cr 635 µg/kg, Co 335 µg/kg and Mo 45 µg/kg.

Case B: A seventy four years female patient suffered from inguinal pain seventy months postoperatively. The HHS at this time was 97. The cup inclination was 58°. Dislocation did not occur. In radiographs local osteolysis was detected in the cranial cup Zone 1 [22]. Revision was refused. Infection lab and Gram`s method were negative. The mean metal concentrations in the effusion after two measurements were: Cr 32 µg/kg, Co 30 µg/kg and Mo 3.1 µg/kg.

Case C: A sixty year old female patient suffered from inguinal and gluteal pain 36 months postoperatively. Radiographs showed no periprosthetic osteolyis. The HHS at this time was 73. The cup inclination was 43°. During revision the cup was loose so a Boesch reinforcementring was implanted with a metal-on-polyethylene articulation. Infection lab and Gram`s method were negative. The metal concentrations in the effusion were: Cr 46095 µg/l, Co 67410 µg/l. The serum metal concentrations were: Cr 5.25 µg/l, Co 7.5 µg/l.

Pathohistological results

At revision surgery the inner layer of the capsule showed macroscopic typically a smooth, slightly red to orange coloured synovial membrane. A necrotic discoloured film could be scratched of the membrane. Microscopic evidence for metallosis derived from the metal-on-metal articulation, was shown in black particle storing macrophages. In all examined cases extended lymphocytic infiltrations which consisted from B and T lymphocytes with relation to secondary follicles could be observed. These were either diffusely distributed or aggregated around capillary vessels and in vascular walls. Little foreign body reactions with mono and multinuclear macrophages were found histomorphologically. Infection was classified histological when more than six neutrophile granulocytes were detected in one high power field area.

Complications (Table 2)

2 periprothetic fractures of the femur around the stem were revised, 1 case had symptomatic metallosis. These fractures were treated with revision stems.
4 late infections (2.3%) with Staphylococcus aureus occurred: 1 cup was revised because of septic loosening six months postoperatively; 1 THA was revised four times until the infection was under control; 1 cup was revised because of septic loosening sixty months postoperatively, 1 patient was revised 72 months postoperatively but stem and cup were stable; and 1 early infection occurred. During revision surgery inlay and head were changed to metal-on-metal and only in one case to ceramic-on-polyethylene.

Complications	n
Infections	5
Fractures	2
Metallosis revisions	18
Metallosis clinical	18
Dislocation	12
Heterotopic ossification	11

Table 2:
Complications of 161 PPF THA`s with metal-on-metal articulation after a mean follow-up of 94.5 months.

Revision surgery because of metallosis was performed in 18 (10.4%) cases. In none of these cases bacteria's could be identified in histopathological analysis, so diagnosis of synovialitis endoprothethica without acute infection sign was postulated. None of the revision cases showed neck impingement. Symptomatic aseptic cup loosening was shown in 7 cups (4%). All these hips were revised at an average of 57.7 months (range 36 to 87 months), postoperatively. 4 hips (3.2%) were revised because of symptomatic dislocation at an average of 49.5 months with a mean cup inclination angle of 48.9°. 6 patients (3.4%) were revised because of inguinal, trochanteric and gluteal symptomatic pain.

At 118 months postoperatively 94.8% of the cups and 98.8% of the stems were still in situ.

Radiological results

Characteristically radiographic findings were seen by comparison of the anteroposterior and lateral radiographs. In most cases radiolucent areas around the femoral stem were seen in zone 1 and 7 [21]. Mild radiolucent areas (< 1 mm) with sclerosis were found in 20.4% of cases in zone 1 and in 5.8% in zone 7 as well. Moderate radiolucent areas (< 2 mm) were evaluated in 4.4% around the femoral stems in zone 1 and 3.6% in zone 7, progressive radiolucency (> 2-4 mm) was observed in 2.9% in zone 1 and 1.5% in zone 7, and osteolytic areas (> 4 mm) were found in 6.6% in zone 1 and 1.5% in zone 7. All radiolucent areas were already detected on the radiographs made for the 6 and 12 months follow-up. Progressive radiolucent areas were observed only after 24 months follow-up. Osteolytic areas were progressive in all cases (Fig. 1, 3, 4).

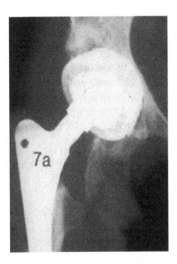

Figure 1:
PPF THA with metal-on-metal articulation seven years after implantation with local osteolysis in the cranial cup area.

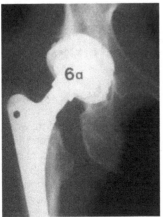

Figure 2:
PPF THA with metal-on-metal articulation six years after implantation with local osteolysis in the caudal cup area and massive bone atrophy between the cup and the inner lamina.

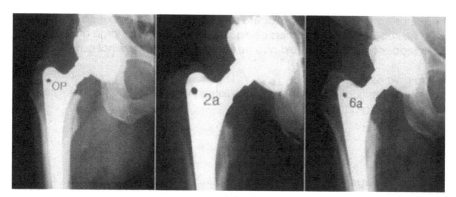

Figure 3:
Series of a PPF THA with metal-on-metal articulation postoperative, two years and six years after implantation with progressive local osteolysis at the calcar.

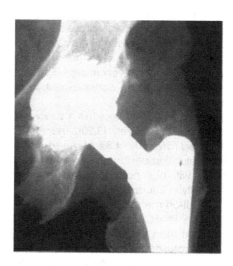

Figure 4:
PPF THA with metal-on-metal articulation seven years after implantation with massive local osteolysis at the trochanter major.

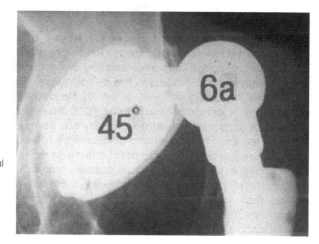

Figure 5:
PPF THA with metal-on-metal articulation six years after implantation. Spontaneous dislocation occurred because of massive joint effusion while the cup inclination was 45°.

The interpretation of radiological acetabulum atrophy is difficult because in some cases postoperatively the authors could identify atrophy as a large effusion filled bursa ileopectinea which could also be interpreted as abdominal gas (Fig. 2).

Heterotopic ossification
Heterotopic ossification grade I was evaluated in 8 cases (13.3%) of THA, grade II in 2 cases and grade IV in 1case [10].

Discussion

In revision surgery we found enlarged bursa ileopectinea`s formed of liquid pressure.In our series of metallosis cases (20.8%) joint effusion was palpatory detected and verified with ultrasound. When effusion was punctured, an orange, turbid and cloudy synovial fluid with a volume up to 90 ml could be aspirated. These purulent imaging fluids had granulocytes but no bacteria's in the bacteriological analysis to grams method and cultures. In a few cases during revision surgery liquid sprayed out by force because of high intracapsular pressure. Joint's effusion because of metallosis is most probably the reason for inguinal pain, especially at initial walking. It occurred at an average time of 30 months postoperatively (range, 5 to 58). Pain in the area of the trochanter major and gluteal can be concomitant. Inguinal pain was interpreted by patients as muscle disorder.

Reported cementless THA`s survival rate ranged from 90.6% to 100% at a 4-10 years postoperatively [3,20]. The survival rate in the present series is within the reported rate with 94.8% of the socket and 98.8% of the stem at the latest follow-up evaluation performed on an average of 94.5 months postoperatively. Results of THA with high carbide metal-on-metal articulation series must also be analysed carefully in future.

Metal-on-metal bearings in THA have experienced a resurgence of popularity in recent times, because many of the early metal-on-metal prostheses functioned for more than two decades without serious signs of wear [11,12]. Advantages in manufacturing technology have enabled more precise tolerances and surface finish which makes metal-on-metal particularly attractive in THA and surface arthroplasties because of ultra-low wear rates exhibited in numerous in vivo and in vitro studies [1-5,11-13,19].

Metal-on-metal devices release metal ions as a byproduct. But they are also released from every metallic implant. Researchers have been trying to define what amount of cobalt and chromium ions are acceptable in THA and to reveal the toxic significance. Workers in the metal industry exposed to chromium and cobalt have much higher levels of ions in the body than of a metal-on-metal implant. Their blood ions values can be 15-20 times higher than that of a metal-on-metal bearing and no systemic toxicity has been established [14-16,29]. It is also reported that metal-on-metal articulation is safe for woman of childbearing age because the placenta acts as an effective barrier for chromium and cobalt [16]. It is also evidenced that loose cobalt chromium stems exhibit equivalent blood ion levels compared to that of a THA metal-on-metal bearing [17]. Studies showed that low and high carbide Co-alloy articulations caused specific macrophagic reactions accompanied by a lymph-cell response [18]. This type of tissue reaction is thought to be a local or systemic immune reaction [7]. All revised cases in this study showed necrosis and extended lymphocytic infiltrations around capillary vessels and in vascular walls. This can be summarized with the clinical results as the typical diagnostic facts for metallosis, being in accordance with so far found patho-histological facts by other studies [4,7-9]. In our, and equal to other authors, revised THA`s with polyethylene-on-ceramic articulation these lymphocytic infiltrations were missing [7]. Authors also attempt to eliminate polyethylene because more reported adverse biologic responses are occurring to polyethylene than to metal in THA [14].

Metal level identification was not done routinely. The analyzed effusions of three patients had extremely high metal concentrations far above normal values for serum. We suppose that these toxic metal concentrations can initiate, eventual concomitant, with an immune reaction, a chronic inflammation and necrosis of the joint capsule that produces massive effusion. Cobalt toxicity after McKee hip arthroplasties are well known since 1975 with all clinical signs we observed: spontaneous dislocation, bone necrosis and progressive pain [27]. Experimental lung research in vitro showed that cobalt and metallic carbides interact with oxygen to produce toxic activated oxygen species (AOS) when inhaled that can produce an interstitial hard metal lung disease, but only in a limited portion of exposed workers (1-5%). It is speculated that individuals with lower antioxidant defense are more susceptible to the toxic effect of AOS [26]. Beside the possible involvement of an immunological sensitization we must include other hypotheses for metallosis in THA like toxokinetic factors, biological defense dysfunctions and the propensity of individuals to develop an inflammation under genetic and environmental control, too [26,28,30,31].

Reports on the metal-on-metal articulation suggest that these tribosystem represent a good alternative for young and active patients [2,3,6,20]. The results of our analysis provide that the PPF total hip replacement with low carbide metal-on-metal articulation were not as satisfactory as those of a conventional polyethylene-on-ceramic or polyethylene-on-metal articulations. Since 2003 we do not implant or recommend metal-on-metal for total hip replacement anymore.

Because of the multifactorial nature of periprosthetic osteolysis with subsequent aseptic loosening in few cases with modern metal-on-metal articulation it needs further clinical and experimental research. It should lead to better mechanism-based prevention strategies, early detection of, and in vivo therapy for this condition. Meanwhile close radiographic monitoring with high mark on typical osteolysis and exact clinical evaluation is recommended for all patients after total hip arthroplasty with metal-on-metal bearing postoperatively.

References

1. McKee GK. Total hip replacement – past, present and future. Biomaterials 1982; 3:130-5.
2. Weber BG. Experience with the metasul total hip bearing system. Clin Orthop Relat Res 1996;329S:569-77.
3. Wagner M, Wagner H. Medium-term results of a modern metal-on-metal hip replacement. Clin Orthop Relat Res 2000;379:123-33.
4. Willert H-G, Buchhorn GH, Göbel D, Köster G, Schaffner S, Schenk R, Semlitsch M. Wear behavior and histopathology of classic cemented metal on metal hip endoprostheses. Clin Orthop Relat Res 1996;329S:160-86.

5. Chan FW, Bobyn JD, Medley JB, Krygier JJ, Tanzer M. Wear and lubrication of metal-on-metal hip implants. Clin Orthop Relat Res 1999;369:10-24.

6. Beaule PE, Campell P, Mirra J, Hooper JC, Schmalzried TP. Osteolysis in a cementless, second generation metal-on-metal hip replacement. Clin Orthop Relat Res 2001;386:159-65.

7. Willert H-G, Buchhorn GH, Fayyazi A, Lohmann CH. Histolopathologische Veränderungen bei Metal/Metall-Gelenken geben Hinweise auf eine zellvermittelte Überempfindlichkeit. Osteologie 2000;9(3):165-69.

8. Doorn PF, Mirra JM, Campell PA, Amstutz HC. Tissue reaction to metal on metal total hip prostheses. Clin Orthop Relat Res 1996;329S:187-205.

9. Justy M, Goetz DD, Bragdon CR, Lee KR, Hanson AE, Elderi JR, Harris WH. Wear of polyethylene acetabular components in total hip arthroplasty. J Bone Joint Surg. Am. 1996;79:349-58.

10. Brooker AF et al. Ectopic ossification following total hip replacement. J Bone Joint Surg. Am. 1973;55:1629-1632.

11. Schmidt et al. Cobald Chromium Molybdenum Metal Combination for Modular Hip Prostheses. Clin Orthop Relat Res 1996;329:35-47.

12. Mc Kellop et al. In vivo war of 3 types of metal on metal hip prostheses during two decades of use. Clin Orthop Relat Res 1996;329:128-40.

13. Medley JB, Chan FW, Krygier JJ, Bobyn JD. Comparison of alloys and designs in a hip simulator study of metal on metal implants. Clin Orthop Relat Res 1996;329S:148-59.

14. Meritt et al. Distribution of cobalt chromium wear and corrosion products and biologic reactions. Clin Orthop Relat Res 1996;329:233-43.

15. Jacobs et al. Cobalt chromium concentrations in patients with metal on metal total hip replacements. Clin Orthop Relat Res 1996;329:256-63.

16. Brodner et al. Elevated serum cobalt with metal on metal articulating surfaces. J Bone Joint Surg. Br. 1997;79:316-21.

17. Kriebich et al. Systemic release of cobalt and chromium after uncemented total hip replacement. J Bone Joint Surg. Br. 1996;78:18-21.

18. Boehler M, Kanz F, Schwarz B, Steffan I, Walter A, Plenk H Jr, Knahr K. Adverse tissue reactions to wear particels from Co-alloy articulations, increased by alumina-blasting particle contamination from cementless Ti-based total hip implants. J Bone Joint Surg. Br. 2002;84:128-36.

19. Reinisch G, Judmann KP, Lhotka Ch, Lintner F, Zweymüller KA. Retriviel study of uncemented metal-metal hip prostheses revised for early loosening. Biomaterials 2003;24:1081-1091.

20. Korovessis P, Petsinis G, Repanti Maria. Zweymüller with metal-on-metal articulation: clinical, radiological and histological analysis of short-term results. Arch Orthop Trauma Surg 2003;123:5-11.

21. Gruen TA, Mc Neice GM, Amstutz HC Modes of failure of cemented stem-type femoral components. Clin Orthop 1979;141:17-27.

22. DeLee JC, Charnley J Radiological demarcation of cemented sockets in total hip replacement. Clin Orthop 1976;121: 20.

23. Tönnis D, Arning A, Bloch M, Heinecke A, Kalchschmidt K. Triple pelvic osteotomy. J Paediatr Orthop Part B 1994;3:54-67.

24. Harris W H. Traumatic arthritis of the hip after dislocation and acetabular fracture – Treatment by mold arthroplasty. J Bone Joint Surg 1969;51-A:737-755.

25. Bertram. Spurenelemente Analytik, ökotokikologische und medizinisch-klinische Bedeutung. Verlag Urban&Schwarzenberg.

26. Lison D, Lauwerys R, Demendts M, Nemery B. Experimental research into the pathogenesis of cobalt/hard metal lung disease. Eur Respir J 1996;9:1024-1028.

27. Jones DA, Lucas HK, O`Driscoll M, Price CH, Wibberley B. Cobalt toxicity after McKee hip arthroplasty. J Bone Joint Surg Br. 1975;57(3):289-96.

28. Huk OL, Catelas I, Mwale F, Antoniou. J, Zukor DJ, Petit A. Induction of apoptosis and necrosis by metal ions in vitro. J Arthroplasty 2004;19(8Suppl):84-7.

29. Schaffer AW, Pilger A, Engelhardt C, Zweymüller K, Ruediger HW. Increased blood cobalt and chromium after total hip replacement. J Toxicol Clin Toxicol. 1999;37(7)839-44.

30. Haynes DR, Rogers SD, Hay S, Pearcy MJ, Howie DW. The differences in toxicicty and release of bone-resorbing mediators induced by titanium and cobalt-chromium-alloy wear particles. J Bone Joint Surg Br. 1975;75(6):825-34.

31. Nemery B, Bast A, Behr J et al. Interstitial lung disease induced by exogenous agents: factors governing susceptibility. Eur Respir J 2001;18:30-42.

5B.2 Results of 10 Years' Follow-Up of Ceramic-Ceramic Couples in Total Hip Replacement

M. Azizbaig Mohajer, F. Plattner and R. Graf

Introduction

Coxarthrosis is not only observed in patients beyond the age of 70, but also more and more frequently in younger patients who are still gainfully employed. The rate of prevalence and incidence of coxarthrosis which can be treated surgically is 10 - 15% in patients aged between 35 and 85. Etiologically speaking, the majority of coxarthrosis in younger patients results from hip dysplasia, femoroacetabular impingement, necrosis of the femoral head or from Perthes disease. Since the average life expectancy of people in Central Europe is as high as 80 years, and since THR is needed by ever-younger patients, today's implants must comply with increased requirements. The couples used in THR are required to last at least 20 years, provided they are perfectly suited for the application. The couples used most frequently today are metal-metal, metal-PE, ceramic-PE and ceramic-ceramic couples. According to the state of the art in research, the process of loosening of stems and acetabular cups is due to osteolysis which is caused by decomposition products. A revision rate of 7% or higher observed for metal-metal couples, and an abrasion rate of 0.1 mm per year observed for conventional metal-PE or ceramic-PE couples must be considered as critical. The benefit offered by ceramic-ceramic couples lies in their low abrasion rate of 0.001 mm per year [1]. For this reason, such couples are especially suited for younger and active patients. Although there hasn't been any age limit defined, it is recommended by specialists to restrict the use of ceramic-ceramic couples to patients below the age of 70. Moreover, ceramic implant materials are superior by the fact that they will not attract bacteria, which makes them particularly suited for use in revision surgery. Among the contraindications first of all count the more general directives such as for articular empyema and juxta-articular osteomyelitis. If intraoperatively suspicion of impingement should arise (e.g. in the event of implantation of a cup outside the safe zone), it is recommended to implant a PE inlay in order to prevent rupture of the ceramic inlay.

Material and Methods

Meanwhile, the initial experience obtained from the use of ceramic-ceramic couples at our hospital dates back 11 years. In the period between 1st September 1996 and 28th February 1997 (6 months), a number of 247 primary THRs were implanted. For 49 THRs thereof, we used ceramic-ceramic couples (the THRs were implanted on one side in 48 patients, and on both sides in one single patient). The THRs were followed up and analyzed consecutively during 10 years after surgery. The prosthetic systems listed below were implanted:
1. anatomic SBG stem (by Plus Orthopedics, Switzerland) (Fig. 1)
2. Lima cup (by Lima, Italy) (Fig. 2)
3. ceramic femoral head of 28 mm in diameter (by CeramTec) (Fig. 1)

4. ceramic inlay on poylethylene bed - sandwich construction -
(by CeramTec, Lima) (Fig. 2)

40 of the THRs were followed up retrospectively in 39 patients during 10 years after surgery.

25 of these THRs were followed up both clinically and radiologically, whereas the remaining 15 THRs could only be followed up radiologically and over the phone (HHS). Follow-up was not possible for 9 of the patients (deceased, could not be located).

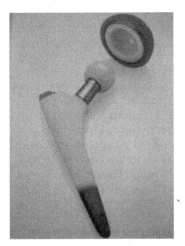

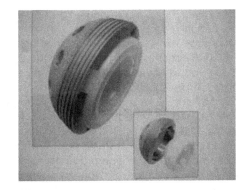

Figure 1:
Anatomic SBG stem (Plus Orthopedics).

Figure 2:
Lima cup (Lima), ceramic inlay on polyethylene (sandwich).

The average follow-up period was 122.5 months (120 months min., 125 months max.). The average age of the patients at the time of surgery had been 52 years (33 years min., 69 years max.). Share of male and female patients: 21 (54%) female and 18 (46%) male patients.

Prior to surgery, the diagnosis specified below had been made:
1. 22 cases of primary coxarthrosis (55%)
2. 9 cases of coxarthrosis resulting from dysplasia (22,5%)
3. 7 cases of secondary coxarthrosis resulting from femoral head necrosis (17.5%)
4. 2 cases of posttraumatic secondary coxarthrosis (5%).

The patients' situation prior to surgery and the postsurgical clinical results were evaluated using the Harris Hip Score (HHS) [2]. The ap and axial II (Sven-Johanson) radiographs taken of the hip joints were taken using a magnification factor of 1.15 as a standard. To evaluate the areas of lysis between the implant and the bone, and osteolysis and bone remodeling in the area of the stem, the area classification system according to Gruen et al [3], and in the area of the acetabulum the area classification system according to DeLee and Charnley [4] were used. For the axial radiographs, the area classification system according to Zweymüller and Samek [5,6] was used. For the assessment of ectopic ossifications, we used the classification system according to Brooker et al [7]. The quantitative measurement of cup migration was described by Nunn et al [8]. Implanted cups must definitely be considered to have loosened if the migration level established for the cup exceeds 3 mm or if measurement of the cup's version or inclination angle yields a change of more than 5°. The surgical approach used was an anterolateral approach according to Watson-Jones [9]. Postsurgically, the patients were administered Indomethacin 90 mg two times a day for a period of one week for the purpose of ectopic ossification prophylaxis, and low molecular heparin (Lovenox) once a day subcutaneously for a period of 6 weeks after the operation for the purpose of thrombosis prevention as described by Wurnig et al [10]. The indirect measurement of inlay wear on the basis of the degree of decentering of the femoral head in the ap radiograph was described by Pieringer et al [11]. This method provides for the distance between the center of the femoral head and the acetabular convexity to be measured on the equator of the acetabular entrance (a, b). The difference between a and b shows the degree of decentering of the femoral head, and serves as an indirect indicator of the degree of inlay wear (Fig. 3).

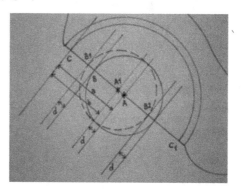

Figure 3:
Removal.
B2C1-B1C=2d=2(AC-A1C).

Clinical results

Presurgical HHS was 36 at average (21 min., 45 max.), and postsurgically (for a period of 10 years) was 86.5 (63 min., 100 max.), which means that there had been an increase by 50.5 notches.

Radiological results

Ectopic ossification (degree I acc. to Brooker) was detected in 4 patients (10%). Minor to moderate osteolysis in the area of the proximal stem was detected in 6 patients (2 times in zone 1, 3 times in zone 8 and 3 times in zone 14 according to Gruen [3]. There weren't any massive areas of osteolysis observed. Formation of seams (radiolucent lines) in the area of the proximal stem was observed in 6 patients (6 times in zone 1, 4 times in zone 13, 1 time in zone 14 according to Gruen [3]). In the area of the stem, there wasn't any stresshilding observed, and in the area of the cup there wasn' t any osteolysis or formation of seams detected (Fig. 4a, b). We did not find any correlation to exist between the formation of seams around the prosthetic stem and the HHS.

In the radiographs, decentering of the femoral head in account of the magnification factor was found to range below 0.5 mm in 3 THRs, and at 0.8 mm in one THR. None of the THRs in this series was subject to revision.

Osteolysis	None		Yes	
Formation of seams	0 mm	1mm	2mm	higher

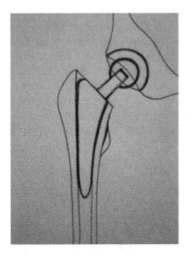

Figure 4a:
Diagrammatic view of lysis zone
classification acc. to Gruen.

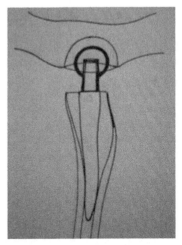

Figure 4b:
Diagrammatic view of lysis zone
classification acc. to Zweymüller and
Samek.

Zone 1:

None	38	Yes	2
39	1	0	0

Zone 8:

None	37	Yes	3
34	6	0	0

Zone 13:

None	40	Yes	0
36	4	0	0

Zone 14:

None	37	Yes	3
39	1	0	0

Discussion

The survival rate of the prosthesis is one of the most important parameters when it comes to evaluation of the materials and design of the prosthesis. If aseptic loosening of the THR is considered to be the final point, the survival rate of both, the stem and the cup after an average period of 120 months has been 100% in our postsurgical examinations. A survival rate of 95.5% was reported by Teloken et al [12] for Monobloc Trilock stems (Depuy, Warsaw, Ind.) and cobalt-chromium femoral components after 10 to 15 years. Pieringer et al [12] reported a survival rate of 98.4% for CSF cups (Centerpulse, Winterthur, Switzerland) and of 100% for SL stems (Centerpulse, Winterthur, Switzerland) which were used together with ceramic-PE couples. In their retrospective comparison of 28 mm and 32 mm femoral heads of the Alloclassic Hip Arthroplasty System, Pieringer et al [12] detected a larger number of osteolysis and seam formations in the area of the proximal stem for 32 mm femoral heads.

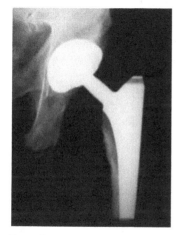

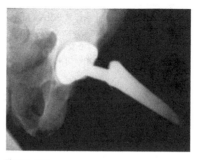

Figure 5b:
Postop. x-ray (axial) of THR (SBG/ Lima) after 10 years.

Figure 5a:
Postop. x-ray (ap) of THR (SBG/ Lima) after 10 years.

Conclusion

The clinical and radiological results obtained from 120 months' follow-up of ceramic-ceramic couples are excellent (Fig. 5a, b). The survival rate obtained for both, the stem and the cup was 100%. Only in as little as 4 cases, minor decentering of the femoral head was observed. Our investigations did not allow for answering the question whether such decentering of the femoral heads was due to ceramic wear or to the ceramic ("sandwich") shell's polyethylene bed.

Reference

1. Pflüger G. Die Wahl der optimalen Gleitpaarung, Jatros Orthopädie 5/2004.
2. Harris WH. Traumatic arthritis of the hip after dislocation and acetabular fractures; treatment by mold arthroplasty. J Bone Joint Surg Am 1969;69:737.

3. Gruen TA, Mc Neice GM, Amstutz HC. „Modes of Failure" of cemented stem-type femoral components. Clin Orthop 1976;141:17.

4. DeLee JG, Charnley J. Radiological demarcation of cemented sockets in total hip replacement. Clin Orthop 1976;121:20.

5. Zweymüller K, Samek V. Radiologische Erkenntnisse der Titaniumpfanne. In: Zweymüller K, editor. 10 Jahre Zweymüller-Hüftendoprothese. Bern: Verlag Hans Huber; 1990:35.

6. Zweymüller K, Samek V. Radiologische Grundphämonene des Titanium-Gradschaftes. In: Zweymüller K, editor. 10 Jahre Zweymüller-Hüftendoprothese. Bern: Verlag Hans Huber; 1990:23.

7. Brooker AF, Bowerman JW, Robinson RA, et al. Ectopic ossification following total hip replacement. J Bone Joint Surg Am 1973;55:1629.

8. Nunn D, Freeman MAR, Hill PF, et al. The measurement of migration of the acetabular component of hip prosthesis. J Bone Joint Surg Br 199;71:629.

9. Bauer R, Kerschbaumer F, Poisel S. Operative Zugangswege in Orthopädie und Traumatologie, 2. Aufl.:Thieme,1990.

10. Wurnig C, Eyb R, Auersperg V. Indomethacin for prevention of ectopic ossification in cementless hip arthroplasties. Acta orthop Scand 1992;63:628.

11. Pieringer H, Auersperg V, Böhler N. Long-term Result of the cementless ALLOCLASSIC hip arthroplasty system using a 28 mm ceramic head. J Arthroplasty 2006 Oct;21(7):967-74.

12. Pieringer H, Auersperg V, Grießler W, et al. Longterm result with the cementless ALLOCLASSIC hip arthroplasty system. J Arthroplasty 2003;18:321.

5B.3 Mid-Term Results of Ceramic-on-Ceramic Bearing Extensively Porous Coated AML® Total Hip Arthroplasty

K.-H. Moon, J.-S. Kang, D.-J. Lee, S.-H. Lee and K.-H. Kim

Abstract

Purpose: This study evaluated the mid term results of primary total hip arthroplasty using a ceramic-on-ceramic bearing extensively porous coated implant.

Materials and Methods: Between April 2001 and August 2004, THA using a ceramic on ceramic bearing cementless implant was performed on 140 cases (131 patients). Among these cases, 138 hips form 129 patients, who were followed up for more than three years were evaluated. The average age was 51.2 years (19-84). The initial diagnosis included osteonecrosis of the femoral head in 87 cases, primary osteoarthritis in 9 cases, pyogenic arthritis sequelae in 9 cases, traumatic osteoarthritis in 8 cases, acetabular dysplasia in 7 cases, femoral neck fractures in 6 cases, an ankylosed hip in 5 cases, and others diagnoses in 7 cases.

Results: On the last X-ray, there was no sign of loosening of the acetabular cup. However, one femoral stem was definitely loose and four femoral stems were possibly loose. The other femoral stems were fixed well by bone ingrowth, and there was no case of osteolysis. Chip fracture of the ceramic liner occurred intraoperatively in 2 cases.

Posterior dislocation occurred 3 weeks after surgery in one case, anterior dislocation with a ceramic liner dissociation occurred 6 weeks after surgery in one case and fracture of the ceramic head occurred 15 months after surgery in one case.

Conclusion: The mid-term results of ceramic-on-ceramic bearing extensively porous coated implant were reasonable. However, a long term follow up will be needed to determine the overall results.

Introduction

Osteolysis is a serious complication that develops after total hip arthroplasty, and has been reported to be a common cause of treatment failure. This is primarily the result of biological reactions caused by wear particles from the polyethylene liner within the acetabulum [23,24]. There are three methods for reducing the amount of ware particles, highly cross-linked polyethylene, metal on metal articulation, and ceramic-on-ceramic articulation. Metal-on-metal has been used since the early 1960s but the early cases did not show a good result. Recently, numerous metal-on-metal articulations have been developed and are used frequently [30]. Nonetheless, the potential local or systemic side effects of the metals are of some concern. It has been reported that metal particles at low concentrations stimulate macrophages and the release of various intracellular mediators [18]. Moreover, chrome particles have been detected in the lymph nodes in the vicinity of the aorta [30], and cardiomyopathy has been also reported [28]. The period of the clinical applications of highly cross-linked polyethylene is short. Therefore, substantial time will be required to determine its effectiveness.

Ceramics have advantages in that it is biomechanically stable, hard and the friction coefficient of its contact areas is low. In addition, the wear of ceramic-on-ceramic articulation is quite low, and it has been reported that even if wear occurs, is the particles produced are inert in vivo, which suggests few if any systemic side effects [1,27]. Ceramic implants have been used in the articulation of artificial hip joints since the early 1970s. However, during the early period, problems such as the loosening of prosthesis, ceramic head fracture, etc. were encountered [4]. Recently, improved ceramics have been used in clinics with satisfactory results [21]. This study reports the mid-term follow up results after the primary total hip arthroplasty using the ceramic-on-ceramic bearing cementless extensively porous coated implants.

Materials and Methods

The patient group

From April 2001 to August 2004, total hip arthroplasty was performed consecutively on 140 hip joints of 131 patients using a ceramic-on-ceramic bearing extensively porous coated implant (AML® ,Dupey, Warsaw, Indiana).

Their preoperative diagnosis was as follows: 89 cases of avascular necrosis of the femoral head, 9 cases of primary degenerative osteoarthritis, 9 cases of septic hip sequelae, 8 cases of traumatic arthritis, 7 cases of acetabular dysplasia, 6 cases of femoral neck fracture, 5 cases of an ankylosed hip, 3 cases of rheumatoid arthritis, 2 cases of LCP sequelae, and 2 cases of tuberculosis hip sequelae.

The 2 cases of avascular necrosis of the femoral head, who were unavailable for a follow-up of more than 3 years, were excluded. Overall, 138 cases (129 patients) were analyzed. There were 80 males and 49 females with a mean age at the time of surgery of 51.2 years (19 years – 84 years). The mean follow up period was 45.6 months (36 months – 76 months).

Prosthesis

In all cases, the extensively porous coated cobalt chrome alloy cementless type AML® implants were used as the femoral stem.

Dularoc® option cups (Dupey, Warsaw, Indiana) were used as acetabular cups. The material was a titanium alloy and was mixed with a ceramic liner using the Sensor locking-ring method. The external surface of the acetabular cup was coated extensively with a porous layer, had 3 screw holes, and no screws were used except in 2 cases.

The third generation ceramics BIOLOX® forte (Ceramtec, Plochingen, Germany) was used as the ceramic liner and femoral head.

Surgical methods and postoperative treatments

In all patients, the first author performed surgery through the posterolateral approach.

For 6 weeks after surgery, the abduction of the hip joint was maintained, and adduction and internal rotation and more than 90 degrees flexion were avoided.

From one week after surgery, walking using crutches and partial weight bearing were permitted, and weight bearing was increased up to 6 weeks using crutches and walking aids. Unless special complications had developed, full weight bearing was allowed from 3 months. Follow ups were performed by an physical examination and simple radiography at the outpatient clinic 6 weeks, 3 months, 6 months and 1 year after surgery, and every year thereafter.

Clinical evaluation

The Harris hip score was measured before surgery and at the last follow up and compared. The cases with more than 90 points were classified as excellent, between 80 points and 90 points as good, between 70 points and 80 points as fair, and lower than 70 points as poor.

In addition, the presence of limping, whether walking aids were required, the presence of the thigh pain were evaluated at the last follow up.

Radiological evaluation

At the last follow up, the level of stress shielding on the simple radiographs was classified into 4 levels according to the standard established by Engh et al [8]. The demarcation radiolucent line in the vicinity of the femoral prosthesis, osteolysis were analyzed by dividing it into 14 areas according to Gruen et al [10]. Osteolysis in the vicinity of the femoral prosthesis was defined as a case with a progressive lesion on the follow up radiographs that was absent immediately after surgery and a radiolucent line contacting the prosthesis more than 2 mm continuously [15].

The fixation condition of the femoral prosthesis was classified as stable bone ingrowth, stable fibrous ingrowth, and unstable fixation using the method reported by Engh et al [8].

Demarcation radiolucent lines and osteolysis in the vicinity of the acetabular cup were classified by dividing the cup into 3 areas according to DeLee and Charnley [7].

Osteolysis in the vicinity of the acetabular cup was defined as a case with continuous radiolucent line more than 2 mm [15]. The wear of the articular surface was measured by comparing the radiographs taken immediately after surgery with the radiographs taken during the recent follow up by applying the computer assisted vector wear analysis program (University of Chicago, Orthopedic Surgery, Hip analysis program version 4.0) developed by Martell et al [19].

Results

Clinical evaluation

The Harris hip score was improved from an average 53.6 points (35-75) preoperatively to an average 95.3 points (78-98) at the last follow up, and 126 cases (91.3 %) were excellent, 10 cases (7.2 %) were good, and 2 cases (1.5 %) were fair. Nine patients (6.5 %) showed limping at the last follow up and 3 patients (2.2 %) presented with thigh pain. None of the patients required walking aids.

Radiological results

A change in bone density caused by stress shielding of the femoral prosthesis was detected in 58 cases (42 %). According to the classification reported by Engh et al., there were 57, 2 and 1 case of grade 1, 2 and 3, respectively. There was no case of grade 4.

Radiolucent lines in the vicinity of the femoral prosthesis were detected in 47 cases (34.1 %), and primarily in the zone 1, 4, and 11. In 1 case (0.7 %), significant aseptic loosening and instability of the femoral prosthesis was detected, possible loosening or stable fibrous ingrowth findings was detected in 4 cases (2.8 %), and bone ingrowth was observed in the remaining cases.

A radiolucent line in the acetabular side was detected in 1 case (0.7 %), and there was no case of osteolysis or the migration of the acetabular cup. In addition, there was no case of detectable wear of the articular surface.

Complications

There were 2 cases (1.4 %) of chip fracture of the ceramic liner (Fig. 1); the acetabular cup and the liner were exchanged in one case. In one case, the chip fracture was not associated with the articulation, and was used without exchanging.

Posterior dislocation occurred in 1 case 3 weeks after surgery, which was treated by a closed reduction under general anesthesia and the wearing of an abduction brace for 6 weeks. No redislocation occurred during the 45 months follow up period.

In 1 case (0.7 %), anterior dislocation with the concomitant dissociation of the ceramic liner developed 6 weeks after surgery (Fig. 2), which was treated by revision surgery of the hip joint, and an exchange of the acetabular cup, the ceramic liner and the artificial ceramic head. In 1 case (0.7 %), a ceramic head fracture developed 15 months after surgery (Fig. 3) without a trauma history. The ceramic liner and the artificial ceramic head were exchanged by revision surgery.

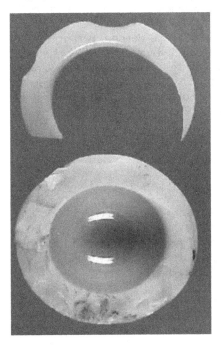

Figure 1:
Intraoperative chip fracture of ceramic liner.

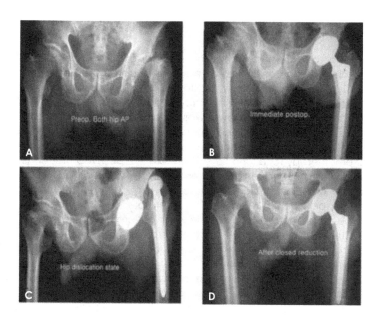

Figure 2:

56 year-old man with secondary coxarthrosis.
A: Initial radiograph reveals finding of sequela of pyogenic coxarthrosis.
B: Immediate postoperative radiograph.
C: Anterior dislocation with liner dissociation of the right hip occured 6 weeks after operation.
D: Radiograph after revision of ceramic head and liner.

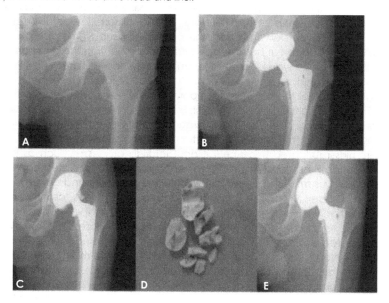

Figure 3:

64 year-old man with avascular necrosis of left femoral head.
A: Initial radiograph reveals finding of avascular necrosis of left femoral head.
B: Immediate postoperative radiograph.
C: Fracture of ceramic femoral head occured 15 months after operation.
D: Photograph shows the fractured ceramic femoral head.
E: Radiograph after revision of ceramic head and liner.

Discussion

It has been reported that the stable fixation of the implant fixation can be obtained using cementless type extensive porous coated total hip arthroplasty. [14,17,20,22]. In this study, unstable aseptic loosening of the femoral stem developed in 1 case (0.7 %), fibrous stable fixation was obtained in 4 cases (2.9 %), and stable bony ingrowth was obtained in the remaining 133 cases (96.4%). One case, which showed aseptic loosening of the femoral implant, was diagnosed with a lymphoma 6 weeks after surgery and had been receiving chemotherapy for a long time. Therefore, it is believed that bone ingrowth could not be achieved due to the chemotherapy. It was difficult to measure the wear of the articular surface because the required shadow of the femoral head overlapped with the liner shadow. Therefore, new measurement methods need to be developed to measure the wear of ceramic-on-ceramic articulation.

Currently, there are two types of ceramic acetabular liner used. One is a one piece type in which a ceramic liner is bound directly to the metal cup, and the other is a so called sandwich type in which the ceramic liner is coated with polyethylene, and polyethylene contacts the metal cup directly [15]. Ceramics have the advantage of less abrasion due to their strong hardness. However, such strong hardness means that the excessive dynamic stress delivered from the joint accessory to the bone during each gait cycle cannot be absorbed by the implant. Therefore, good outcomes of ceramic one piece type liner have only been reported in young patients with good bone quality [25,26]. On the other hand, according to Dalla et al. [5] the hardness of the sandwich type decreased by more 30 times compared with the one piece type because of the intercalation of the polyethylene layer. Therefore, it can absorb impact by releasing the excessive tension delivered from the acetabular cup to the acetabulum during walking. In addition, it has the advantage of preventing the main disadvantage of the one piece type in terms of jamming of the liner in cases with a margin area that is damaged during surgery or an erroneous direction. Nevertheless, cases with a dissociation of the ceramics and polyethylene have been reported [29].

The ceramic particles of the first generation and the second generation ceramics used in the past were large. Therefore, the hardness of the ceramics was weak and the rate of destruction was high. However, the third generation ceramics fabricated using new manufacturing processes, such as hot isostatic processing, the laser marking, a nondestructive proof-testing have been produced as small size ceramic crystals with high purity and density.

The incidence of the ceramic fracture in previous ceramic-on-ceramic articulation were of considerable concern [15]. Before 1985, it was reported that ceramic femoral head fracture occurred in 13.4 % of cases [16]. However, this was considered to be due to problems that developed during the ceramic manufacturing process and the incompatibility of the moth taper. The cause of the previous ceramic breakage of ceramic-on-ceramic articulation was the low quality ceramics, the use of a skirt type femoral head, the poor location of the acetabular cup. Therefore, the risk of ceramic breakage of artificial joints made from the improved ceramics is anticipated to be low. However, ceramic fractures have been reported studies.

Hasegawa et al. [13] reported ceramic fracture concentrated in the stress of the liner rim 16 months after surgery, and Garino et al. [9] reported ceramic fracture in 3 cases out of 35 follow up cases. Yoo et al. [33] reported that ceramic fracture occurred only in 1 out of 93 cases after a motorcycle accident. Technical problem involving inadequate placement of the ceramic insert and a difficult intraoperative reduction due to high soft tissue can cause a chip fracture of the ceramic insert [6,9,32]. In addition, the impingement of the ceramic head and the liner caused by frequent subluxation and dislocation might be another cause of segmental fracture [11]. Small pieces generated can induce excessive abrasion and ultimately increase the possibility of ceramic fracture [33]. It is believed that the ceramic head fracture that developed in this study was caused by excessive muscle force due to sudden standing. In the 2 cases of chip fracture of the ceramic liner, the rim of the cup was hit hard by a cup impactor to alter the position of the acetabular cup during the stability test after inserting the titanium metal cup. Hence, it was considered that the shape of the metal cup was altered. Therefore, hitting the rim of cup with a cup impactor should be avoided. The dissociation of the ceramic liner that developed simultaneously with the anterior dislocation of the joint is believed to be caused by the gravity generated by continuous walking of the patient after the anterior dislocation of the hip joint.

Conclusion

The result of a mid-term follow up of ceramic-on-ceramic total hip arthroplasty showed relatively satisfactory outcomes but a longer term follow up will be needed.

References

1. Archibeck MJ, Jacobs JJ and Black J : Alternative bearing surface in total joint arthroplasty: Biologic consideration. Clin Orthop, 379: 12-21, 2000.
2. Bands R, Pelker RR, Shine J, Bradburn H, Margolis R and Leach J : The noncemented porous-coated hip prosthesis. Clin Orthop, 269:209-219, 1989.
3. Bhler M, Mochida Y, Bauer TW, Plenk H and Salzer M : Wear debris from two different alumina-on-alumina total hip arthroplasties. J Bone Joint Surg, 82-B: 901-909, 2000.
4. Clarke IC and Willmann G: Structural ceramics in orthopedics. In: Cameron(ed). Bone Implant Interface. St Louis, Mosby:203-252, 1994.
5. Dalla PP and Bregant L Di MF: Stiffness of the acetabular cup: A comparative study using the finite element method. Proceedings of the 2nd Symposium on Ceramic Wear Couple, Stuttgart. Enke, Stuttgart:136-138, 1997.
6. D. Antonio J, Capello W, Manley M and Bierbaum B : New experience with alumina-on-alumina ceramic bearing for total hip arthroplasty. J arthroplasty, 17:390-397, 2002.
7. DeLee JG and Charnley J: Radiological demarcation of cemented sockets in total hip replacement. Clin Orthop, 121:20-32, 1976.
8. Engh CA, Bobyn JD and Glassman AH: Porous-coated hip replacement. The factors governing bone ingrowth, stress shielding, and clinical results. J Bone Joint Surg, 69-B:45-55, 1987.
9. Garino JP : Modern ceramic-on-ceramic total hip system in the United States. Clin Orthop, 379:41-47, 2000.
10. Gruen TA, McNeice GM and Amstutz HC: "Modes of failure" of cemented stem-type femoral components: a radiographic analysis of loosening. Clin Orthop, 141:17-27, 1979.
11. Hannouche D, Nich C, Bizot P, Meunier A, Nizard R and Sedel L : Fracture of ceramic bearings: history and present status. Clin Orthop, 417:19-26, 2000.

12. Harris WH: The problem is osteolysis. Clin Orthop, 311: 46-53, 1995.

13. Hasegawa M, Sudo A, Hirata H and Uchida A : Ceramic acetabular liner fracture in total hip arthroplasty with a ceramic sandwich cup. J arthroplasty, 18:658-661, 2003.

14. Keisu KS, Oronzco F, Sharkey PF, Hozack WJ and Rothman RH : Primary cementless total hip arthroplasty in octogenerians. J Bone Joint Surg, 83-A:359-363, 2001.

15. Kim YM and Kim SR: Short term Results of Ceramic-on-Ceramic Bearing Bicontact Total Hip Arthroplasty. J Korean Hip Society, 13:1-7, 2001.

16. Knahr K, B Hler M, Frank P, Plenk H and Salzer M: Survival analysis of an uncemented ceramic acetabular component in total hip replacement. Acta Orthop Trauma Surg, 106:297-300,1987.

17. Konstantoulakis C, Anastopoulos G, Papaeliou A, et al : Uncemented total hip arthroplasty in the elderly. Int Orthop, 23:334-336, 1999.

18. Lee SH,Brennan FR, Jacobs JJ, Urban RM, Ragasa DR and Glant TT: Human moncyte/macrophage response to cobalt-chromium corrosion products and titanium particles in patients with total joint replacement. J Orthop Res, 15:40-49, 1997.

19. Martell JM, Berdia SM : Determination of polyethylene wear in total hip replacements with use of digital radiographs. J Bone Joint Surg, 79-A:1635-1641, 1997.

20. McAuley JP, Moore KD, Culpepper WJ 2nd and Engh CA : Total hip arthroplasty with porous-coated prosthesis fixed without cement in patients who are 65 years of age or older. J Bone Joint Surg, 80-A:1648-1655, 1998.

21. Nizard RS, Sedel L, Christal P, Meunier A, Soudry M and Witvoet J: Ten-year survivorship of cemented ceramic-cermic total hip prosthesis. Clin Orthop, 282:53-63, 1992.

22. Purtill JJ, Rothman RH, Hozack WJ and Sharkey PF : Total hip arthroplasty using two different cementless taperd stems. Clin Orthop, 393:121-127, 2001.

23. Santacirta S, Nordstrom D, Metsarinne K and Konttinen YT : Biocompatibility of polyethylene and host response to loosening of cementless total hip replacement. Clin Orthop, 297:100-110, 1993.

24. Schmalzried TP, Jasty M and Harris WH: Periprosthetic bone loss in total hip arthroplasty. Polyethylene wear debris and the concept of the effective joint space. J Bone Joint Surg, 74-A: 849-863, 1992

25. Sedel L : Ceramic hips. J Bone Joint Surg,74B:331-332, 1992.

26. Sedel L, Nizard R, Bizot P and Meunier A: Perspective on a 20-year experience with ceramic-on-ceramic articulation in total hip replacement. Semin Arthroplasty, 9:123-134, 1998.

27. Sharkey PF, Barrack RL and Tvedten DEL: Five year clinical and radiologic follow up of the uncemented long-term stable fixation total hip arthroplasty. J arthroplasty, 13:645-551, 1998.

28. Sullivan JF, George R, Bluvas R and Egan JD: Myocardiopathy of beer drinker. Subsequent course, Ann Intern Med, 70:277-282, 1969.

29. Hwang SK, Jeon JS and Lee BH: Ceramic on sandwich ceramic bearing primary cementless total hip arthroplasty. J Korean Orthop Assoc. ;39:679-85, 2004.

30. Urban R, Jacobs J and tomlinson M : Particles of metal alloys and their corrosion products in the liver, spleen and para-aortic lymph nodes of patients with total hip replacement prostheses. Trans Orthop Res Soc, 20:241-248, 1995.

31. Wagner M and Wagner H: Medium-term results of a modern metal-on-metal system in total hip replacement. Clin Orthop, 379:123-133, 2000.

32. Yoo JJ, Kim HJ, Kim YM : Damage of an alumina-on-alumina bearing surface from a difficult reduction of a total hip arthroplasty. A report of three cases. J Bone Joint Surg, 86-A:376-378, 2004.

33. Yoo JJ, Kim YM, Yoon KS, Koo KH, Song WS and Kim HJ : Alumina-on-alumina total hip arthroplasty. J Bone Joint Surg, 87-A:530-535, 2005.

5B.4 Alumina-on-Alumina Total Hip Arthroplasty in Patients with Osteonecrosis less than 50 Years Old

S.-Y. Kim

Introduction

The results of total hip arthroplasty (THA) in patients with osteonecrosis less than 50 years old are less durable. The purpose is to report the 5-year minimum follow-up results of THA with contemporary alumina-on-alumina bearing.

Methods

TWe evaluated the results of a consecutive series of 68 alumina-on-alumina THAs that had been performed with use of a metal-backed cementless socket and a cementless stem in 59 patients by a single surgeon. The mean age of the patients was less was 39 years old (range, 16-49). The mean duration of follow-up was 6 years (range, 5 to 9 years). Preoperative associated factors included idiopathic in 21 hips, alcohol abuse in 28, steroid induced in 11, and posttraumatic in 8 hips.

Results

The mean Harris hip score was 95 points at the time of the latest follow-up evaluation. Noises were found in 3 patients. There was no squeaking in any patient. All acetabular and femoral components demonstrated radiographic evidence of stable by bony ingrowth. Ceramic wear was not detectable. Periprosthetic osteolysis was not observed in any hip. There was no fracture of the alumina head or peripheral chip fracture of the alumina insert. There were 2 nonrecurrent dislocations.

Conclusion

The results of contemporary alumina-on-alumina THA with a metal-backed socket and a cementless stem were perfect after 5-year minimum follow-up. We believe contemporary alumina-on-alumina bearing offer a promising option for younger, active patients with osteonecrosis of the femoral head.

5B.5 Total Hip Arthroplasty using third Generation Alumina-on-Alumina Articulation

K.-H. Koo

In 1970, Boutin introduced ceramic-on-ceramic total hip arthroplasty (THA) [1]. The ceramic-on-ceramic articulation has the lowest wear rate among various articulations [2]. Ceramic particles induced less macrophage reaction and decreased cytokine secretion compared with particles of high-density polyethylene [3] and THA with use of the ceramic-on-ceramic articulation showed little periprosthetic osteolysis [1].

Early ceramic prostheses combined an alumina head and conically-threaded 'monobloc' or spherical press-fit cup. However, insufficient fixation of the acetabular component appeared to be a problem of the early ceramic prostheses. Besides, early generations of ceramic articulations frequently were associated with ceramic implant fracture and excessive wear [1]. In 1990's, modular acetabular system with a taper fixation between the metal shell and ceramic liner has been introduced to obtain sound acetabular component fixation. In addition, hot isostatic pressing has been introduced to improve the material property of ceramic implants [1].

In our department, third generation alumina-on-alumina articulations have been used in total hip arthroplasty since 1997.

In 2005 and 2007, we reported the results of 178 total hip arthroplasties with use of third generation alumina-on-alumina articulation after a minimum duration of follow-up of five years. The acetabular component was a hemispherical titanium and the femoral component was a porous coated titanium stem.

A 28-mm alumina femoral head and alumina acetabular insert (BIOLOX® forte, CeramTec AG) were used. At the final followup evaluation, all acetabular and femoral components were bone-ingrown, and neither pelvic nor femoral osteolysis was identified. Wear of the ceramic components was undetectable. A fracture of the alumina femoral head and a peripheral chip fracture of the alumina insert occurred in one hip following a motor-vehicle accident [4,5]. I was very encouraged with the early results of the third generation alumina-on-alumina articulations and continued to use this bearing surface in THA.

Between July 1999 to June 2001, I used sandwich-type acetabular components in 157 primary cementless THA. The sandwich-type acetabular components (BIOLOX® forte, CeramTec AG) had polyethylene between a ceramic liner and metal shell and was expected to reduce the rigidity of the ceramic-on-ceramic bearing and absorb excessive loads on articulation [6]. The acetabular cup was a porous-coated hemispherical titanium cup and the femoral component was a tapered, rectangular, grit-blasted, titanium alloy stem. A 28 mm diameter alumina head (BIOLOX® forte, CeramTec AG) was used in all patients. One hundred and forty-four hips had follow-up study for an average of 45 months. All acetabular cups and femoral stems were radiographically stable at last followup. Five hips in five patients (3.5%) were revised because of the ceramic liner fracture. Ceramic liner fractures occurred at a mean of 35 months (range, 24–48 months) postoperatively. These ceramic liner fractures seemed to be associated with impingement associated with excessive anteversion of the acetabular cup in patients who habitually squatted [7].

Betwen July 2001 and October 2003, we performed a multicenter study including 312 patients (367 hips) who underwent cementless alumina-on-alumina THA with the use of 28-mm BIOLOX® *forte* femoral head and BIOLOX® *forte* liner at four participating centers. Three hundred and five patients (359 hips) were evaluated at a mean of 45 months postoperatively. All of the acetabular cups and femoral stems had radiographic evidence of bone ingrown stability. Periprosthetic osteolysis was not detected around any implant. However, five hips (1.4%) were revised because of the ceramic head fracture during the follow-up period. The fracture was detected during normal daily activities from 12 to 31 months (mean, 22.6 months) after the index THA and no patient had any unusual impact loading or trauma. All five fractures occurred in hips that had short neck alumina heads, while there was no fracture in hips that had medium or long neck head. The fracture pattern suggested that the mechanism of ceramic head fracture is a brittle fracture after the use of the short neck head.

During last ten years we have used contemporary alumina-on-alumina THA and we believe that this articulation offers a promising option for younger, active patients. However, we are still concerned about the possibility of ceramic component fracture.

References

1. Sedel L. Evolution of alumina-on-alumina implants: a review. Clin Orthop Relat Res. 2000;379:48-54.
2. Dorlot JM: Long-term effects of alumina components in total hip prostheses. Clin Orthop Relat Res. 1992;282:47-52.
3. Catelas I, Petit A, Marchand R, Zukor DJ, Yahia L, Huk OL: Cytotoxicity and macrophage cytokine release induced by ceramic and polyethylene particles in vitro. J Bone J Surg Br. 1999;81:516-521.
4. Yoo JJ, Kim YM, Yoon KS, Koo KH, Song WS, Kim HJ: Alumina-on-alumina total hip arthroplasty. A five-year minimum follow-up study. J Bone Joint Surg Am. 2005;87:530-535.
5. Ha YC, Koo KH, Jeong ST, Joon Yoo J, Kim YM, Joong Kim H. Cementless alumina-on-alumina total hip arthroplasty in patients younger than 50 years: a 5-year minimum follow-up study. J Arthroplasty. 2007;22:184-188.
6. Hannouche D, Nich C, Bizot P, Meunier A, Nizard R, Sedel L. Fracture of ceramic bearings. History and present status. Clin Othop Relat Res. 2003;417:19-26.
7. Ha YC, Kim SY, Kim HJ, Yoo JJ, Koo KH. Ceramic liner fracture after cementless alumina-on-alumina total hip arthroplasty. Clin Orthop Relat Res. 2007;458:106-110.

5B.6 Ceramic on Ceramic in Hybrid THR (Cemented Femoral Stem) – A five to seven year evalution

S.-J. Yim

Between 2000 and 2002, We implanted 89 hybrid alumina-on-alumina hip arthroplasties in 85 consecutive patients. The prostheses involved a cemented stainless steel (orthinox®) stem, 28, 32mm alumina head, and a porous coated metal-backed socket with an alumina insert.

We evaluated survival rate, implant- and non-implant-related complications. Clinical outcomes included the Merle d'Aubigné score. We assessed radiographs for the signs of osteolys, component loosening, and implant wear. No patients had osteolysis and there were no hip dislocations. One patient (one hip) died from unrelated causes. Three hips had revision surgery for either deep infection, unexplained pain or aseptic loosening of the socket. The six-year survival rate was 96.6% with revision for any cause as the end-point There was a 2.3% incidence of implant-related complications. Our data showed low aseptic revision rates and low revision rates for instability. Total hip arthroplasty using alumina ceramic-on-ceramic implant is a safe and reliable procedure. Especially these hybrid arthroplasty gave satisfactory mid-term results. The porous coated metal-backed socket appeared to have reliable fixation in alumina ceramic-on-ceramic hip arthroplasty. The excellent resulls using cemented fixation of the stem may be related the low production of wear debris.

Hybrid total hip arthroplasty (THA), combining a cemented stem and a cementless socket, is an alternative to a fully cemented or cementless arthroplasty. The main argument for the hybrid configuration is concern about the long-term fixation of the cemented all-polyethylene cup. Although progress in cementing techniques has significantly improved the fixation of implants, this improvement has been more significant for the stem than for the socket. A survival rate for a cemented slem of over 90% after more than seven years' follow-up is common. Other arguments include the uncertainty about the long-term result of modern uncemented stems and the promising results obtained with the new generation of cementless metal-backed socket. With the increasing durability of fixation, polyethylene wear has become a major limiting factor, especially in young and active patients.

The alumina-on-alumina couple was introduced in the 1970s in order to suppress wear and its consequences. Initially, the main limiting factors were the failure of fixation of the socket and the risk of fracture of the component. During the last decade the quality of the materials has improved significantly and the risk of fracture reduced. Consequently, fixation of the socket became the weak link of an alumina-on-alumina arthroplasty. Since 2000, we have used a press-fit metal-backed socket with an alumina insert.

The aim of our study was to present the results of this hybrid alumina arthroplasty, comprising a press-fit metal-backed socket and a cemented collarless stem, which was implanted between 2000 and 2002 in a active patients.

Materials and Methods

Between 2000 and 2002, we implanted 89 hybrid alumina-on-alumina hip arthroplasties in 85 consecutive patients, The criteria for exclusion from the study were a history of infection of the hip or failure of a previous THA. Four procedures were bilateral. The mean age of the patients at the time of surgery was 63 years (37 to 78.)

The pre-operative diagnosis is shown in Table 1. There were all primary procedures. The prostheses were a cemented stainless steel (orthinox®) stem, 28, 32mm alumina head and a metal-backed socket with an alumina insert.

We evaluated survival rate, implant-and non implant-related complications.

Diagnosis	Number of patients
Atraumatic osteonecrosis	34
Osteoarthritis	18
Sequelae of a congenital dislocated Hip	8
Fracture of the proximal femur	6
Inflammatory disease	4
Sequelae of fracture of the acetabulum	3
Sequelae of LCP	3

Table 1:
The pre-operative diagnoses for the 85 patients (89 hips), aged less than 63 years, who received a hybrid alumina THA using porous coated metal-backed socket.

The main diagnosis was atraumatic osteonecrosis (34 patients), which 18 patients had primary osteoarthritis or osteoarthritis secondary to minimal hip dyslpasia (18 patients).

THA was all primary procedure the operation was undertaken through the modified Hardinge lateral approach.

All patients received the same design of prosthesis (Exeter®), manufactured by Howmedica (Benoist-Girard, France). The prostheses comprised a cemented, collarless, Smooth polished stem of stainless steel alloy (orthinox®), a 28, 32mm alumina head and porous coated hemispheric metal-backed socket with an alumina insert (Secure fit®).

The stem was cemented with low viscosity cemented after insertion of an intramedullary polyethylene plug. The cement was introduced with cement gun and pressurised about 5 minutes using proximal seal before inserting the stem. The socket comprised a titanium shell with screw holes covered with HA coated porous coated. Partial weight-bearing was allowed on the second post-operative day, and full weight-bearing after four to six weeks.

Clinical results were analysed with the Merle d'Aubigné and Postel function score [24]. Radiological analysis included radiolucent lines around both the socket and the stem according to DeLee & Charnley Zone and Gruen Zone respectively. Migration of the components and periprosthetic osteolysis were also recorded. For the survival analysis we used both the actuarial and Greenwood methods in order to calculate the confidence between different groups was calculated using the log-rank test with a probability level of $p < 0.05$.

Results

One patient (one hip) with excellent result at the last follow-up, died at two years post-operatively from unrelated causes. Early complications included one patient with deep vein thrombosis, one with a femoral nerve palsy with complete recovery, and two with dislocation which did not recur.

Three patients (three hip: 3.4%) underwent revision of their THA. A 60-year-old man with a destructive hip lesion of unknown origin developed a deep infection due to Staphylococcus aureus within three months of surgery and underwent a two-stage revision.

Another patient underwent a revision of the socket 2 years after THA for persistent pain which may have been caused by anterior impingement of the shell with iliopsoas.

The socket was well fixed, but was changed to porous coated metal backed cup.

A 62-year-old obese woman sustained aseptic loosening of the socket about 3 years. At revision, the porous coated cup, although broken was partially integrated into the acetabular bone. The stem was well fixed and was retained. The socket was changed to porous coated metal backed cup with bone graft with a very good result 2 years post operatively.

Survival analysis

Taking revision for any reason as the end-point the overall survival rate was 96.6% at six years. Taking revision for aseptic loosening as the end-point, the overall six-years survivorship was 98.9% with a survival rate of 98.9% for the socket and 100% for the stem (Fig.1a, b).

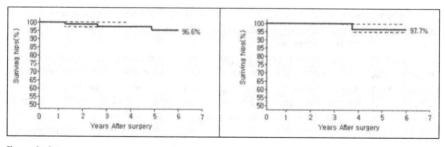

Figure 1a,b:
Actuarial survivorship curves with the upper and lower limits of the 95% confidence interval.
a: Revision for any reason as the end-point and
b: revision for aseptic loosening as the end-point

Clinical and radiological outcomes

The results were assessed in the surviving patients with a minimum following of years. Excluding those who died (one patient, one hip), and those who underwent revision (three patients, three hips), 81 surviving patients (85 hips) were available for final assessment. All had clinical and radiological assessment at the last follow-up.

The mean follow-up, the mean Merle d'Aubigné and Postel score was 14.58 (13 to 15) compared with 8.65 (6 to 9) pre-operatively.

The outcome was excellent in 57 hips (67.1%), very good in 12 (14.1%), good in 16 (18.8%).

At the last follow-up 60 patients remained employed, and 25 patients were unemploved.

Radiological data were documented in 81 patients (85 hips), There were no abnormalities in 54 sockets but 31 (37%) had a thin and partial lucent line, mainly localized to Charnley and DeLee zone III. One patient, with an excellent result at six years, has a non-progressive complete lucency around the socket.

It was less than 1mm thick, and there was no detectable migration, acetabular osteolysis. Five stem (6%) had isolated and partial lucencies that involved two to four zones.

In one hip with an excellent clinical result there was femoral osteolysis.

This was in a 64-yaer-old man who had undergone THA for post-traumatic osteoarthritis and had required acetabular reconstruction with an autograft fixed with screws. Six years post-operatively, femoral osteolysis was visible in Guren Zone II and III, associated with partial lucencies around the stem. He was symptom-free.

Discussion

Despite improvements in technique and design of the components, the results of THA are less satisfactory in younger patients. Accelerated polyethylene wear due to increased activity in the younger patient is assumed to be the principal mechanism of failure.

One can argue that age and levels of activity vary widely in any series of arthroplasty in younger patients, so that correlations between age, activity and polyethylene wear are not precise. We have used this femoral component with the same cementing technique since 1995. The overall survival rate, 95% after 10 years, is even better in younger patients.

The use of the so-called second generation cementing technique offers excellent results which compare favourably with other series. This demonstrates the optimal design of the stem and the greater resistance to wear of alumina.

The hybrid alumina-on-alumina hip prosthesis, which uses a porous coated metal-backed excellent results in the medium-term. A significant improvement in fixation of the alumina socket has been obtained with the use of a hemispheric porous coated metal-backed component. The differences in the initial diagnosis between older and younger patient may also influence the final outcome. Many studies into the use of cemented or cementless designs have reported a higher rate of osteolysis in young people and have recognised polyethylene wear as the principal cause of long-term failure in these patients. Our results support this conclusion. Compared with conventional THA in younger patients, the reduction of wear achieved by using alumina appears to give better results. These results are comparable to those reported at a similar follow-up for older patients. A flaw in our study may be the limited follow-up and the age limit of 55 years, as this may represent a middle-aged rather than a younger population. All the patients were active and the majority were either employed or involved in some sporting activities.

Alumina wear was impossible to measure on serial radiographs and special attention was, therefore, paid to the occurrence of osteolysis. Individual instances of femoral osteolysis after alumina hip replacement have been reported in the literature, although all were associated with the Mittlemeier design. Yoon et al have reported a high rate of so-called linear femoral osteolysis. These were thick radiolucent lines or bone-implant demarcation which corresponded to a fibrocytic reaction without osteoclastic activity on histological analysis. This might reflect the poor design of the prosthesis with poor fixation and high contact alumina stresses due to impingement with the mushroom-shaped alumina head. In our study, no osteolysis occurred around the acetabluar component and femoral osteolysis was only seen in one patient who had undergone massive acetabular reconstruction. Animal studies and histological analysis of pseudomembranes from loosened alumina cups suggest that this unexpected osteolysis was probably particles. Metal abrasion might occur between the shell and the screws which hold the acetabular graft or be due to fretting of the stem.

The main consideration when using a hybrid combination was concern about the fixation of the alumina socket. In the past, failure of this fixation was the commonest indication for revision of an alumina hip replacement. Many methods of fixation have been explored, both cemented and cementless, and it was concluded that failure was not wear-dependent, but was related to poor design or to the material, especially its high rigidity and biologically inert nature. This compromised the fixation of cemented or press-fit, plain alumina socket. Press-fit metal-backed sockets have been introduced in order to obtain durable fixation through direct bone ingrowth and to reduce the peak stresses in both the acetabular bone and the liner. Promising results have been reported in metal-polyethylene hip replacements with the use of hemispherical, porous-coated metal backed shells, although additional problems due to modularity of the socket have been noted. Our results are satisfactory and show a significant improvement in fixation of the socket when compared with earlier series of alumina-on-alumina arthroplasties. We encountered no problems related to the modularity of the socket. The locking mechanism of the alumina insert with its conical sleeving appeared to be safe and reliable, provided that a careful technique was used. The latter thus required a more horizontal position of the shell in order to reduce peak stresses in the alumina insert and to minimize wear. Great attention was paid to cleaning the interior of the metal-backed shell, and to position the insert correctly before seling it by gentle hammering.

Excellent results were obtained with the cemented stem. The excellent wear resistance of alumina suggest that these results may be maintained in the longer term. Hybrid alumina-on-alumina hip arthroplasty appears to be a good alternative to other, more conventional arthroplasty.

References

References at the author.

5B.7 Mechanical Effect of the Articulating Materials on the Proximal Femur and the Femoral Stem in Total Hip Arthroplasty

Y.-Y. Won, K.-H. Moon, Y.-S. Yu, L.-S. Hyup and W.-Q. Cui

Introduction

Many factors contribute to failure of a hip arthroplasty. These include infection, instability, fracture and loosening of implants, and malalignment of the artificial joint component. Recently, many clinical reports have demonstrated that osteolysis and aseptic loosening are associated with wear debris from the articulating surface [7,13,14,17,19]. Therefore, research over the past several decades have focused on the reduction of the particle debris. For example, many types of materials have been used as artificial joint components. However, little information is available concerning the stress distribution pattern and the micromotion of the proximal femur and the femoral stem associated with the use of these materials in total hip arthroplasty. Therefore, the purpose of this study is to evaluate the effect of three different articulating materials used in total hip arthroplasty on the stress and micromotion of the proximal femur and femoral stem.

Materials and Methods

Three different modules were used for the geometry of the Finite Element Mesh (Fig 1): Part I: Shell and Insert, Part II: Stem and Ball Head, Part III: Spongy and Cortical Bone. The type and properties of the materials used for the head , insert and metal shell are shown at Tables 1 and 2. The femur modeled for this study consists of cortical and cancellous bone.

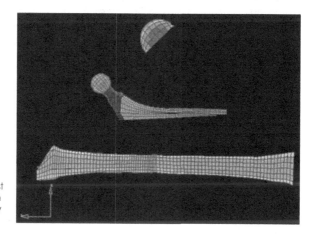

Figure 1:
The component models consist of shell and insert (part I), stem and ball head (part II), spongy and cortical bone (part III).

	Ball head	Insert	Shell
CECE	Ceramic (Alumina base)	Ceramic (Alumina base)	Metal backing (Titanium)
CEPOLY	Ceramic (Alumina base)	Polyethylene	Metal backing (Titanium)
MEME	Metal (Co-Cr Base)	Metal (Co-Cr Base)	Metal backing (Titanium)
MEPOLY	Metal (Co-Cr Base)	Polyethylene	Metal backing (Titanium)
MEMEPO	Metal (Co-Cr Base)	Metal & Poly (Co-Cr Base)	Metal backing (Titanium)

Table 1:
Matching Type.

	Elastic modulus, (GPa)	Poisson's ratio	Reference
Cancellous bone	14.7	0.3	Moroi [8], 1993
Cortical bone	0.49	0.3	Moroi [8], 1993
Titanium	110	0.3	Ye-Yeon Won [18], 1999
Co-Cr Alloy	210	0.3	Ji-Hoon Shin [16], 1999
Ceramic (alumina)	350	0.3	Joon B. Park [11], 1992
Polyethylene	1.2	0.3	Joon B. Park [11], 1992

Table 2:
Material properties.

Three different values for the coefficient of friction between the femoral bone and the Omnifit femoral stem were used. They are: M=0.3, M=0.4, M=2.0 [6, 10]. The boundary conditions were applied to the most distal portion and the acetabular component to prevent stress concentration: 1) The fixed (zero displacement) most distal section of the femoral main stem. 2) Every nodal point at the articulating surface of the acetabular component has the same amount of displacement (multiple point constraints). The femoral main stem modeled was Omnifit HA #9 (Osteonics, UK). The femoral head size and the outer diameter of the metal backing used for this study were 54 mm and 28 mm, respectively. The thickness of the polyethylene was 11.4 mm.

Non-liner contact analysis was made in patients with body weight exceeding 70 kg; the analysis was made in patients standing on one leg and climbing stairs. Considering the force exerted by the abductors, the effective body weight in patients standing on one leg was assumed to be oriented at a 16 degree angle with respect to the vertical axis. For climbing stairs, the methods described by Masao et al. [1] was used (Table 3). These geometric data were incorporated into the Hypermesh 3.1 as pre/post processor of FEM. Then, using the nonliner three-dimensional contact option in ABAQUS 5.8, the Finite Element calculations on the above geometry were performed to evaluate stress distribution and micromotion of the proximal femur and femoral stem.

	Head force					Abductor force	
	Fx	Fy	Fz	Mx	Mz	Fx	Fz
One-leg standing	-447.5	0	-1670	0	0	-697.4	-831.6
Stair climbing	-709.2	-600.8	-1553.2	-123.9	-25	0	0

Table 3:
Loading condition.

Results

The Z-direction stress, which is oriented along the longitudinal direction of the femur, was analyzed first. A specific number was assigned to each condition: 01 for one leg standing, and 02 for stair climbing. For example, CECE01 refers to the use of ceramic femur head on ceramic insert while the patient is standing on one leg whereas MEPOLY02 refers to the use of metal femur head on polyethylene insert while the patient is climbing stairs. The stress distribution in Z-direction for MEPOLY01 was shown in Figure 2, in which the medial aspect of mesh model underwent the compressive stress while the lateral aspect underwent the tensile stress. Similar stress distribution pattern was also observed in CECE, CEPOLY and MEME, suggesting that the modeling and finite element analysis for various materials was theoretically adequate. The Z-direction stress is shown in Table 4 and Figure 3 (standing on one leg) and in Table 5 and Figure 5 (stair climbing). In Figure 3 and 4, max(+) and min(-) represent the compressive stress and the tensile stress, respectively.

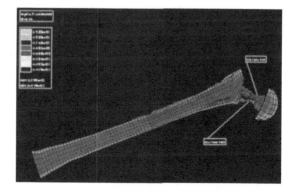

Figure 2:
Z-direction stress of MEPOLY under one-leg standing condition.

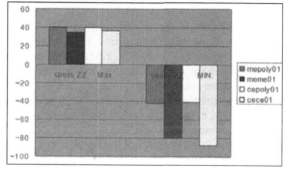

Figure 3:
Z-direction stress contour under one-leg standing condition (N/mm²).

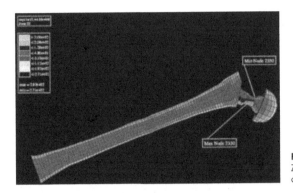

Figure 4:
Z-direction stress under stair climbing condition.

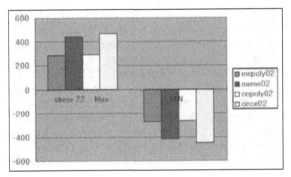

Figure 5:
Z-direction stress contour under stair climbing condition (N/mm²).

		MEPOLY	MEME	CEPOLY	CECE	MEMEPO
Stress Z-Z	Max.	39.9	34.7	40.1	36.1	41
	Min.	-41.9	-80	-41.2	-87.4	-43.1

Table 4:
Z-Z direction stress in the case of one-leg standing (N/mm²).

	MEPOLY02	MEME02	CEPOLY02	CECE02	MEMEPO02
stress ZZ max.	287	446	288	469	288
stress ZZ min.	-271	-416	-264	-450	-270

Table 5:
Z-direction stress (stair climbing, N/mm²).

The maximal yield stress associated with standing on one leg and on stair climbing is shown in Tables 6 and 7. The mises stress contour for each case is shown at Figure 6, 7 and 8. In both conditions (standing on one leg and stair climbing), the maximal yield stress was higher in hard-hard coupling (MEME and CECE). In hard-hard coupling, the site of maximal yield stress was on the loading point of the articulating surface measured while the patient was standing on one leg. However, in the case of stair climbing, the site of maximal yield stress is at the contact surface between the femoral head and the insert component In contrast, the lateral aspect of the neck of the femur was the site of maximal yield stress in hard-soft coupling (MEPOLY and CEPOLY).

While standing on one leg, there is no big change in the mises stress contour secondary to changes in material property; stress to the proximal portion of the femur increased by 13N/mm². The stress on the femur associated with stair climbing was higher in hard-hard couple (MEME and CECE); stress on the proximal portion of the femoral bone decreased by 80N/mm².

In the case of MEMEPO, the biomechanical effect was similar to that of MEPOLY. In each case (standing on one leg and stair climbing), the micromotions between the proximal femur and femoral stem were higher in hard-hard coupling (Table 8).

	MEPOLY01	MEME01	CEPOLY01	CECE01	MEMEPO01
Max. Mises stress	110	141	93.4	149	110
Location	Loading point	Loading point	Loading point	Loading point	Loading point

Table 6:
Maximal Mises stress (one-leg standing, N/mm²).

	MEPOLY02	MEME02	CEPOLY02	CECE02	MEMEPO02
Max. Mises stress	435	465	436	507	435
Location	Lateral neck	Surface of ball & insert	Lateral neck	Surface of ball & insert	Lateral neck

Table 7:
Maximal Mises stress (stair climbing, N/mm²).

	MEPOLY	MEME	CEPOLY	CECE	MEMEPO
Stair climbing	67.3	96.6	67.5	98.7	68.9
One-leg standing	125.3	173.9	149.8	187.5	126.8

Table 8:
Maximum micromotions (μm).

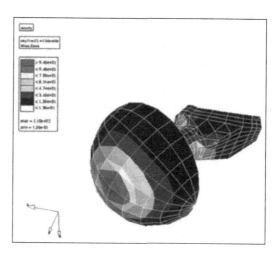

Figure 6:
Mises stress contour under
one-leg standing for MEPOLY.

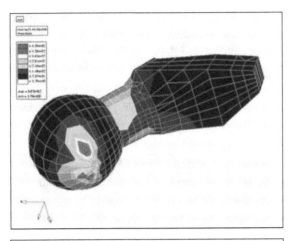

Figure 7:
Mises stress contour under stair climbing for CECE.

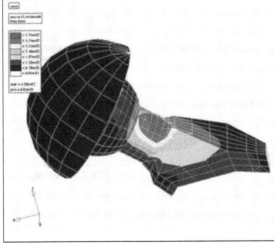

Figure 8:
Mises stress contour under stair climbing for CEPOLY.

Discussion

Osteolysis induced by wear debris and aseptic loosening is the major problem limiting clinical success of total hip arthroplasty. Several biomaterial combinations for total hip implants have been used to reduce wear debris. These include ceramic femur head on polyethylene liner and metal shell couple, ceramic femur head on ceramic liner and metal shell couple, metal femur head on metal-polyethylene liner (sandwich type), and metal shell couple. However, few studies have examined the effects of the articulating material used in total hip arthroplasty on the stress and micromotion of the proximal femur and femoral stem.

Ceramics are wear-resistant and have great compression strength. However, they are very brittle and are susceptible to cracking, and therefore must be chosen carefully for specific implant applications [2,3,15]. When measured in patients standing on one leg, the maximal yield strength was higher in MEME and CECE than in MEPOLY and CEPOLY. The site of maximal yield strength was the loading point of articulating surface. However, in stair climbing, the maximal yield strength was higher in MEME and CECE than in MEPOLY and CEPOLY. The site of maximal yield strength was at the same site as in MEME and CECE, but was at the lateral aspect of the neck of the femur main stem in MEPOLY and CEPOLY. This finding suggests that in patients standing on one leg, the longitudinal load affects the femoral bone as compressive forces, and the site of maximal yield stress is at the loading point.

On stair climbing, the flexion force of the hip joint was the dominant load applied to the femoral bone; here, the site of maximal yield stress is at the lateral aspect of the neck of the femoral main stem. The site of maximal stress applied was at the articulating surface of the joint component in hard-hard coupling (MEME and CECE). But in hard-soft coupling, the site of maximal stress applied was at the lateral aspect of neck of femur. These data suggest that the center of the flexion force moved to the distal portion secondary to deformation of the polyethylene material; this means that liner displacement of the femoral component may affect the direction of the load. These results suggest that fatigue fracture may occur at the neck of the femur main stem in the hard-soft coupling (MEPOLY and CEPOLY), which is thought to be overcome using current material technology. Based on our results, it is possible to produce femoral head components with decreased diameter which will have proper mechanical stability and reduce wear debris from the contact surface of the femoral head and the rim of the ceramic cup. Therefore, hard-hard coupling component (CECE and MEME) are more resistant to wear than hard-soft coupling component (CEPOLY and MEPOLY), as viewed from the standpoint of stress produced from the articulating surface. As a known fact, the stress distribution around the implants can affect bone remodeling. Kim et al compared the bone mineral density around cementless acetabular and femoral components which were identical in geometry and had the same alumina modular femoral head, but differed in regard to the material of the acetabular liners (alumina ceramic or polyethylene) in 50 patients who had undergone bilateral simultaneous primary total hip replacement (THR), demonstrating that there was no significant difference in the bone remodeling of the acetabulum and femur five years after THR in those two groups [5]. Another clinical report shows that the newer component (Metasul, Allopro, Swiss), which has polyethylene between the ceramic liner and the metal shell provides a more uniform distribution of stress to the acetabular component. The latter author also examined the biomechanical effect of polyethylene-inserted metal-banked metal shell component and showed that the biomechanical effect of the component was similar to that of MEPOLY. Also, the micromotion of the femur main stem increased by 20% in hard-hard couple (CECE and MEME) compared to hard-soft couple (MEPOLY and CEPOLY).

It is generally known that the amount of bone in-growth, which is more important in cementless total hip arthroplasty, depends on an optimal primary stability of the femur main stem. In addition, bone in-growth wound not occur within 150 μm or more of the interface micromotion; this interface micromotion causes fibrous in-growth which is responsible for the osteolysis of the bone around the femur main stem [4,9,12]. Viewed from the fact that 150 μm or more of the interface micromotion may occur in hard-couple (CECE and MEME) in a patient standing on one leg, more caution must be exercised in the use of hard-hard couple components in total hip arthroplasty, with considerations given to adequate bone in-growth during the rehabilitation period. But given the fact that finite element analysis has certain limitiations, they required the follow-up experimental and clinical studies. There are no changes in the pattern of stress distribution of the femur secondary to changes in the material properties.

Acknowledgement: This study was supported by ''2000 grant from School of Medicine, Inha University''.

References

1. Ando M, Imura S, Omori H, et al (1999) Nonlinear Three Dimensional Finite Element Analysis of Newly Designed Cementless Total Hip Stems. Artificial Organ, 23(3):339-346.
2. Bergmann G, Graichen F, Rohlmann A (1993) Hip joint loading during walking and running, measured in two patients. J Biomech 26:969-690.
3. Clarke I, Willmann G (1994) Structural ceramics in orthopedics. In : Cameron HU (ed) Bone Implant Interface. St Louis, Mo: Mosby, pp203.
4. Kim SK (1997) Comparative stress analysis of the straight and the curved stem on stress shielding-A three dimensional finite element analysis. J of Korean Hip 9(1):82-91.
5. Kim YH, Yoon SH, Kim JS (2007) Changes in the bone mineral density in the acetabulum and proximal femur after cementless total hip replacement. J Bone Joint Surg 89-B:174-179.
6. Kupier JH, Huiskes R (1996) Friction and Stem Stiffness Affect Dynamic Interface Motion in Total Hip Replacement. J Orthop Res 14;36-43.
7. Maloney WJ, Peters P, Engh CA, Chandler H (1993) Osteolysis of the pelvis in association with acetabular replacement without cement. J Bone Joint Surg 77-A:1301-1310.
8. Moroi HH, Okimoto K, Moroi R Terada Y (1993) Numeric approach to the biomechanical analysis of thermal effects in coated implants. Int J Prosthodont 6:564-572.
9. Otani T, Whiteside LA, White SE, McCarty DS (1993) Effect of femoral component material properties on cementless fixation in total hip arthroplasty. J Arthrop 8:67-74.
10. Otani T, Whitesode LA, White SE (1993) Strain Distribution in the Proximal Femur with Flexible Composite and Metallic Femoral Components under Axial and Torsional Loads J. Biomed Materials Res 27;575-585.
11. Park JB and Lakes RS (1992) BIOMATERAL An Introduction Second Edition, Pleum Publishing Corporation.
12. Pilliar RM, Lee JM, Maniatopoulos C (1986) Observations on the effect of movement on bone ingrowth into porous-surfaced implants. Clin Orthop 208:108-113.
13. Santavirta S, Hoikka V, Eskola A, Konttinen YT, Paavilainen T, Tallroth K (1990) Aggressive granulomatous lesions in cementless total hip arthroplasty. J Bone Joint Surg 72-B:980-984.
14. Schmalzried TP, Justy M, Harris WH (1992): Periprosthetic bone loss in total hip arthroplasty. Polyethylene wear debris and the concept of the effective joint space. J Bone Joint Surg 74-A:849-863.
15. Semlitsch M Dawihl W (1994): Basic requirements for alumina ceramic in artificial hip joint balls articulation with polyethylene cups. In: Buchhorn GH, Willer HG, eds. Technical Principles, Wash: Hogrefe & Huber Publ.
16. Shin JH Lee KH (1999) Metals as Biomaterials. Biomaterial Research 3(1):28-33.
17. Tanzer M, Maloney WJ, Jasty M Haris WH (1992) The progression of femoral cortical osteolysis in associated with total hip arthroplasty without cement. J Bone Joint Surg 74-A:404-410.
18. Won YY, Ahn JI, Yoo SH, Byun CJ, Choi WS Cho JH (1999) Finite Element Analysis for Micromotion of Femoral Stem and Stress Concentration of Femur after Removal of DHS System, J of Korean Hip Society, 11(1), June.
19. Xenos JS, Hopkinson WJ, Callaghan JJ, Heekin RD SavoryCG (1995) Osteolysis around an uncemented cobalt chrome total hip arthroplasty. Clin Orthop 317:29-36.

SESSION 6

Market Trends and Future Applications

6.1 Surface Characteristics and Biocompatibility of Micro Arc Oxidized (MAO) Titanium Alloy

S.-Y. Kwon, Y.-S. Kim, D.-H. Sun, S.-S. Kim and H.-W. Kim

Abstract

The aim of this research was to characterize micro arc oxidized titanium (MAO-Ti), accompanied by biocompatibility test in vivo as well as in vitro in comparison to the different types of surface modification; machined, blasted and plasma spray.

XRD and SEM investigations were performed in order to assess the structure and morphology. Biologic and morphologic responses to the osteoblast cell lines (Saos-2) were then examined, using Promega® proliferation assay, alkaline phosphatase activity, $\alpha v \beta 3$ integrin expression and cytoskeleton staining (Rhodamine-Phallodine). The analysis of gene expression for osteocalcin and collagen I was done through RT-PCR. In addition, differential histologic evaluation and interfacial strength at the bone-implant interfaces were then evaluated in the distal femur of 4 beagle dogs.

In summary, MAO-Ti appears to exhibit more favorable biocompatibility than the compared groups in vitro and in vivo as well.

Introduction

The majority of implants in orthopedic and dental fields are fabricated from titanium alloy owing to their minimal tissue reaction, strength and especially acceptable biocompatibility to result in strong osseointegration with osteoblasts [1,2,3,17]. For promoting and accomplishing osseointegration, the thermo-dynamically stable oxide film naturally formed on the surface is regarded as the most influential factor and surface modification as well to allow for a mechanical bonding with bone tissue [8,12,14]. Among the methods used to alternate the property of oxide layer, the microarc oxidation (MAO) procedure has been reported to be a preferred method to provide a good combination of porous and thick oxide films with a well characterized biocompatible Ca and P substrate. The TiO2 layer generated by the MAO treatment was found to significantly improve the cellular activities of Ti in vitro and the bone-implant bonding properties in vivo [18,23,24]. These improvements were attributed the increase in the surface roughness, as well as to the incorporation of Ca and P into the coating layer. The porous and rough morphology produced by MAO process increased the cell attachment and mechanical interlocking of the tissue and implant. Moreover, the Ca and P source, incorporated from the electrolyte in the coating layer, improved the osteoblast cell responses and further osseointegration [4,9,14,26,27]. The aim of this research was to characterize micro arc oxidized titanium (MAO-Ti), accompanied by biocompatibility test in vivo as well as in vitro in comparison to the different types of surface modification; machined, blasted and plasma spray.

Materials and Methods

Characterization of substrates surface treatment

EDS X-ray dispersion energy (EDS) were carried out in order to evaluate the chemical composition in the surface of the MAO-Ti and the compared groups as well.

Surface observation of substrates

The morphological comparison of surface was studied by means of scanning electron microscope (SEM, JEOL JSM-6700F, JEOL Ltd.) after the test specimens had been coated with platinum in order to evaluate qualitatively the effect of the different surface treatment: machining, grit-blasted, plasma spray, and anodizing surface treatment.

Cell Culture

Osteoblast-like SaOs-2 (ATCC, HTB-85) were cultured in RPMI 1640 (Gibco, Gran Island, NY, USA), with 10% fetal bovine serum (Gibco, Gran Island, NY, USA), 10U/ml penicillin/streptomycin (Gibco, Gran Island, NY, USA). The cells were then cultured on the different specimens for time periods ranging from 4 to 72 hours before analysis. With the separately prepared titanium substrates with the thickness of 1mm X 10mm X 10mm, the following biological analysis and cytological morphology observation were performed. Human osteoblast-like cell line, Saos-2 (ATCC, HTB-85) was incubated under the condition of 5% CO_2 at 37°C on the RPMI 1640 media (Gibco, Gran Island, NY, USA) which included 10% Fetal Bovine Serum (Gibco, Gran Island, NY, USA) and 10U/ml of penicillin/streptomycin (Gibco, Gran Island, NY, USA). After changing to a fresh media and incubating at 3 days interval, when the cell had grown 80 – 90%, it was isolated using Trypsin-EDTA (Gibco, Gran Island, NY, USA), and was cultivated/incubated on the prepared titanium and tested for the the biological assays as described below at each time point,

Preparation for observing the cell using SEM

Saos-2 was seeded by 1 X 10^5 cells/ml on the Titanium, and after 8 hours of incubation, the media was removed. PBS was added and irrigated 2-3 times. After adding 2% Glutaraldehyde-PBS solution, cells were left for 2 hours to be stabilized. The fixative solution is removed after 2 hours and irrigated with distilled water 3 times. 50, 70, 90 and 100% of the ethanol acceptor solution were added in sequence by 30 minutes interval and dehydrated. Lastly, the ethanol was removed and left at a normal temperature (room temperature) to vaporize the ethanol completely.

Cell Proliferation assay

For proliferation assays, Saos-2 cell was seeded by 5 X 10^4 cells/ml on the Titanium sample and was incubated at intervals of 4, 24, 48, 72 hours and 1 week, and was changed to a fresh media before measuring the proliferation (37°C, 5% CO_2 and 95% humidity) using CellTiter 96 non-radioactive cell proliferation kit from Promega as described by the manufacturer.

The CellTiter 96 non-radioactive assay is colormetric method for determining the number of viable cells in proliferation assays. The assay uses a novel tetrazolium compound with an electron coupling reagent. The tetrazolium compound is converted into a soluble formazan, the end product of the assay, by the action of dehydrogenases present in living cells. The amount of formazan formed can be measured by its absorbance at 450 nm using a plate reader. The amount of formazan formed is directly proportional to the number of viable cells in culture.

Using the Cell Titer 96® Non-Radioactive Cell Proliferation assay kit (Promega Corporation, Madison, WI), 15 µl of Dye Solution was added on the titanium and incubated in 5% CO_2 at 37°C for 4 hours. After 100µl of Stop solution was added, each 100µl of pipetted cell was transferred onto a 96well plate (NUNC, Roskilde, Denmark). The cell proliferation was measured at 450nm of optical density using the spectrophotometer (EL 312e, Bio-Tek instrument, Winooski, Vermont, USA).

Measurement of Alkaline phosphatase activity

On the Titanium sample prepared for a medical experiment, 5×10^4 cells/ml of Saos-2 was seeded and incubated for 21 days; the media was then removed and irrigated with PBS 3 times to remove the serum in culture fluid as much as possible. 1ml of 0.02% Triton X-100 was added on each Titanium sample and dissolved the cell. Cytolytic solution was transferred into a 1.5ml tube, and the cell was crushed by sonication. It was then centrifuged by 14,000 rpm at 4°C for 15 minutes, and the supernatant was transferred to a new 1.5ml tube. 100µl of 1M Tris-HCl, 20µl of 5mM $MgCl_2$ and 20µl of 5mM p-nitrophenyl phosphate were added to the supernatant. Then, it was left to react at 37°C for 30 minutes, and 50µl of 1N NaOH was added to stop the reaction. Using the p-nitrophnol, used as standard along with each spectrophotometer (EL 312e, bio-Tek instrument, Winooski, Vermont, USA), the optical density was measured at 410 nm wavelength. Measured Alkaline phosphatase activity was expressed with the value of p-nitrophenol production quantity divided by reaction time and the protein synthesis quantity, measured by the Bio-rad Protein assay kit (Bio-Rad Laboratories, San Jose, CA).

Visualization of actin cytoskeleton and αVβ3 integrin using confocal microscopy

Actin cytoskeleton

After Saos-2 by 1×10^5 cells/ml was seeded on a Titanium sample for 6 hours, it was irrigated with PBS 3 times and stabilized with 4% Paraformaldehyde for 10 minutes. After the stabilized cell was irrigated with PBS 3 times and treated with 0.1% Triton X-100 for 10 minutes, it was again irrigated with PBS. Rhodamine phalloidin (Molecular Probes inc.) was diluted by 1:100 and left to react for 1 hour at 37°C avoiding any lights. It was irrigated with PBS 3 times and included by the aqueous mount. Using confocal & multiphoton microscope system (Bio-Rad Laboratories, Mississauga, ON, Canada), the actin filament structure (cytoskeleton of cell) was observed.

αVβ3 integrin

After Saos-2 by 1×10^5 cells/ml was seeded on a Titanium sample for 6 hours, the media was removed and washed 3 times with PBS. It was then stabilized by 4% Paraformaldehyde for 10 minutes. It was again irrigated with PBS after stabilizing and treated by 0.1% Triton X-100 for 10 minutes. After blocking with 5% serum, mouse anti-human αVβ3 monoclonal antibody (MAB 1976, Chemicon Temecula, CA) was left to react for 16 hours at 4°C. The following day, Alexa Fluor 488 goat anti-mouse IgG (Molecular Probes Inc.) was reacted and irrigated with

PBS; the pattern of the cell adhesion agent, integrin, was comparatively observed using the confocal & multiphoton microscope system (Bio-Rad Laboratories, Mississauga, ON, Canada).

RT-PCR

Saos-2 by 1×10^5 cells/ml was seeded on a Titanium sample and incubated for 4 days. The media was exchanged to a fresh one before extracting RNA. The media was removed from the incubated cell and irrigated with PBS twice; then, TRIzol reagent (Invitrogen, Carlsbad, CA, USA) was added. Each 0.5ml was placed in a 1.5ml tube and chloroform (Sigma, St. Louis, MO, USA) was added, followed by strongly vortex for 20seconds, centrifuged by 13,000 rpm.

After Isopropanol (Sigma, St. Louis, MO, USA) was added and strongly shaken, it was left to react for 10 minutes at a normal temperature and the supernatant was removed through the centrifugation by 13,000rpm at 4°C for 15 minutes. It was then again centrifuged by adding 1ml of 70% ethanol to the sediment, and after removing the ethanol, the sediment was melted by adding the diethlpyrocarbonate-treated (DEPC) distilled water; and the RNA was measured using spectrophotometer.

1ug of total RNA, separated to synthesize cDNA was admixed with 50uM of Oligo $(dT)_{20}$ and 10mM of dNTP (dATP, dGTP, dCTP and dTTP), and reacted at 65°C for 5 minutes. Again 200units/ul of SuperScript III reverse transcriptase (Invitrogen, San Diego, CA), 5X First-Strand buffer, 40units/ul of RNase inhibitor and 0.1M of DTT were admixed and reacted at 50°C for 1 hour; it was left at 70°C for 15 minutes and stopped the reaction. PCR of osteonectin, osteopontin, osteoprotegerin were performed from this synthesized cDNA. The synthesized cDNA was admixed with each sense, 1ul of antisense primer and RT-PCR premix (Bioneer, Chungbuk, Korea) and repeated the circulation process of denaturation at 94°C for 1 minute, annealing at 55°C for 1 minute and extension at 72°C for 1 minute for 30 times. After the electrophoresis of PCR products at 1.5% agarose gel (Invitrogen, San Diego, CA), it was dyed with ethidium bromide to validate/identify (Table 1).

RT-PCR primer set	Sequence	AT(°C)	Product length(bp)
Osteonectin	5'-GATGAGGACAACAACCTTCTGAC-3' 5'-TTAGATCACAAGATCCTTGTCGAT-3'	55	369
Osteopontin	5'-AAATACCCAGATGCTGTGGC-3' 5'-AACCACACTATCACCTCGGC-3'	65	348
Osteoprotegerin	5'-TGCTGTTCCTACAAAGTTTACG-3' 5'-CTTTGAGTGCTTTACTGCGTG-3'	62	435
GAPDH	5'-ACC ACA GTC CAT GCC ATC AC-3' 5'-TTC ACC ACC CTG TTG CTG TA -3'	56	452

Table 1:
Primer pairs used for RT-PCR experiments.

Preparation of specimen for animal study

The metal material, Ti-6Al-4V (Titanium, 6% Aluminum, 4% Vanadium) alloy in 10 mm in length and 4±0.45 mm in diameter was manufactured in circular bar structure. These 32 metal poles were divided into 4 groups and were treated with different surfacing methods: machined, grit-blasted, anodized and plasma sprayed.

Animal experiment
Eight full-grown beagles over 15 kg in weight (mean weight of 16.5±0.75 kg) were assigned as the experiment animal, and 2 of them were for the histomorphometry.

There was approximately 1 week of adaptation period before the experiment began. The operation was performed once experiment animals were intravenously injected with the general anesthesia. The painting & draping was done using the aseptic technique after the skinpreparation of the thigh. The femus shaft metaphysic was obtained by the anterolateral approach resecting the femoral illiotibial band and the musculus vastus lateralis; and meticulous hemostasis was performed. A drill with 4 mm in diameter was used for the lateral cortical bone of the femur; and was drilled with caution in order to avoid medial cortical bone damage. The depth of drilling was maintained at 6 mm and the produced bone fragments were removed by irrigating with normal saline. When inserting specimen, the sequence was decided by random sampling for statistical reliability and was press-fitted.

After the surgery, cefazolin 25 mg/kg was intramuscularly injected for 1 week to prevent infection, and acetachlorphenac sodium 0.5 mg/kg was intramuscularly injected for 24 hours postoperative to minimize pain. Eight beagles were then each sacrificed; and the simple radiologic examination, push-out test and histologic test were carried out.

The femur in which the specimen was implanted for histomorphometry was fixated in 70% ethanol and was kept in Villanueva bone stain solution for 72 hours. After dehydrating the ethanol, prepolymerized embedding medium was used to penetrate. 100 ml of methyl-methacrylate monomer, 40 g of poly-methyl-methacrylate bead and 1 g of benzoyl peroxide were admixed into solution and used for the tissue embedding. Once consolidated/hardened in the thermostat for 40 days, it was made into slices of 100 – 150 μm in thickness by microtome, and polished again to make less than 10 μm in thickness. It was then observed through a microscope (Bone Science Institute, Niigata, Japan).

Push-out biomechanical analysis for interfacial strength
For the biomechanical analysis, the soft tissue sample was removed from the femur of 9 months postoperative; the proximal contact tissue including the metal material was amputated by 20 mm of the major axis. The amputated sample was inferiorly fixated with the bone cement.

The substance tester, INSTRON 6022 (Instron, Canton, MA) was used to assess, and to prevent the dry-out of the sample; the normal saline was applied during test. After placing the specimen on the test strip, the machine, metal intrusion/extrusion velocity of 0.5 mm/hr was set up. By measuring the load-displacement curve, the bone-metal interfacial shear strength was measured.

Results

Characterization of substrates surface treatment

The highest surface roughness (Ra-values) of the plasma sprayed group was statistically significant, and the order of groups was as followed: grit blasted, MAO and machined.

From the microstructure surface observation of test specimens: machined, grit-blasted, plasma sprayed, MAO though the SEM (Scanning Electron Microscopy), Al_2O_3 particles were found to adhere on the surface of grit-blasted, and micropores were observed remarkably on MAO. The equivalent observation finding of Al_2O_3 was confirmed by the EDS spectrum result of surface chemical characterization using EDS X-ray dispersion energy (EDS).

Cell Proliferation assay

Among 4 test specimens and the result of Cell Titer 96® Non-Radioactive Cell Proliferation assay kit (Promega Corporation, Madison, WI) for the cell proliferation, incubation interval of 4, 24, 48, 72 hours and 1 week, respectively. All groups showed satisfying results however, the difference was not statistically significant.

Cell Differentiation

By measuring Alkaline phosphatase activity, the cell differentiation was compared on each sample; the mean and standard deviation of the activity measurement were resulted.

The activity of alkaline phosphatase was increased in the plasma sprayed and MAO groups but the result of quantitative analysis was not statistically significant.

Cell Morphology

Through the morphological study using SEM (Scanning Electron Microscopy) of the cell after 6 hours of incubation, the increased pattern of the cell spreadness was shown in the MAO group, and could confirm the significant activation of the cell adhesion of micropore area.

Confocal Microscopy Examination

Actin filament differentiation and organization using Rhodamine phalloidin (Molecular Probes inc.) staining was evenly distributed compared to the MAO group, the cell adhesion area intensity showed the increased pattern, these findings were also observed in the expression and distribution of the integrin using the mouse anti-human $\alpha V\beta 3$ monoclonal antibody (MAB 1976, Chemicon Temecula, CA), the activated pattern of cell adhesion related cellular microstructure was observed in the MAO group.

RT-PCR

The molecular biologic analysis using the primer pair of osteocalcin and collagen I, the gene expression of osteocalcin and collagen I was observed in 4 groups; the increased pattern was indicated in the plasma sprayed and MAO groups but the result of quantitative analysis was not statistically significant.

Radiologic examination

Through the radiologic study done at 9 months postoperatively, there was no finding of osteoporosis, bone resorption or osteolysis around the implant, There was no particular difference among 4 groups of metal materials.

Histomorphometry

From the femur obtained 9 months postoperatively, the non-decalcified histomorphometry analysis was evaluated. Through the phase contrast microscope, the new bone formation could be seen around the areas of metal materials, and the findings of lamellar bone formation and peri-implant osseointegration were observed from the dye sample. These osseointegration findings were particularly significant in the MAO group, and a favorable pattern was found in the grit blasted and plasma sprayed groups.

Push-out biomechanical analysis

The measurement of interfacial shear strength was statistically higher in the grit-blasted, anodized and plasma sprayed groups compared to the machining group (P< 0.05). However, there was no statistically significant difference between the plasma sprayed and MAO groups (P> 0.05).

Discussion

The initial responses of osteoblasts and other mesenchymal cells to implanted orthopedic biomaterials can play a critical role in the future extent of osseointegration of the implant. Early substrate-surface receptor interactions are altered by the surface characterization of implant [4,5,7,10,11,12].

The alteration of surface treatment on titanium implant determines the nature and extent of cytoskeletal and extracellular matrix protein production and organization, and, subsequently, the degree of cell spreading, adhesion, differentiation on the different substrates and bone-implant interfacial interaction as well; machined, blasted plasma spray and MAO [2,6,10,18,20].

A recent study for MAO has found that MAO induced showed a favorable biocompatibility in vitro and in vivo. However, very little data exists on the nature of direct cellular interaction with MAO treatment surfaces. More information is needed about the early factors involved in the osseointegration process and the importance of osteoblast spreading and adhesion to MAO, especially in comparisioin to different surfaces. This study have analyzed comparatively the alteration of osteoblast proliferation, differentiation, and matrix production in vitro as well as interfacial shear strength biomechanically on different types of surface modification [18,23,24].

The anodizing surface treatment method has already been used industrially for treating titanium or aluminum of aircraft parts in Soviet Union; metals such as titanium which can form an oxidation layer is added in the low concentration alkali solution, containing calcium and phosphate, the surface of the metal is oxidized by applying high-voltage and inducing electric arc.

Once the surface of titanium is oxidized through this method, a titanium oxide (TiO_2) layer which is ceramic is formed on the surface; this surface layer and titanium are known to have a very strong bonding strength (80 – 90% of the body) [14,24].

In addition, depending on the added electric pressure level, application method and type of electrolyte, the surface demonstrates different appearances. Composition components of the surface are commonly consisted with calcium and phosphate, and contain the porous structure with the size of micron or submicron [9,14,15,16,19].

This special structure facilitates the osseointegration. Despite of mentioned structural characteristics or chemical advantages, it is scarcely used in the orthopaedic field, however unlike artificial hip joints, dental implants in which the initial bone stability is crucial has reported outstanding results compared to other preexisting surface treatment methods by the clinical application continued by active researches.

A pore formed by the anodizing method is less than 5 um in size, extremely small compared to 150 – 400 μm, the pore size of porous coated stem purposing bone ingrowth. According to the cell adhesion study using the osteoblast, the initial adhesion of the osteoblast is reported to be better in the microporous structure than in the macroporous structure [2,18,26].

In other words, if the surface has the microporous structure, the filopodia extension of the osteoblast to the microporous structure makes it easier to attach. The porous structure has advantages of maximizing the surface of artificial joints other than these initial cell adhesion and the calcium and phosphate, the composition components of surface are thought to provide a good environment for the bone stability.

These findings, like the experiment done, could confirm the excellent result of the cell proliferation, morphology, differentiation, adhesion molecule gene and gene expression compared with the currently used surface treatment methods; especially, biomechanical push-out test through the animal experiment was a meaningful result indicating the excellent biocompatibility and osseointegration inducement.

At present, the artificial joints used in human body has adapted the technical method of MAO and demonstrated outstanding clinical results; it is expected to be even widely applied to implants of human body. However, MAO doesn't contain the perfect composition component, hydroxyapatite like the human bones. Therefore, the modified surface treatment method technique will be developed through researches combing the described advantages of anodizing and HA coating.

Conclusion

High success rates have been reported in the cases of currently used cementless artificial joints or dental implants; it could be stated that there is no hitch in bone stability. However, when the bone quality is not as good like for the revision surgery, the surface treatment which can achieve or induce strong initial stability is essential. In this aspect, the development of MAO with enhanced biocompatibility compared to the conventional surface treatment methods suggested through the cell test and animal experiment of this study may greatly contribute, and, it is expected to open new area of surface treatment through the MAO method with appropriate surface roughness application and new technology using HA as a composition component.

References

1. Annaz B, Hing KA, Kayser M, Buckland T and Di Silvio LJ (2004) Porosity variation in hydroxyapatite and osteoblast morphology: a scanning electron microscopy study. Microsc 215:100-110.
2. Anselme K (2000) Osteoblast adhesion on biomaterials. Biomaterials 21:667-681.
3. Brunette DM, Tengvall P, Textor M, Thomsen P (2001) Titanium in medicine. Berlin: Springer.
4. Buser D, Schenk RK, Steinemann S, Forellini JP, Fox C, Stich H (1991) Influence of surface characteristics on bone integration of titanium implants. A hisomorphometric study in miniature pigs. J Biomed Mater Res 25:889-902.
5. Callen BW, Sodhi RN, Griffiths K (1995) Examination of clinical surface preparations on titanium and Ti-6Al-4V by X-ray photoelectron spectroscopy and nuclear reaction analysis. Prog Surf Sci 50:269-279.
6. Clark EA, Brugge JS (1995) Integrins and signal transduction pathways: the road taken. Science 268:233-239.
7. De Groot, K., Geesink, R.G.T., Klein, C.P.A.T., and Serekian, P (1987) Plasma sprayed coating of hydroxyapatite. J Biomed Mater Res 21:1375-1387.
8. Feng B, Weng J, Yang BC, Qu SX, Zhang XD (2003) Characterization of surface oxide films on titanium and adhesion of osteoblast. Biomaterials 24:4663-4670.
9. Fu Liu, Ying song, Fuping Wang, Tadao Shimizu, Kaoru Igarashi, Liancheng Zhao (2005) Formation characterization of hydroxyapatite on titanium by microarc oxidation and hydrothermal treatment. J biosci bioeng 100:100-104.
10. Groessner-Schreiber B, Tuan RS (1992) Enhanced extracellular matrix production and mineralization by osteoblast cultured on titanium surfaces in vitro. J Cell Sci 101:209-217.
11. Hacking SA, Bobyn JD, Tanzer M and Krygier JJ (1999) The Osseous response to corundum blasted implant surfaces in a canine hip model. Clin Orthop 364:240-253
12. Hazan R, Brener R, Oron U (1993) Bone growth to metal implants in regulated by their. surface chemical properties. Biomaterials 14:570-574.
13. Hure G, Donath K, Lesounrd M, Chappard D, Basle MF (1996) Dose titanium surface treatment influence the bone-implant interface? SEM and histomorphometry in a 6-sheep study. Int J Oral Maxillofac Implants 11:506-511.
14. Ishizawa H, Ogino M (1995) Formation and characterization of titanium anodic oxide film containing Ca and P. J Biomed Mater Res 29:65-72.
15. Johansson, C. Albrektsson, T (1987) Integration of screw implants in the rabbit: A 1-year follow-up of removal torque of titanium implants. Int J Oral Maxillofacial Implants 2:69-75.
16. Lee IS, Whang CN, Kim HE, Park JC, Song JH and Kim SR (2002) Various Ca/P ratios of thin calcium phosphate films. Materials Science and Engineering 22:15-20.
17. Lee TM, Tsai RS, Chang E, Yang CY and Yang MR (2002) The cell attachment and morphology of neonatal rat calvarial osteoblasts on the surface of Ti-6Al-4V and plasma-sprayed HA coating: Effect of surface roughness and serum contents. J Mater Sci Mater Med 13:341-350.
18. Li LH, Kong YM, Kim HW, Kim YW, Kim HE, Heo SJ, Koak JY (2004) Improved biological performance of Ti implants due to surface modification by microarc oxidation. Biomaterials 25:2867-2875.
19. Nie X, Leyland A and Matthews A (2000) Deposition of layered bioceramic hydroxyapatite/TiO2 coatings on titanium alloys using a hybrid technique of micro-arc oxidation and electrophoresis. Surface and Coatings Technology 125:407-414.
20. Ong JL, Prince CW, Raikar GN, Lucas LC (1996) Effect of surface topography of titanium on surface chemistry and cellular response. Implant Dent 5:83-88.
21. Raymond PR, Gaston RD and Thomas MG (1996) Uncemented total hip arthroplasty using the CLS stem: A titanium alloy implant with a corundum blast finish: Results at a mean 6 years in a prospective study. J Arthroplasty 11:286-292.

22. Sitting C, Textor M, Spencer ND, Wieland M, Valloton PH (1999) Surface characterization of implant material CP Ti Ti-6Al-4V with different pretreatments. J Mater Sci Mater Med 10:35-46.

23. Son WW, Zhu X, Shin HI, Ong JL, Kim KH (2003) In vivo histological response to anodized and anodized/hydrothermally treated titanium implants. J Biomed Mater Res B 66:520-525.

24. Sul YT (2003) The significance of the surface properties of oxidized titanium to the bone response: special emphasis on potential biochemical bonding of oxidized titanium implant. Biomaterials 24:3893-3907.

25. Van NR (1987) Titanium: the implant material of today. J Mater Res 22:3801-3811 Zhu X. Kim KH, Jeong Y (2001) Anodic oxide films containing Ca and P of titanium. Biomaterials 22:2199-2206.

26. Zhu X, Chen J, Scheideler L, Altebaeumer T, Geis-Gerstorfer J and Kern D (2004) Cellular reactions of osteoblasts to micron- and submicron-scale porous structures of titanium surfaces. Cells Tissues Organs 178:13-22.

6.2 Reasons for our Preference for Ceramic over Metal Bearing – clinical, radiological and biological evidences

J.-Y. Lazennec, P. Boyer, J. Poupon, M. A. Rousseau, F. Laude, Y. Catonné and G. Saillant

Introduction

The second generation of metal on metal prosthesis benefited from improvements in industrial manufacturing and optimisation of the articular movement [1-3]. Short term clinical results are promising [4-7]. However concerns remain about radiological and biological aspects [8-14]. The questions surrounding "ideal" articular clearance still haven't been answered and the influence of the mode of lubrication seems essential today [15-19]. Release of chromium and cobalt from the bearing couple is one of the problems [20-24].

Since 1994 serum cobalt, chromium and titanium levels have been analysed in parallel to clinical and radiological evolution of more than 400 hip prosthesis using Metasul® metal on metal bearing couples in 28mm diameters. The prospective follow up of the first 97 implanted prosthesis was centred on three themes:

- The evolution of the cobalt and chromium ratios after running in phase.
- The consequences of a bilateral arthroplasty on the cobalt, chromium and titanium levels.
- The evaluation of these ratios as markers of prosthetic functioning or defection.

Material und Methods

Population

The series counts 97 prosthesis for 76 patients (21 bilateral implants) with an average 9 years follow up (7-12 years).

The cemented femoral stem is collarless, oval in cross section and straight (Alizé® Fournitures Hospitalières, Quimper, France). The implant is made of titanium alloy (TiA16V4) with a polished surface coated with titanium oxide (TiO2) obtained by anodic oxidation [16,18].

The modular stem is combined with a 28 mm Metasul® femoral head (Centerpulse-Zimmer, Warsaw, Indiana, U.S.) using a 12 – 14 taper.

Tapers were inspected individually before micro threading, using an electro pneumatic system (High pressure electronic pneumo transducer 150015, Solex Metrologie, La Boisse, France) for the taper angle (precision 1 minute), the diameter at the base and the diameter at the summit (precision 1 micron). This inspection was counterchecked by a unit control on a tridimensional machine with 1-micron precision. The micro threading was inspected using a projected side view with an enlargement x20 for the pace, profile and dimension of the threading (Pexit 14 VS Profile Profector, Pixit Dorsey Gage, Cambridge, UK) Compatibility between cones and heads have been controlled and guaranteed by the manufacturers.

All of the sockets were cemented Metasul® cups, Weber cups (Centerpulse-Zimmer, Warsaw, Indiana, U.S.). Palacos Genta® cement (Scherring Plough, Brussels, Belgium) was used.

In our institution, the standard procedure was an antero-lateral approach on a Judet orthopaedic table [25]. The femoral cementing technique used pressurisation and a resorbable femoral plug (Synplug®, Zimmer, Warsaw, Indiana, U.S) in order to obtain a complete and thick cement mantle.

Hip function results were rated according to the Harris Hip Score grading system in preoperative period and latest follow up [26].

A preoperatory renal control was systematically performed in order to eliminate any defection countra indicating a metal on metal bearing couple. Possible intake of medication or vitamin and mineral supplements containing cobalt or vitamin B12 was systematically checked.

Clinical and radiological evaluation

All patients were clinically evaluated after 3 months, 6 months and then every 2 years. Two more parameters were documented through dedicated question-naires.

- The functional profile according to Devane score [27] and the level of physical activity classified in 3 increasing grades in the hour and week previous to the evaluation.
- Subluxation phenomena [8].

All x-rays were reviewed independently by two different observers. We defined radiographic loosening of the cup as the presence of radiolucent lines measuring in at least two DeLee-Charnley zones, axial cup migration of > 5 mm, or > 5° of change in cup inclination on the AP radiographs of the pelvis [28].

Parameters investigated on the femoral side included presence and progression of radiolucent lines according to Gruen et al. [29], calcar resorption or atrophy, subsidence, periprosthetic osteolysis, and cortical hypertrophy. Loosening of the stem was defined as a migration exceeding 3 mm or a continuous radiolucent line wider than 2 mm.

Heterotopic ossifications, if present, were graded according to Brooker et al. [30].

Biological evaluation

The cobalt and chromium were measured using Electrothermal Atomic Absorption Spectrometry. Evaluation of the physiological ratios of Co and Cr inferior to 10 nmol/l required the perfecting of a sensitive method (detection below 1 nmol/l). The titanium was measured using Inductively-Coupled Plasma Atomic Emission Spectrometry. The limit of detection (LD) of titanium is 30 nmol/L of serum. For values below LD it was half LD (15nmol/l) that was used for calculations.

Serum dosages of titanium (Ti), chromium (Cr) and cobalt (Co) were taken before operating and then on regular basis in the post operative period. The dosages were also taken in patients having undergone a prosthetic revision with removal of metal on metal bearing couple.

Results

Radiological and clinical results
Twelve patients present recurrent subluxations.
The principal complications are summarised in 12 revisions with
- 2 because of early recurring dislocations for impingement
- 8 because of clinical and radiological failure (1 femoral stem subsidence due to suboptimal cementing technique and 7 severe acetabular osteolysis).
- 2 because of worrying X-rays presenting osteolysis on the acetabulum (Fig. 1,2).
Three other revisions are programmed because of rapidly evolving radiological alterations. During these revisions we were able to observe 4 severe "metallosis" infiltration, leading us to choose an alumina on alumina bearing couple.
30 implants showed radiological signs of deterioration on the acetabular side:
25 radiolucent lines in zone 1 out of which 11 were worrying
and 5 rapidly evolving osteolysis in zone 1.
Amongst the 30 cases, 8 femoral osteolysis were observed (3 in zone 1 and 5 in zone 7). We did not observe any relationships between the size of the cups and the occurrence of acetabular side deteriorations .

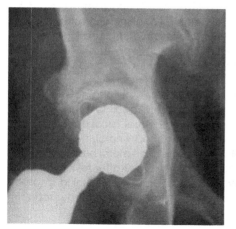

Figure 1:
Evolutionary radiolucent line and acetabular osteolysis.

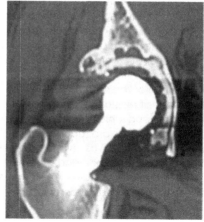

Figure 2:
CT scan evaluation of periacetabular osteolysis.

Biological results
• *Evolution of cobalt levels*
A great stability of the levels is observed in monolateral prosthesis over time, this applies to the median as much as the average, with a running in phase followed by a status phase. During the running-in stage, the median culminates at 33,2 nmol/l (SD 61,3) and the highest levels are found in this period. After 2 years, the values stabilise around 25 nmol/l and remain at this level beyond 5 years. Concerning bilateral prosthesis, our results show an increase in levels (double) as soon as the second prosthesis is implanted.

• *Evolution of chromium levels*

Chromium level graphs of mono and bilateral prosthesis are superimposable to those of cobalt levels. The higher values of the median and average are present in the first 24 months. Then the levels are stable and low for monolateral prosthesis (median around 45 nmol/l through time). The median and average values are much higher for the bilateral prosthesis group.

• *Evolution of titanium levels*

The titanium levels show a different evolution to those of the cobalt and chromium ratios. Indeed the initial running in phase is not observed, this is logical. A real metallurgical silence exists: the median is stabilised at 15nmol/l at this period. An increase in titanium rates has been observed in the case of femoral stem subsidence into the cement mantle and in case of impingement between the neck and the acetabular insert.

• *Relation between unilateral and bilateral prosthesis*

The values of the 3 metallic elements are significantly higher for the bilateral prosthesis group. The average levels are doubled for Co and Cr and quadrupled for Ti.

• *Relation between activity and levels of chromium and cobalt.*

According to Devane's activity score [27] there doesn't seem to be a relation between the measured levels and general activity in the hour or week preceding the blood sampling whether it concerns monolateral or bilateral prosthesis.

• *Relation between the serum ratios and dysfunctioning of the bearing couple*

All detected biological abnormalities had clinical and radiological explanations or were solved during the revision except for one case under close observance.

• *Evolution of the serum metal levels after removal of the bearing couple*

In case of revision with removal of the metal on metal bearing couple, a drop in cobalt and chromium values is observed until normal ratios found in non exposed subjects are reached (respectively below 5 and 9 nmol/l). One case of bilateral prosthesis was revised on one side with a metal on metal bearing couple. No decrease in cobalt and chromium ratios was observed after revision. In one case of bilateral metal on metal prosthesis with acetabular loosening on both sides, the change of bearing couple on one hip entailed significant decrease in serum levels.

Discussion

This series shows the stability of the cemented titanium stem, a combination denounced by certain authors yet widely used in anterior series with equivalent results [31,32,33]. We observed unexpected evolutions and complications singular to the metal on metal bearing couple. Periacetabular bone loss has been the main concern, but metal release is still a problem for us , due to potential relationship with bone resorption and implant loosening.

1- Osteolysis theoretically should be reduced or marginal, in particular with such a follow -up. However osteolysis can occur in hips with metal on metal bearings [9,34] and represents in certain series a frequent complication [4 13]. In our series a radiolucent line, generally precocious and with progressive evolution was seen in zone 1, in 31% of the cases (30 cases out of 97). Dorr [35] also observed a significant number of radiolucent lines in zone 1 over the same amount of time. Eleven of the thirty cases evolved in a worrying way and five cases of visible osteolysis of the roof justify a further revision. We observed 9 severe acetabular osteolysis during revisions. Among non revised cases, we detected 8 limited femoral osteolysis and 5 more worrying acetabular osteolysis. These lesions can be hypothesized as a local reaction to metal bearing.

Although the wear volume is decreased with metal on metal T.H.P., the physical properties of the wear particles from Co-Cr-Mo bearings are different and may have a unique set of consequences, especially regarding regarding macrophages activation and the osteolysis cascade [36]. The size of metal particles reported by scanning electron microscopy studies ranges from 0.1 to 5 μm. Some studies have suggested that large metallic particles observed with light microscopy were agglomerates of the smaller particles [37]. Additional analysis indicates that the particles have several different elemental compositions. There are CoCr-Mo particles, but there is an even greater number of chromium oxide particles [37,38].

It has been hypothesized that the Co-Cr-Mo particles are produced by the wear of the carbides on the bearing surfaces and the prosthesis matrix, and that the chromium oxide particles come from the passivation layer on the implant surface and possibly from oxidized chromium carbides [39].

Several studies tried to demonstrate that one of the mechanisms of osteolysis could be a hypersensitive reaction to metal implants [13]. But are these reactions due to the deterioration of the implant or a consequence of excessive releasing of metal? The smaller wear particles from metal-on-metal articulations may interact with the immune system through different mechanism than those used by the larger polyethylene particles [40].

The increased risk of developing hypersensitivity is a real concern today because of the elevated level of Co and Cr ions in patients with a metal on metal bearing [41,42,43]. Recently, some studies confirmed specific histological changes in the tissues around revised metal on metal prostheses [44,45,46]. In vitro studies have shown a dose-response effect with metal particles with a greater potentiel for cytotoxicity than polyethylene particles [46].

Low to moderate concentrations of metal particles stimulate the release of cytokines that can lead to periprosthetic osteolysis and aseptic loosening [47-49]. At higher concentrations, however Co-Cr have been found to be cytotoxic, altering the phagocytic activity of macrophages and leading to cell death [50-53].

Metal-on-metal hip joints often generate plentiful articular liquid as expressed by the patients, with local swelling and proven by ultrasonographic explorations. We could observe an improvement of the symptoms by the use of anti-inflammatory. In our experience, osteolysis could be linked to diffusion of joint liquid due to articular hyperpressure according to the principle of "effective joint space" [54]. Beaule reported a case of a well-fixed, cementless THR with a Metasul® bearing with progressive diaphyseal osteolysis occurring within 2 years [9]. There was minimal bearing surface wear and only small numbers of inflammatory cells in the tissues. It was hypothesized that this was a case of osteolysis secondary to transmission of joint fluid pressure, rather than particulate-induced osteolysis considering the absent evidence of a foreign-body reaction [40]. We could also detect such an osteolysis behind the acetabular metal back in a more recent series of cementless metal on metal T.H.P. (Fig.3).

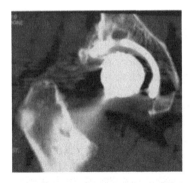

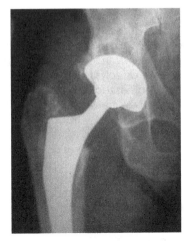

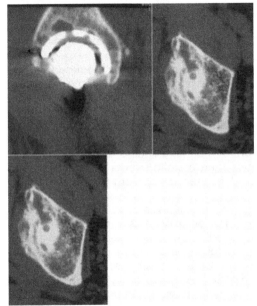

Figure 3:
Cementless metal on metal implants; 5 years follow-up. Osteolysis can be observed behind the acetabular metal back. The increase of the bone loss has been associated with a reduction of the swelling phenomenon for the patient.
Our hypothesis is a fluid joint diffusion process around the metal back according to the "effective joint space" theory.

2 - Many publications have been centred on the release of metallic particles and their serum or blood dosage [20-24,55-62]. But the numbers studied are often low and the follow-up short. The studies report global values with averages without analysing the evolution of each patient. Cobalt diffusing from the implant area is considered to be rapidly eliminated by the urine [36]. However the evacuation cycle of chromium is much slower and passes through a stage of storage in the tissues [42]. The statistical risk of an alteration of the renal function through time is not to be neglected because it can reduce the possibilities of elimination as demonstrated by Brodner [20].

There are few studies concerning chromium and cobalt levels in same subjects [22,59]. There are no studies where serum cobalt, chromium and titanium dosages have been measured in the same series of total metal on metal hip prosthesis.

Studies reporting serum metallic element ratios after revision and suppression of the metal on metal couple are rare [56]. They seem to confirm the decrease of levels and in an indirect way the role of the bearing couple in the production of metallic elements.

Our series brings new elements: it shows the existence of a significant running-in phase in the first 34 months as much for the cobalt as for the chromium levels. These findings are in agreement with the tests done in simulators [2,59] and are in opposition to Brodner's results [24]. Chromium and cobalt levels evolve in an equivalent fashion, and the implant of a second prosthesis increases the values for all metals. Our studies allow us to suppose that certain dysfunctions can be detected through metal ratio variations. Thus increases in titanium ratios peaks were observed in patients presenting a femoral subsidence or an impingement with abrasion of the neck of the titanium prosthesis against the chrome-cobalt insert.

The lesion of the bearing couple in relation to a dislocation has sometimes been incriminated. In our experience no increase of serum chromium or cobalt dosages after dislocation have been observed. The appearance of an articular laxity, with subluxation remains difficult to give evidence for radiologically and clinically. In this series we observed that the patients presenting the highest scores in subluxation increased their cobalt ratios through time.

Like in other studies we haven't proven the relation of the position of the implants and the metal ratios [63]. Activity can increase the ratios but it has been shown that this increase isn't significant [64]. Our results based on the activity questionnaire confirms this tendency [65].

Apart from the 2 cases of repetitive dislocation, 12 patients are invalidated by situations of instability with sensations of catching, limitations or apprehension in the area of the hip. With conflicts [5,66], these instability phenomenons (subluxation, micro separation) are potentially at the origin of a local and systemic releasing of chromium and cobalt [67]. Typical lesions of microseparation with stripe wears have been observed on our metal on metal heads and inserts retrivials . Mapping of stripe wear on the balls and cup rim showed that such wear phenomena appeared to be the natural consequence of edge contact by hard CoCr bearings [68].

Despite very good functional results, certain series report unexplained pain in the hip [6]. During some revisions, an important grey metallosis was observed with no other anomalies and without conflict; we observed the same in one case. Today we still don't have a clear explanation. "Allergy" is evoked without being proven, sometimes a lack of lubrication or phenomenon of piston similar to those described in conventional alumina on alumina bearing couples [18]. These cases cause difficult strategic problems and exclude reimplanting a new metal on metal bearing couple ; resorting to an alumina on alumina bearing couple seems the best solution [69].

Conclusion

This series raises questions concerning the reliability of the metal on metal bearing couple. Osteolysis is an unsolved problem. The cup fixation is a worrying aspect due to the frequency of radiolucent lines that evolve in an unknown fashion over time.

Today cemented fixation is debatable although this series doesn't allow this parameter to be held directly responsible. Nothing points to any shortcomings concerning the taper fixation or the metallurgy of the femoral stem.

The study of the serum metal levels seems a good indicator of the impingement situations and the functioning of the bearing couple.

Certain mechanical complications are far from been anecdotal. We observed phenomenon of articular laxity and subluxation corresponding to micro separations described in "hard on hard" bearing couples. Those phenomenons may have an impact on bearing surfaces deterioration and metal release.

Cementless metal on metal implants; 5 years follow-up. Osteolysis can be observed behind the acetabular metal back. The increase of the bone loss has been associated with a reduction of the swelling phenomenon for the patient. Our hypothesis is a fluid joint diffusion process around the metal back according to the "effective joint space" theory.

References

1. Weber BG. Experience with the Metasul total hip bearing system. Clin Orthop Relat Res, 1996-329 Suppl:S69-77.
2. Rieker CB, Schon R, Kottig P. Development and validation of a second-generation metal-on-metal bearing: laboratory studies and analysis of retrievals. J Arthroplasty, 2004;19-8 Suppl 3:5-11.
3. Sieber HP, Rieker CB, Kottig P. Analysis of 118 second-generation metal-on-metal retrieved hip implants. J Bone Joint Surg Br , 1999;81-1:46-50.
4. Dorr LD, Hilton KR, Wan Z, Markovich GD, Bloebaum R. Modern metal on metal articulation for total hip replacements. Clin Orthop Relat Res , 1996-333:108-17.
5. Delaunay CP. Metal-on-metal bearings in cementless primary total hip arthroplasty. J Arthroplasty , 2004;19-8 Suppl 3:35-40.
6. Hilton KR, Dorr LD, Wan Z, McPherson EJ. Contemporary total hip replacement with metal on metal articulation. Clin Orthop Relat Res , 1996-329 Suppl:S99-105.
7. Migaud H, Jobin A, Chantelot C, Giraud F, Laffargue P, Duquennoy A. Cementless metal-on-metal hip arthroplasty in patients less than 50 years of age: comparison with a matched control group using ceramic-on-polyethylene after a minimum 5-year follow-up. J Arthroplasty , 2004;19-8 Suppl 3:23-8.
8. Lazennec JY, Boyer P, Poupon J, Rousseau MA, Laude F, Catonne Y, Saillant G. [In Process Citation]. Rev Chir Orthop Reparatrice Appar Mot 2007;93-3:298-302.
9. Beaule PE, Campbell P, Mirra J, Hooper JC, Schmalzried TP. Osteolysis in a cementless, second generation metal-on-metal hip replacement. Clin Orthop Relat Res, 2001-386:159-65.
10. Willert HG, Buchhorn GH, Fayyazi A, Flury R, Windler M, Koster G, Lohmann CH. Metal-on-metal bearings and hypersensitivity in patients with artificial hip joints. A clinical and histomorphological study. J Bone Joint Surg Am 2005;87-1:28-36.
11. Ward JJ, Thornbury DD, Lemons JE, Dunham WK. Metal-induced sarcoma. A case report and literaturereview. Clin Orthop Relat Res , 1990-252:299-306.
12. Lewis CG, Sunderman FW, Jr. :. Metal carcinogenesis in total joint arthroplasty. Animal models. Clin Orthop Relat Res , 1996-329 Suppl:S264-8.
13. Park YS, Moon YW, Lim SJ, Yang JM, Ahn G, Choi YL. Early osteolysis following second-generation metal-on-metal hip replacement. J Bone Joint Surg Am , 2005;87-7:1515-21.
14. Doherty AT, Howell RT, Ellis LA, Bisbinas I, Learmonth ID, Newson R, Case CP. Increased chromosome translocations and aneuploidy in peripheral blood lymphocytes of patients having revisionarthroplasty of the hip. J Bone Joint Surg Br , 2001;83-7:1075-81.
15. Dowson D. New joints for the Millennium: wear control in total replacement hip joints. Proc Inst Mech Eng [H] , 2001;215-4:335-58.
16. Hu X. A frictional study of metal on metal hip prostheses with different clearances. 52 nd annual meeting of the Orthopaedic Research Society, 2006. Research Society, 2006.

17. McMinn D, Daniel J. History and modern concepts in surface replacement. Proc Inst Mech Eng [H] 2006;220-2:239-51.

18. Lundberg H. Quantifying fluid ingress to the joint space durinf THA subluxations. 51 th annual meeting of the Orthopaedic Research Society, 2005.

19. Dowson D, Hardaker C, Flett M, Isaac GH. A hip joint simulator study of the performance of metal-on-metal joints: Part I: the role of materials. J Arthroplasty 2004;19-8 Suppl3:118-23.

20. Brodner W, Bitzan P, Meisinger V, Kaider A, Gottsauner-Wolf F, Kotz R. Elevated serum cobalt with metal-on-metal articulating surfaces. J Bone Joint Surg Br , 1997;79-2:316-21.

21. Jacobs JJ, Skipor AK, Patterson LM, Hallab NJ, Paprosky WG, Black J, Galante JO. Metal release in patients who have had a primary total hip arthroplasty. A prospective, controlled, longitudinal study. J Bone Joint Surg Am , 1998;80-10:1447-58.

22. MacDonald SJ, McCalden RW, Chess DG, Bourne RB, Rorabeck CH, Cleland D, Leung F. Metal-on-metal versus polyethylene in hip arthroplasty: a randomized clinical trial. Clin Orthop Relat Res , 2003-406:282-96.

23. Brodner W, Grohs JG, Bitzan P, Meisinger V, Kovarik J, Kotz R. [Serum cobalt and serum chromium level in 2 patients with chronic renal failure after total hip prosthesis implantation with metal-metal gliding contact]. Z Orthop Ihre Grenzgeb 2000;138-5:425-9.

24. Brodner W, Bitzan P, Meisinger V, Kaider A, Gottsauner-Wolf F, Kotz R. Serum cobalt levels after metal-on-metal total hip arthroplasty. J Bone Joint Surg Am , 2003;85-A-11:2168-73.

25. Siguier T, Siguier M, Brumpt B. Mini-incision anterior approach does not increase dislocation rate: a study of 1037 total hip replacements. Clin Orthop Relat Res, 2004-426:164-73.

26. Harris WH. Traumatic arthritis of the hip after dislocation and acetabular fractures: treatment by mold arthroplasty. An end-result study using a new method of result evaluation. J Bone Joint Surg Am 1969;51-4:737-55.

27. Devane PA, Horne JG. Assessment of polyethylene wear in total hip replacement. Clin Orthop Relat Res 1999-369:59-72.

28. DeLee JG, Charnley J. Radiological demarcation of cemented sockets in total hip replacement. Clin Orthop Relat Res , 1976-121:20-32.

29. Gruen TA, McNeice GM, Amstutz HC. "Modes of failure" of cemented stem-type femoral components: a radiographic analysis of loosening. Clin Orthop Relat Res , 1979-141:17-27.

30. Brooker AF, Bowerman JW, Robinson RA, Riley LH, Jr. :. Ectopic ossification following total hip replacement. Incidence and a method of classification. J Bone Joint Surg Am, 1973;55-8:1629-32.

31. Bowditch M, Villar R. Is titanium so bad? Medium-term outcome of cemented titanium stems. J Bone Joint Surg Br 2001;83-5:680-5.

32. Buly RL, Huo MH, Salvati E, Brien W, Bansal M. Titanium wear debris in failed cemented total hip arthroplasty. An analysis of 71 cases. J Arthroplasty 1992;7-3:315-23.

33. Thomas SR, Shukla D, Latham PD. Corrosion of cemented titanium femoral stems. J Bone Joint Surg Br 2004;86-7:974-8.

34. Schmalzried TP, Peters PC, Maurer BT, Bragdon CR, Harris WH. Long-duration metal-on-metal total hip arthroplasties with low wear of the articulating surfaces. J Arthroplasty, 1996;11-3:322-31.

35. Dorr LD, Long WT, Sirianni L, Campana M, Wan Z. The argument for the use of Metasul as an articulation surface in total hip replacement. Clin Orthop Relat Res , 2004-429:80-5.

36. Doorn PF, Campbell PA, Worrall J, Benya PD, McKellop HA, Amstutz HC. Metal wear particle characterization from metal on metal total hip replacements: transmission electron microscopy study of periprosthetic tissues and isolated particles. J Biomed Mater Res 1998;42-1:103-11.

37. Hanlon J, Ozuna R, Shortkroff S, et al. Analysis of metallic wear debris retrieved at révision arthroplsty. Presented at: Implant Retrieval Symposium of thé Society for Biomaterials; 1992; St Charles, IL.

38. Catelas I, Medley JB, Campbell PA, Huk OL, Bobyn JD. Comparison of in vitro with in vivo characteristics of wear particles from metal-metal hip implants. J Biomed Mater Res, 2004;70B-2;167-78.

39. Doorn PF, Campbell PA, Amstutz HC. Metal versus polyethylene wear particles in total hip replacements. A review. Clin Orthop Relat Res, 1996-329 Suppl:S206-16.

40. Willert HG, Broback LG, Buchhorn GH, Jensen PH, Koster G, Lang I, Ochsner P, Schenk R. Crevice corrosion of cemented titanium alloy stems in total hip replacements. Clin Orthop Relat Res 1996-333:51-75.

41. Hallab N, Merritt K, Jacobs JJ. Metal sensitivity in patients with orthopaedic implants. J Bone Joint Surg Am, 2001;83-A-3:428-36.

42. Merritt K, Brown SA. Distribution of cobalt chromium wear and corrosion products and biologic reactions. Clin Orthop Relat Res, 1996-329 Suppl:S233-43.

43. Al-Saffar N. Early clinical failure of total joint replacement in association with follicular proliferation of B-lymphocytes: a report of two cases. J Bone Joint Surg Am 2002;84-A-12:2270-3.

44. Davies A, Willert HG, Campbell P, et al. Metal-on-metal bearing surfaces may lead to higher inflammation. Presented ai: 70th Annual Meeting of the American Academy of Orthopaedic Surgeons; 2003.

45. Willert HG, Buchorn GH, Fayyazi A, et al. Histopathological changes in tissues surrounding metal/metal joints: signs of delayed type hypersensitivity (DTI-I), In: Rieker C, Oberholzer S, Wyss U, eds. World Tribology Forum in Arthroplasty. Bers: 11 ans Nuber, 2001:147-166

46. Haynes DR, Boyle SJ, Roger SD. Variation of cytokines induced by particles from different prosthetic materials. Clin Orthop Relat Res , 1998; 223-230.

47. Haynes DR, Rogers SD, Hay S, Pearcy MJ, Howie DW. The differences in toxicity and release of bone-resorbing mediators induced by titanium and cobalt-chromium-alloy wear particles. J Bone Joint Surg Am, 1993;75-6:825-34.

48. Lee SH, Brennan FR, Jacobs JJ, Urban RM, Ragasa DR, Glant TT. Human monocyte/macrophage response to cobalt-chromium corrosion products and titanium particles in patients with total joint replacements. J Orthop Res 1997;15-1:40-9.

49. Apley AG. Malignancy and joint replacement: the tip of an iceberg? J Bone Joint Surg Br, 1989;71-1:1.

50. Shanbhag AS, Jacobs JJ, Black J, Galante JO, Glant TT. Human monocyte response to particulate biomaterials generated in vivo and in vitro. J Orthop Res 1995;13-5:792-801.

51. Visuri T, Pukkala E, Paavolainen P, Pulkkinen P, Riska EB. Cancer risk after metal on metal and polyethylene on metal total hip arthroplasty. Clin Orthop Relat Res, 1996-329 Suppl:S280-9.

52. Anissian L, Stark A, Dahistrand H, Granberg B, Good V, Bucht E. Cobalt ions influence proliferation and function of human osteoblast-like cells. Acta Orthop Scand, 2002;73-3:369-74.

53. Shanbhag AS, Jacobs JJ, Black J, Galante JO, Glant TT. Effects of particles on fibroblast proliferation and bone resorption in vitro. Clin Orthop Relat Res 1997-342:205-17.

54. Schmalzried TP, Jasty M, Harris WH. Periprosthetic bone loss in total hip arthroplasty. Polyethylene wear debris and the concept of the effective joint space. J Bone Joint Surg Am , 1992;74-6:849-63.

55. Kreibich DN, Moran CG, Delves HT, Owen TD, Pinder IM. Systemic release of cobalt and chromium after uncemented total hip replacement. J Bone Joint Surg Br , 1996;78-1:18-21.

56. Milosev I, Pisot V, Campbell P. Serum levels of cobalt and chromium in patients with Sikomet metal-metal total hip replacements. J Orthop Res , 2005;23-3:526-35.

57. Haudrechy P, Foussereau J, Mantout B, Baroux B. Nickel release from nickel-plated metals and stainless steels. Contact Dermatitis, 1994;31-4:249-55.

58. Damie F, Favard L. [Metal serum levels in 48 patients bearing a chromium-cobalt total hip arthroplasty with a metal-on-polyethylene combination]. Rev Chir Orthop Reparatrice Appar Mot , 2004;90-3:241-8.

59. Savarino L, Granchi D, Ciapetti G, Cenni E, Greco M, Rotini R, Veronesi CA, Baldini N, Giunti A. Ion release in stable hip arthroplasties using metal-on-metal articulating surfaces: a comparison between short- and medium-term results. J Biomed Mater Res A, 2003;66-3:450-6.

60. Schaffer AW, Pilger A, Engelhardt C, Zweymueller K, Ruediger HW. Increased blood cobalt and chromium after total hip replacement. J Toxicol Clin Toxicol , 1999;37-7:839-44.

61. Lhotka C, Szekeres T, Steffan I, Zhuber K, Zweymuller K. Four-year study of cobalt and chromium blood levels in patients managed with two different metal-on-metal total hip replacements. J Orthop Res, 2003;21-2:189-95.

62. Jacobs JJ, Skipor AK, Doorn PF, Campbell P, Schmalzried TP, Black J, Amstutz HC. Cobalt and chromium concentrations in patients with metal on metal total hip replacements. Clin Orthop Relat Res, 1996-329 Suppl:S256-63.

63. Brodner W, Grubl A, Jankovsky R, Meisinger V, Lehr S, Gottsauner-Wolf F. Cup inclination and serum concentration of cobalt and chromium after metal-on-metal total hip arthroplasty. J Arthroplasty, 2004;19-8 Suppl 3:66-70.

64. Heisel C, Silva M, Skipor AK, Jacobs JJ, Schmalzried TP. The relationship between activity and ions in patients with metal-on-metal bearing hip prostheses. J Bone Joint Surg Am, 2005;87-4:781-7.

65. Gleizes V, Poupon J, Lazennec JY, Chamberlin B, Saillant G. [Value and limits of determining serum cobalt levels in patients with metal on metal articulating prostheses]. Rev Chir Orthop Reparatrice Appar Mot, 1999;85-3:217-25.

66. Iida H, Kaneda E, Takada H, Uchida K, Kawanabe K, Nakamura T. Metallosis due to impingement between the socket and the femoral neck in a metal-on-metal bearing total hip prosthesis. A case report. J Bone Joint Surg Am , 1999;81-3:400-3.

67. Mak MM, Besong AA, Jin ZM, Fisher J. Effect of microseparation on contact mechanics in ceramic-on-ceramic hip joint replacements. Proc Inst Mech Eng [H] , 2002;216-6:403-8.

68. Clarke IC, Ishida T, Shirasu H, Shishido T, Yamamoto K, Lazennec JY. A detailed wear mapping of retrieved second-genration metal-on-metal THR 52 nd annual meeting of the Orthopaedic Research Society, 2006. Research Society, 2006.

69. Catonne Y, Lazennec JY, Nogier A, Fourniols E. Metal on metal T.H.A revision with delta ceramic femoral heads using the sleeve technique. Bioceramics 2006.

6.3 Spine: Ceramic Disc – what you should know

M. Grässel

Introduction

In recent years non-fusion techniques in spine surgery using total disc replacement (TDR) for motion preservation and restoring have emerged worldwide, competing with fusion technologies in getting the preferred choice of surgical treatment of degenerative spinal diseases [1,2,7,8,11].

While spinal fusion technology has made impressive advance over the past few decades from rigid plates, pedicle screws and interspinous devices up to dynamic stabilisation it still leaves many problems unsolved. These include limitation of movement, altered spinal kinematics and a more rapid degeneration of adjacent spinal segments [2,3,4,7,9].

Against the background of these disadvantages, attempts with the concept of disc reconstruction with a prosthesis that maintains motion and alignment date back to the 1960s when the first time implanting a stainless steel ball bearing into the lumbar disc space after discectomy (Fernström). However, no long term success was achieved as this implant type was unable to adequately transfer the high intervertebral compressive loads across the bony endplates, and many of them subsequently penetrated into the adjacent vertebral bodies and led to spontaneous fusion. It was not before 1984 when the first TDR system was developed with good short term, mid term, and now limited long term clinical outcomes of about 18 years (SB Charité™) [4-6].

Today, the efficiency of several TDR systems could be confirmed by the latest clinical outcomes of several IDE studies for both lumbar and cervical TDR. Significantly better clinical outcomes of the arthroplasty groups versus fusion could be asserted [17-24].

Taking a look at the figures of the spine market, a big growth of spine surgery in general as well as a transition from TDR to fusion is perceivable indicating also its increasing economic importance. Over the past two decades, the worldwide spine industry has grown dramatically, with annual revenues in 2006 of about EUR 3.5 billion (Fig. 1).

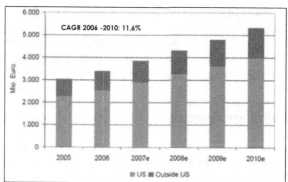

Figure 1:
Worldwide Spine Surgery market 2005-2010 (without market segment „Vertebral Compression Fractures").
* Source: Millennium Research Group, 2004/2005/2006

For spinal motion products an augmentation rate of 10,4 % is assessed from 2006 to 2010, compared to 1,2 % for fusion products (Fig. 2).

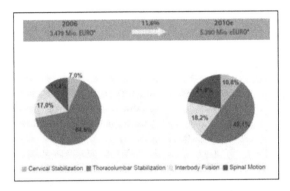

Figure 2:
Worldwide spine surgery market 2006 and 2010 by major product categories (*without market segment "Vertebral Compression Fractures")
Source: Millennium Research Group, 2004/2005/2006

Problems of current TDR solutions

Despite the fact that well over 100 patent applications on TDR devices exist only few systems have been produced for implantation yet [4] and it appears obvious that the complex anatomy and kinematics of the spine makes the design of intervertebral implants an engineering challenge. The following describes problems have retained unsolved so far in the existing TDR solutions independent of the system type but depending on the used implant materials. The currently available designs use metal alloys or combinations of polymers and metal alloys [5,10,11,12].

Wear debris

Factors determining TDR survivability are similar to those for joint replacement technology in hip and knee arthroplasty, and include prosthetic wear, formation of wear debris, and tissue reaction to wear debris [9-11]. Wear is the physical process caused by motion across the bearing surface, not to forget backside wear when modularly systems are used. It is associated with loss of joint height and ultimately failure. More important, the particulate debris can induce hypersensitivity associated with allergic reactions and inflammatory response of its surrounding tissue. An inflammatory response can lead to pain, osteolysis and to aseptic loosening of the prosthesis [6,9-11,16]. There is limited, and only short term information regarding the amount of wear in TDR. But to date wear seems to be lower than in hip and knee arthroplasty [9,10,13].

It is a concern however, that wear debris and any resultant inflammatory reaction would occur in close proximity to neural structures.

Metal ion release

Systemic metal ion release is a problem associated with metallic implants, especially in metal-on-metal bearings. In total hip arthroplasty (THA) with metal-on-metal combinations it is a well described phenomenon, proven many times [14,15,26].

Significant systemic release of metal ions can also be detected in metal-on-metal TDR and evidently persist throughout the patient's lifetime [10,15]. The amount of systemic metal ion release in TDR is discussed controversially and is stated between ten times lower, equal or even higher than the values given in literature about THA [15,25,26].

MRI artefacts

A modern non-invasive postoperative imaging includes MR scanning, e.g. to assess adjacent segments, but it is accompanied by artefacts with every metal alloy (Fig. 3) [5,10,11]. This severe disadvantage of all described TDR implant devices constrains the physician to use diagnostic treatments of the "second choice" like computed tomography. Additionally, there are still no in-vitro data provided by the manufacturers about possible heating or moving of the implants when MRI is in use [7,10].

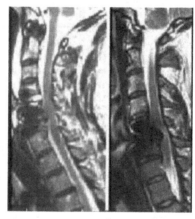

Figure 3:
Sagittal T2-weighted MR scanning of two implants showing the relative amount of artefact seen after artificial disc implantation. The metal blooming artefact of the titanium alloy (left) and even worse with the cobalt chromium alloy (right) hinder the clear interpretation of MR images [11].

Requirements of future TDR generations

There is an ongoing scientific discussion about the advisability of constrained or unconstrained TDR with mobile or fixed centre of rotation [6,7]. Only mid and long term clinical outcomes can bring clarification.

Implants have to be biocompatible and mechanically stable to ensure durability of up to 40 years [7] as patients getting younger and have longer life expectancy than ever. Therefore, a number of requirements have to be fulfilled: Both wear debris (including its amount, shape and composition) with all its possible negative consequences as described above and metal ion release should be reduced up to zero. This also in respect of the fact that like in THA no hydrodynamic lubrication sets up in TDR as it is physiological the case, and thus increasing the wear amount additionally.

Another factor determining the long term durability of TDR is its secure and enduring fixation in the vertebral endplates protecting it against migration. Thus, especially secondary stability with full osseointegration in the implant needs to be optimized. MR imaging with excellent contrast and the absence of artefacts will help to ensure optimum post operative surveillance of the patient.

The risk of fracture should be reduced to a minimum. This is possible with the right choice of material and a validated implant design. Providing the surgeon with a biocompatible TDR solution also applicable for patients with a metal ion allergy or renal insufficiency tops the list of requirements.

Future spine solutions from CeramTec

The choice of material for TDR prosthesis should consider the needs of both the articulating surface and the interface between prosthesis and vertebral body. CeramTec has gathered experience over the past 30 years in the development and manufacturing of ceramic total hip and recently knee joint replacement bearings. The composite Biolox® *delta* is a superior ceramic material which is able to face the challenging requirements of future TDR solutions. Excellent biocompatibility, wear behaviour and resistance against fracture can ensure durability of the TDR during patient's lifetime with superiority in radiography and MR imaging for post operative surveillance [27].

The following solutions, to be developed with partners from industry and university indicate the way CeramTec sees the future of superior TDR.

Modular ceramic TDR

The first generation of ceramic TDR will be a hybrid solution consisting of bearing surfaces made of Biolox® *delta* and non-ceramic endplates for anchorage in the vertebral endplates as discussed schematically in Figure 4 (right). The interface between ceramic inlay and endplates may be implemented by mechanical interlocking or positive locking (form-fit). Due to the limited dimensions taper fit between endplates and ceramic inlay may not be possible. Alternatively, a ceramic sliding core can be applied between concave shaped vertebral endplates with inferior wear characteristics compared to the ceramic-on-ceramic articulation.

At this stage of development design of the ceramic components is concentrated on rotational symmetry.

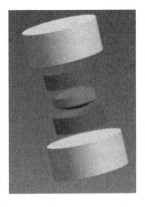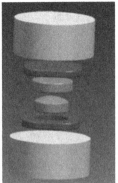

Figure 4:
Modular ceramic TDR solutions with mobile (left) and fixed centre of rotation. Fixation to the vertebral endplates is provided by non-ceramic components.

Monolithic ceramic TDR

A monolithic ceramic TDR solution is the logic consequence of the above stated requirements (Fig. 5), avoiding any negative side effects resulting from the use of metal alloys for vertebral endplates. Beside the advantage of the excellent behaviour in diagnostic imaging it is the absence of metal ion release and possible backside wear which qualifies the monolithic ceramic solution as the next generation of TDR. With a monolithic design for cervical applications, an overall implant height of less than 8mm can easily be realised with superior fracture resistance compared to modular solutions.

Primary stability can be provided by e.g. spikes or macro structuring machined into the ceramic. Secondary stability needs to be realised by a thin plasma sprayed or vapour depositioned coating of titaniumdioxide. This can be combined with a micro hydroxyapatite coating applied on the rough surface of the sintered ceramic body. Preliminary test results regarding the adhesion and shear strength of the coating layers as well as the fracture resistance and fatigue behaviour of surface roughened Biolox® *delta* ceramic are promising.

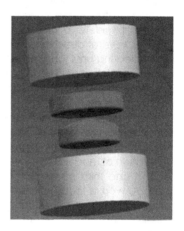

Figure 5:
Monolithic ceramic TDR solution. Fixation to the vertebral endplates is provided by a thin coating layer of titaniumdioxide, if applicable in combination with hydroxyapatite.

Direct to bone monolithic ceramic TDR

A further improvement of surface coated monolithic ceramic TDR is a ceramic solution directly in contact with the bone, ensuring full bony in-growth for long-lasting secondary stability. With the absence of coating layers, and thus an additional interface between ceramic and vertebral endplate, no theoretically imaginable chip off of the coating is possible. A three dimensional macro structured surface as seen in Figure 6 is realised by sintering processes with embedded organic spacers in the ceramic greenbody surface. This generates cavities with sufficient space for osteoblasts not to be sheared off by micromotion of the implant and diffusion processes for osteoblast nutrition. Currently, mechanical and biological characteristics of the pore sizes and volume are optimized. In addition bioactivation, with polylactide or hydroxyapatite for faster osseointegration is tested.

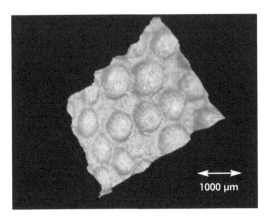

Figure 6:
Three dimensional view of Biolox® *delta* surface structure with a mean pore size of 800µm and a porosity of ~ 40%. Pore depth is variable with its maximum at about 500-600µm.

Summary

TDR as a relatively new field in spine surgery is on its best way getting the gold standard in the surgical treatment of degenerative spinal diseases. With good short and mid term clinical outcomes of currently on the market available solutions several disadvantages still exist with negative consequences probably not appearing until long term outcomes are available. With the ceramic matrix composite Biolox® *delta* and proper engineered and tested designs, requirements of future TDR solutions can be accomplished. However, this is a challenge and an ongoing process.

The development activities at CeramTec together with our partners from the orthopaedic industry aim to provide the surgeon with superior TDR solutions especially for younger, high active or hypersensitive patients. For the first generation of modular ceramic TDR approval is planed for the near future. For the second and third generation of monolithic ceramic TDR made of Biolox® *delta* intensive work is focused on the design optimisation and manufacturing of small rotational and non-rotational symmetric geometries with surface structuring and coating. The development results will also be applicable for other future applications like osseointegrative knees, acetabular shells for THA or furthermore fields in the arthroplasty surgery.

References

1. Krämer J et al (2005) Artificial Discs: Review, Current Status, Outlook. Z Orthop 143: 281-286.
2. Papavero L (2007) Developments in Spine Surgery – Non-fusion Technology. European Musculoskeletal Review, Touch Briefings 1:50-52.
3. Bertagnoli R et al (2005) Why spine arthroplasty? In: Mayer HM, Marnay T, Bertagnoli R (eds) Total disc replacement for degenerative disc disease in the lumbar spine. Synthes, Oberdorf, pp 5-13.
4. Büttner-Janz K (2003) History. In: Büttner-Janz K, Hochschuler SH, McAffee PC (eds) The Artificial Disc. Springer, Berlin, Heidelberg, New York, pp 1-10.
5. Podichetty VK et al (2007) The History of Spinal Fusion Surgery. And: Kim DH et al (2007) History of Disk Replacement Surgery. In: Vaccaro AR, Papadopoulos S et al (eds) Spinal Arthroplasty: The Preservation of Motion.: Saunders, Philadelphia, pp 21-51.

6. Mayer HM (2005) Total lumbar disc replacement. J Bone Joint Surg Br 87-B:1029-1037.

7. Mayer HM (2005) Degenerative disorders of the lumbar spine. Total disc replacement as an alternative to lumbar fusion? Orthopäde 34:1007-1020.

8. Dominkus C (2005) Siegeszug der Bandscheibenprothese. Pressekonferenz anlässlich des 2. internationalen Bandscheibenoperationskurses, 3.Juni 2005, Anatomisches Institut Wien.

9. Anderson P et al (2004) Intervertebral Disc Arthroplasty. Spine, vol 29, 23:2779-2786.

10. Oskouian R J et al (2004) The Future of Spinal Arthroplasty: a Biomaterial Perspective. Neurosurg Focus 17, E2:10-14.

11. Sekhon L H S. et al (2005) Artificial cervical disc replacement: Principles, types and techniques. Neurology India, vol 53, 4:445-450.

12. Aspenber P et al (1996) Periprosthetic bone resorption, Particles versus movement. J Bone Joint Surg Br 78: 641-646.

13. Popoola O et al(2007) In Vitro Wear of UHMWPE Inlays in Dynardi™ and Prodisc® Spine Disc Replacement Implants. Zimmer Inc.. SAS 7, Berlin. Poster P014.

14. Brodner W et al (2003) Serum cobalt levels after metal-on-metal total hip arthroplasty. J Bone Joint Surg Am 85:2168-2173.

15. Zeh A et al (2007) Release of Cobalt and Chromium Ions Into the Serum Following Implantation of the Metal-on-Metal Maverick-Type Artificial Lumbar Disc (Medtronic Sofamor Danek). Spine, vol 32, 3:348-352.

16. Van Ooij A et al (2007) Polyethylene wear of Charité artificial discs. Macroscopic and microscopic wear and inflammatory reaction in peri-prosthetic tissue of 23 retrievals in 19 patients. EFORT, Florence. Abstract F758.

17. Burkus J K et al (2007) Two-Year Results from a Prospective, Randomized IDE Study of the Prestige ST Cervical Disc. SAS 7, Berlin. Abstract Book, Paper PA-WE01.

18. Assietti R et al (2007) Clinical and Radiological Outcome after Double-Level Cervical Arthroplasty with the Bryan Prosthesis. Two-Years Follow-Up. SAS 7, Berlin. Abstract Book, Paper PA-WE02.

19. Datta J et al (2007) Cervical Disc Arthroplasty: Preliminary Results of a Randomized Prospective Study of ACDF Versus Prodisc-C for the Management of Cervical Spondylosis. SAS 7, Berlin. Abstract Book, Paper PA-WE03.

20. Delamarter R B et al (2007) 3 to 4-Year Prospective Results of 1,2, and 3-Level Cervical Arthroplasty with the Prodisc-C Device at a Single Institute. SAS 7, Berlin. Abstract Book, Paper PA-WE04.

21. Phillips F M et al (2007) Initial Outcomes Following PCM Arthroplasty for the treatment of Symptomatic Cervical Spondylosis: Results of a Prospective, Randomized, Multi-Center Study. SAS 7, Berlin. Abstract Book, Paper PA-WE05.

22. Delamarter R B et al (2007) Up to 5-Year Prospective Results of 1,2, and 3-Level Lumbar Arthroplasty with the Prodisc-L Device at a Single Institute. SAS 7, Berlin. Abstract Book, Paper PA-TH02.

23. Geisler F H et al (2007): Evidence for One-Level Lumbar Arthroplasty or Arthrodesis for Degenerative Disc Disease: A Comparison of Two Lumbar Arthroplasty IDE Studies with 2-Year Follow-Up. SAS 7, Berlin. Abstract Book, Paper PA-TH03.

24. Theofilos C et al (2007) Segmental Motion at and Adjacent to a 1-Level FlexiCore® and Fusion. SAS 7, Berlin. Abstract Book, Paper PA-TH06.

25. Burkus J R et al (2007) Serum Metal Ion Levels in Patients with Metal-on-Metal Cervical Disc Replacements. SAS 7, Berlin. Abstract Book, Paper PA-WE13.

26. Sargeant A et al (2006) Ion concentrations from hip implants. J Surg Ortop Adv. 2006 Summer 15(2):113-4.

27. Merkert P et al (2006): Future applications in ceramics. Benazzo F, Falez F, Dietrich M (eds.) Bioceramics and Alternative Bearings in Joint Arthroplasty. 11th Biolox®-Symposium Proceedings. Steinkopff-Verlag, Darmstadt, pp 283-288.

6.4 Trend: Bigger Ball Heads: Is Bigger Really Better?

K.-H. Widmer

Size matters! This is not only true in most parts of today's life but also in total hip arthroplasty in recent years. The head size of the femoral prosthesis has been increased over the years up to the normal femoral head size. But the question arises whether total hip arthroplasty will meet the same fate as the dinosaurs in former times since size seems not to be the only parameter that is important. Looking at the short history of total hip arthroplasty there was a trend to smaller head sizes which was inaugurated by Sir John Charnley in the sixties. He introduced the low friction arthroplasty which is characterized by a smaller head diameter and high density polyethylene as the articulating surface of the cup demonstrating lower friction characteristics. Such, he was able to gradually replace the metal-on-metal arthroplasty of that time. In the latter large head diameters have been used and unfortunately these arthroplasties suffered from friction problems because of unresolved clearance incompatibilties.

Besides low friction smaller heads demonstrated another very important advantage: a lower rate of debris was observed with smaller heads. Since time did show that debris does play a major role in the aseptic loosening process of a total hip arthroplasty using small head size has become a kind of paradigm in total hip arthroplasty, at least for components made out of polyethylene. Small head sizes exert a smaller sliding distance on the articulating surface thus reducing the machining effect of any surface roughness. This is probably the main cause for the reduced debris in smaller heads.

But smaller head sizes did not show favorable effects only but also detrimental ones. Smaller prosthetic head sizes are linked to a higher rate of prosthesis dislocations [1,4,7] whereas larger heads did show a higher resistance against dislocation [2,3]. Since dislocation is still a major concern in total hip arthroplasty any mean to reduce the dislocation rate is an attractive option per se. In former times gaining higher resistance against dislocation by using larger head sizes had to be trade-off against the higher rate of debris associated with larger heads. With the advent of hard-on-hard bearing like ceramic-on-ceramic and metal-on-metal large diameter heads have become applicable without additional draw-backs and therefore the use of larger diameters has become more popular. The rate of dislocation could be reduced dramatically by this mean in accordance with former clinical experience. As soon as highly cross-linked polyethylene has become available the use of large diameter head has become even more popular [5], a real boom has started. One has to point out that by using larger diameter heads articulating against cross-linked polyethylene a remarkable part of the gain in debris reduction is lost again. So, in arthroplasties with polyethylene there is still this trade-off between stability and debris.

Larger head sizes have also become popular because of the increased range of motion. The risk for prosthetic impingement is reduced when a higher head to neck ratio is achieved. This reduces the risk for damage at the rim of the cup and at the prosthetic neck [6]. The rate for dislocation due to neck-to-cup impingement is reduced too resulting in a more stable total hip arthroplasty.

Larger heads increase the stability of a total hip not only by reducing the risk for impingement but also by increasing the distance the head has to be lifted out of the cup when the patient sustains such an undesirable event. The higher the distance the higher the resisting force exerted by the surrounding soft-tissue. This force is counteracting against dislocation forces. Larger heads in total hip resurfacing arthroplasties achieve the same increase in joint stability as large heads in a standard type of a total hip arthroplasty. It should be noted that in hip resurfacing the use of larger heads does not necessarily increase the range of motion since the head-to-neck ratio is decessive for a good range of motion not the pure diameter alone.

What are the downsides of large diameter heads? Well, increasing the head size does increase the range of motion, but the gain in increase becomes smaller and smaller at larger diameters. So, stepping from a 22mm head to a 32mm head is more beneficial than stepping from a 32mm head to a 42mm head.

Furthermore, there is a leveling-off at a certain head-to-neck ratio since the range of motion is not limited by prosthetic impingement alone but also by bone-to-bone impingement, i.e. from a specific head-to-neck ratio on the impingement that limits the range of motion switches from prosthetic to bone-to-bone impingement. In other words, increasing the head size is not reflected by an increase in range of motion any more in larger heads and hence increasing the head diameter is not beneficial any more and therefore is not needed.

Additionally, larger head diameters limit the wall thickness of the acetabular socket, especially of the acetabular liner in modular implants. Decreasing the wall thickness in these implants may put both type of components, those made out of polyethylene and ceramic, at risk for breakage or exessive deformation.

Larger head diameters pose an additional task when reducing the hip during surgery since a larger distance is needed for reduction. This might be overcome by exerting higher pulling forces, but one has to consider that higher forces may also act during slippage of the head over the rim of the cup. In hard-on-hard bearings this edge loading may lead to surface damage putting the arthroplasty at an additional risk.

After all, larger diameter heads do show a couple of advantages in the clinical setting but the benefits are becoming smaller and smaller in the upper diameter range. Therefore, there exists a reasonable limit for the upper head diameter. Time and clinical experience has to tell where this limit has to be placed. There is increasing evidence that a maximum 44mm diameter head turns out to be a good compromise with respect to joint stability and range of motion. In any case, minimal wall thicknesses will dictate the maximum head diameter especially in smaller sized hips like in women or in the asian population. In these cases smaller heads than 44mm have to be accepted.

References

1. Alberton GM, High WA, Morrey BF. Dislocation after revision total hip arthroplasty: an analysis of risk factors and treatment options. J Bone Joint Surg Am. 2002 Oct;84-A(10):1788-92.
2. Amstutz HC, Le Duff MJ, Beaule PE. Prevention and treatment of dislocation after total hip replacement using large diameter balls. Clin Orthop Relat Res. 2004 Dec;(429):108-16.
3. Beaule PE, Schmalzried TP, Udomkiat P, Amstutz HC. Jumbo femoral head for the treatment of recurrent dislocation following total hip replacement. J Bone Joint Surg Am. 2002 Feb;84-A(2):256-63.
4. Berry DJ, von Knoch M, Schleck CD, Harmsen WS. Effect of femoral head diameter and operative approach on risk of dislocation after primary total hip arthroplasty. J Bone Joint Surg Am. 2005 Nov;87(11):2456-63.
5. Geller JA, Malchau H, Bragdon C, Greene M, Harris WH, Freiberg AA. Large diameter femoral heads on highly cross-linked polyethylene: minimum 3-year results. Clin Orthop Relat Res. 2006 Jun; 447:53-9.
6. Kluess D, Martin H, Mittelmeier W, Schmitz KP, Bader R. Influence of femoral head size on impingement, dislocation and stress distribution in total hip replacement. Med Eng Phys. 2007 May;29(4):465-71.
7. Woolson ST, Rahimtoola ZO. Risk factors for dislocation during the first 3 months after primary total hip replacement. J Arthroplasty. 1999 Sep;14(6):662-8.

Hip Revision

7.1 Strategies for Head and Inlay Exchange in Revision Hip Arthroplasty

K. Knahr and M. Pospischill

Introduction

Revision surgery has become more and more important because of the increased number of total hip arthroplasties performed during the past three decades and their limitation of long-term survival mainly due to polyethylene wear [1].

A recent study formulating projections for the number of primary and revision total hip and knee arthroplasties that will be performed in the United States through 2030 predict a demand for primary total hip arthroplasty to grow by 174% from 208.600 in 2005 to 572.000 by 2030. Overall, the total number of revision arthroplasty procedures performed in 2005 is expected to double by the year 2026 for revision total hip arthroplasty [2].

One of the most important concerns of long term survival of total hip arthroplasty is wear. In conventional wear couples polyethylene wear and its biologic reaction to wear debris lead to osteolysis and subsequent loosening of the implant [3]. Therefore, several attempts have been made in the past to solve this problem including cross-linked polyethylene, and the so called hard-on-hard bearings, metal-on-metal and ceramic-on-ceramic [4-7]. Beside the dramatically improved wear rate of all these new articulations we are still faced with problems related to each single combination [8,9].

The aim of this paper is to present strategies if joint replacement fails either because of failure of the articulation material or of other reasons necessating revision hip arthroplasty.

Strategies for metal/ceramic-on-polyethylene articulations

The major reason for revision of these couplings is increased polyethylene wear, with subsequent osteolysis (Fig. 1a,b). As the annual wear rate of metal-on-polyethylene is approx. 0.1 – 0.3 mm/y and the rate for ceramic-on-polyethylene is about 0.05 – 0.15 mm/y [10], the onset of visible wear and osteolysis occurs later in ceramic articulations than in metal articulations [11].

In case of revision there are no limitations concerning the use of subsequent implant materials or revision surgery as the only debris material found is polyethylene and no metal or ceramic particles of relevant amount.

Strategies for revision of metal-on-metal articulations

Metal-on-metal bearings have been reintroduced by Weber in 1988 as an alternative to metal/ceramic-on-polyethylene bearings due to improved wear behavior of high carbon implants [12]. However, there are several reports in literature that show hypersensitivity to metal wear particles leading to early

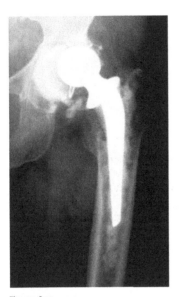

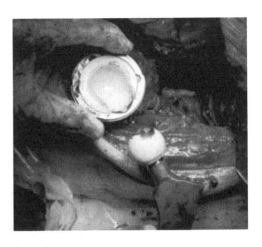

Figure 1b:
Implant loosening due to polyethylene wear
(ceramic-on-polyethylene).

Figure 1a:
Implant loosening due to
polyethylene wear (metal-on-
polyethylene).

osteolysis and aseptic loosening of components (Fig. 2) [13-15]. Clinical data suggest an association with a delayed hypersensitivity type IV to metal, mainly cobalt. It is still unclear whether the allergy to metal alloys is preexisting preoperatively or the patients became hypersensitive secondary to metal particles. As a consequence, in patients with postoperative persisting or early recurrent, load-dependent thigh pain - with or without radiographic signs of osteolytic lesions - a possible hypersensitivity to metal should be considered.

In case of revision surgery, all bearing couples except metal-on-metal are suggested.

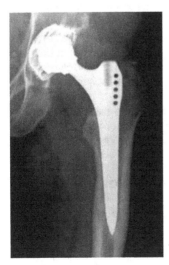

Figure 2:
. Early osteolysis of low-carbide metal-on-metal articulation
3 years postoperatively.

Strategies for revision of ceramic-on-ceramic articulations

As ceramic-on-ceramic bearings produce very few wear debris, revisions mainly are not caused by osteolysis and secondary loosening of the implant. The serious problems of ceramics are wear of the material f.e. due to impingement or recurrent dislocation or in very rare cases fracture of the material.

Alumina ceramic is a very hard and resistent material with excellent wear characteristics. The linear wear rate is very low and described in literature about 0.003 mm/year [16]. Nevertheless the elasticity of the material is also low and does not allow any deformation under load. High punctual stress can lead to fracture. Exact positioning of the cup is necessary to avoid edge loading by impingement at the rim of the liner [17].

The revision of ceramic components is not as straightforward as of the other bearing partners and requires certain considerations. Therefore, different failure modes need different approaches to manage revisions of ceramic implants.

Revision of the femoral head

Loose cup – stable stem

In many cases it is necessary to remove the ceramic ball head of a well fixed stem either to improve the exposure or to vary the length of the neck after the cup revision. It is recommended to perform cup exchange with the original ball head in place as long as possible to protect the taper. A rough removal can damage the surface structure of the taper. If a ceramic head would be used on a damaged taper once again, high stress concentration can develop leading to a breakage of the ball. For this reason the removal should be done with special tools and under protection of a swab to avoid any scratches on the taper. In principle if the surface structure is macroscopically not damaged a new ceramic head can be used. Only the surgeon is responsible when re-using the taper of a stable stem. Manufacturers state that tapers are never to get re-used with a ceramic ball head because of the danger of damage of the taper during removal which is not in their control. If the surgeon is uncertain or unwilling to take over responsibility, he has to remove the stem which often complicates the surgical procedure.

In the last several years new concepts were developed to solve this problem. Recently, CeramTec offers a metal sleeve that can be put on the original taper to create a smooth surface where a new ceramic ball head can be attached (Fig. 3a,b).

Stable implants – recurrent dislocation

Recurrent dislocations may be the reason of abductor muscle weakness because of less tension of the muscle. This problem can be solved just by exchange of the femoral head using a longer neck size. Again one is faced with the possible damage of the taper during removal of the original head. Therefore careful removal described above as well as using the ceramic revision ball heads with an inner metal sleeve is recommended.

Another problem is the possible limitation of neck length increase for joint stabilization. As the use of ceramic skirted balls is not advisable because of possible impingement leading to fracture, modern ceramic head systems do not exist in the sizes XL or XXL. These issues can limit the ability of ceramic heads for use in revision cases with dislocation. One solution is again the use of the revision ball heads system including an inner metal sleeve allowing longer neck length sizes.

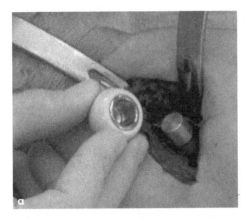

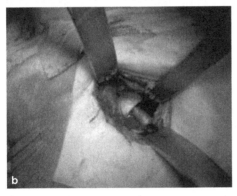

Figure 3a, b:
Revision ball heads system by CeramTec. Inner metal sleeves allow ceramic XL neck sizes.

Revision of fractured ceramic implants

Fracture of the liner

Fracture can be caused either by intraoperative rim chipping due to malinsertion by the surgeon (Fig. 4a) or by impingement between the rim of the liner and the taper, especially when skirted balls are used. Similar to the revision of the femoral ceramic head it is important to remove the ceramic liner without damage of the inner surface of the cup. This is usually managed by a perpendicular impact to the rim of the metal shell of the cup resulting in a loosening of the conical press fit. By use of a suction cup instrument the ceramic liner can be removed easily without any damage of the inner surface (Fig. 4b). Again, the one and only choice of articulation type is renewal of a ceramic wear couple to reduce the risk of third-body-wear.

Fracture of the ceramic head

Despite of the substantial improvement in clinical performance the concern of fracture still continues. This may be caused either by a substantial trauma of the patient, it may be related to dislocation or probably to poor intraoperative

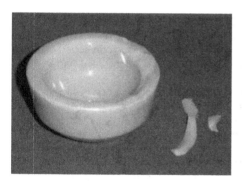

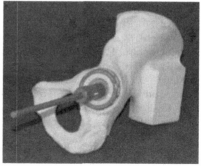

Figure 4a:
Rim fracture due to incorrect insertion of the
ceramic liner.

Figure 4b:
The suction cup instrument.

handling when implanting the ceramic head to the metallic cone of the stem. In case of fracture many ceramic particles of different sizes can be found during revision. Despite meticulous synovectomy and extensive joint lavage there are always small particles left. This remaining debris is harder than metal and leads to third-body-wear. Therefore it is absolutely necessary to avoid an exchange to a metal head after fracture of a ceramic articulation. Especially if a polyethylene liner is used the small ceramic wear particles get pressed into the soft poly which works like a sandpaper leading soon to massive abrasion of the metal head [18]. The one and only choice of articulation type for revision is renewal of a ceramic wear couple to reduce the risk of third-body-wear.

Prevention of ceramic failure

To avoid any damage to the ceramic liner during insertion a special suction cup instrument was created [19]. It allows a simple and secure fixation.
Concerning the fixation of the ceramic ball to the taper, similar precaution should be taken. The ceramic head should be placed to the taper in rotating movement to achieve already primary fixation. Only a single blow with the impactor not too heavy should be added for the definite stability.

Conclusion

Revision of a total hip arthroplasty needs comprehensive knowledge of the characteristics of the articulating materials. A wrong re-implanted wear couple can lead to early re-failure.
Selection of articulation in primary THA can be influenced by possible revision scenarios. Today the new XL-PE, metal-on-metal and ceramic-on-ceramic articulations offer excellent wear behaviors. Concerning the amount of wear, ceramic-on-ceramic seems to be the favourite. Nevertheless, a certain amount of risk for fractures has to be considered.

References

1. Pospischill, M. and K. Knahr, Cementless total hip arthroplasty using a threaded cup and a rectangular tapered stem. Follow-up for ten to 17 years. J Bone Joint Surg Br, 2005. 87(9): p. 1210-5.

2. Kurtz S, Ong K, Lau E, Mowat F, Halpern M, Projections of primary and revision hip and knee arthroplasty in the United States from 2005 to 2030. J Bone Joint Surg Am, 2007, 89: p. 780-5.

3. Harris WH, Wear and periprosthetic osteolysis: the problem. Clin Orthop Relat Res, 2001. 393: p. 66-70.

4. Santavirta S, Bohler M, Harris WH, Konttinen YT, Lappalainen R, Muratoglu O, Rieker C, Salzer M, Alternative materials to improve total hip replacement tribology. Acta Orthop Scand, 2003. 74 (4): p. 380-8.

5. Harris WH, Highly cross-linked, electron-beam-irradiated, melted polyethylene: some pros. Clin Orthop Relat Res, 2004. 429: p. 63-7.

6. Silva M, Heisel C, Schmalzried TP, Metal-on-metal total hip replacement. Clin Orthop Res, 2005. 430: p. 53-61.

7. Hamadouche M, Boutin P, Daussange J, Bolander ME, Sedel L, Alumina-on-alumina total hip arthroplasty: a minimum 18.5 year follow-up study. J Bone Joint Surg Am, 2002. 84-A(1): p. 69-77.

8. MacDonald, Metal-on-metal total hip arthroplasty: the concerns. Clin Orthop Relat Res, 2004. 429: p. 86-93.

9. Barrack RL, Burak C, Skinner HB, Concerns about ceramics in THA. Clin Orthop Relat Res. 2004. 429: p. 73-9.

10. Zichner, L. and T. Lindenfeld, [In-vivo wear of the slide combinations ceramics-polyethylene as opposed to metal-polyethylene]. Orthopade, 1997. 26(2): p. 129-34.

11. Urban JA, Garvin KL, Boese CK, Bryson L, Pedersen DR, Callaghan JJ, Miller RK. Ceramic-on-polyethylene bearing surfaces in total hip arthroplasty. Seventeen to twenty-one-year results. J Bone Joint Surg Am 2001;83-A-11:p. 1688-94.

12. Rieker, C., M. Windler, and U. Wyss, Metasul - A Metal-on-Metal Bearing. 1999, Bern: Hans Huber.

13. Park, Y.S., et al., Early osteolysis following second-generation metal-on-metal hip replacement. J Bone Joint Surg Am, 2005. 87(7): p. 1515-21.

14. Willert, H.G., et al., Metal-on-metal bearings and hypersensitivity in patients with artificial hip joints. A clinical and histomorphological study. J Bone Joint Surg Am, 2005. 87(1): p. 28-36.

15. Baur, W., et al., [Pathological findings in tissue surrounding revised metal/metal articulations]. Orthopade, 2005. 34(3): p. 225-6, 228-33.

16. Skinner, H.B., Ceramic bearing surfaces. Clin Orthop Relat Res, 1999(369): p. 83-91.

17. Mittelmeier, H. and J. Heisel, Sixteen-years' experience with ceramic hip prostheses. Clin Orthop Relat Res, 1992(282): p. 64-72.

18. Kempf, I. and M. Semlitsch, Massive wear of a steel ball head by ceramic fragments in the polyethylene acetabular cup after revision of a total hip prosthesis with fractured ceramic ball. Arch Orthop Trauma Surg, 1990. 109(5): p. 284-7.

19. Knahr, K. and R. Beck, An Instrument for the Insertion of Ceramic Liners, in Bioceramics in Joint Arthroplasty - Proceedings 7th international BIOLOX Symposium, J.P. Garino and G.

7.2 Live-Time Prediction of BIOLOX® *delta*

M. Kuntz

Introduction

In the last 7 years more than 250.000 artificial hip joints with components of the high performance ceramic composite BIOLOX® *delta* have been successfully implanted. Due to the unique strength and toughness of this material the risk of fracture has been drastically reduced when compared to BIOLOX® *forte*.

However, one should keep in mind that the outstanding properties of BIOLOX® *delta* rely on complex reinforcing mechanisms. Therefore, it is necessary to assess if reinforcement is maintained throughout the live-time of the artificial joint which is anticipated to exceed more than 20 years.

Like any other material which is intended for surgical applications, the suitability must be evaluated based on multiple approaches:

1. Intrinsic mechanical material properties
2. Biocompatibility
3. System compatibility
4. In-vivo scoring of the surgical outcome

The basis of all progress in material development for surgical applications are the intrinsic material properties. When the surgeon decides to replace a known material by a new one, there must be sufficient indication for a substantial benefit. The most challenging question is to predict the reliability of the material after many years of service life.

Within the scope of this paper, the intrinsic material properties of the composite ceramic BIOLOX® *delta* are analysed. Live time can be traced back to basic principles, i.e. how can a material be damaged after many years of service. Every material degrades after many years loading in an aggressive environment. It is the challenge to create a material which preserves sufficient residual reliability even under worst case conditions for many years.

Due to the chemical stability ceramics obviously provide an intrinsic advantage in comparison to other materials like metals and polymers. Ceramics are produced in the state of a fully saturated chemical bonding. There is no driving power left for further chemical interaction with the environment. Thus, typical live time limiting problems like corrosion or water adsorption are not relevant for high performance and high purity ceramics.

However, it must be considered whether there are other mechanisms which may limit the live time of ceramics. It is well known that like all other materials also ceramics may suffer degradation from following distinguished events:

- Fatigue   resistance against long time static and alternating load
- Ageing   resistance against hydrothermal or other chemical attack
- Wear   durability under abrasive conditions

In this paper, the live time limiting mechanisms and the relevance for the application as a surgical implant are discussed. It is shown how live time of the ceramic material BIOLOX® delta can be described and evaluated. The unique microstructure and reinforcing mechanisms of the material not only support the short term performance like fracture toughness and strength but also improve substantially the long term reliability.

Description of BIOLOX® delta

BIOLOX® delta is an alumina based composite ceramic. 80 vol % of the matrix consist of fine grained high purity alumina which is very similar to the well known material BIOLOX® forte. As it is the case in any other composite material, the basic physical properties like stiffness, hardness, thermal conductivity etc. are mainly predetermined from the dominating phase. It was the basic idea for the development of the new material to preserve all the desirable properties of BIOLOX® forte which has millions of components in service but to increase its strength and toughness.

These properties are rigorously improved by implementation of reinforcing elements. Figure 1 shows the microstructure of BIOLOX® delta.

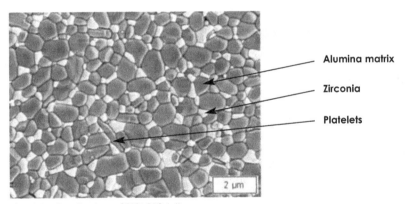

Figure 1: Microstructure of BIOLOX® delta.

Two reinforcing components are integrated in BIOLOX® delta. 17 vol % of the matrix consist of tetragonal zirconia particles. The average grain size of the zirconia is around 0.2 µm. As a further reinforcing element, apprx. 3 vol % of the matrix are built by platelet shaped crystals of the ceramic composition strontiumaluminate. The platelets stretch to a maximum length of apprx. 3 µm with an aspect ratio of 5 – 10. The reinforcing ability of these ingredients is explained below.

Additionally to the reinforcing components, there are also stabilizing elements doped to the material. Chromium is added which is soluble in the alumina matrix and which increases the hardness of the composite. The minor amount of chromium is the reason for the mauve colour of the material. Furthermore, some yttrium is added to the composite which is solved in the zirconia and which supports the stabilization of the tetragonal phase.

The reinforcing elements, i.e. the zirconia and the platelets, substantially increase fracture toughness and strength of the material [1-2]. Fracture toughness (K_{IC}) is a measure for the ability of the material to withstand crack extension. Strength (σ_c) is defined as the maximum stress within a structure that causes failure of the component. Consequently, when the fracture toughness of the alumina is increased also the strength is directly improved. This basic principle is the concept of the development of BIOLOX® delta. The microstructure is designed in order to provide a maximum of resistance against crack extension.

The benefit in crack resistance which is obtained from either incorporating zirconia or platelets into an alumina matrix are well known in the science of high performance ceramics. However, the material BIOLOX® delta represents an unique combination of both mechanisms, which is shown in Figure 2.

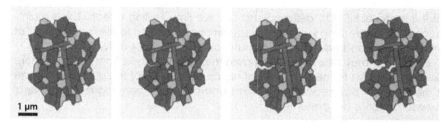

Figure 2:
Reinforcing mechanism in BIOLOX® delta at crack initiation and propagation.

The figure represents a realistic part of the microstructure. In the case of severe overloading crack initiation and crack extension will occur. High tensile forces in the vicinity of the crack tip trigger the tetragonal – monoclinic phase transformation of the zirconia particles. The accompanied volume expansion leads to the formation of compressive stresses which are very efficient for blocking the crack extension. Furthermore, the crack path is deflected by the platelets, thus activating bridging forces and crack shielding. As it is schematically shown in Figure 2 the crack extension also leads to higher yield of phase transformation in the immediate vicinity of the microcrack.

As it is shown all these reinforcing mechanisms are fully activated within a region of a few micrometers. For the macroscopic performance of the material it is extremely important that immediately at the beginning of crack initiation also the reinforcing mechanisms are activated. Regarding Figure 2 one should keep in mind that the average distance between the reinforcing zirconia particles is apprx. 0,2 µm, i.e. similar to the grain size. Thus, the reinforcement is activated immediately when any microcrack is initiated.

The ability of zirconia particles to reinforce is derived from the phase transformation, i.e. the spontaneous change from the tetragonal to the monoclinic phase. The phase transformation is accompanied by a volume change of 4 % of the zirconia particle, i.e. a linear expansion of 1,3%. Spontaneous phase transformation is a well known principle in material science. For example, the properties of high performance steels also rely on spontaneous phase transformation from austenite to martensite.

It should be emphasized that the ability of phase transformation is the precondition for any benefit of the zirconia within the material. The composite is designed such that phase transformation occurs when it is needed, i.e. in the case of microcrack initiation. In contrast to pure zirconia (which draws its high strength from the same principle) the main source of the stability of the tetragonal phase is the embedding of the zirconia particles in the alumina matrix. In contrast, the stability of pure zirconia only relies on the chemical stabilisation (i.e. doping with yttria) and the grain size, which should not exceed a certain range. This is the most important distinction of the composite material BIOLOX® delta to pure zirconia. In particular, the mechanical stabilization of the stiff alumina matrix is not sensitive to any ageing effect.

Comparison of component and material testing

As described above, it is the objective of this paper to show the intrinsic stability of the material BIOLOX® delta against any live-time limiting effects. This is mainly accomplished by using well defined specimens according to the requirements of international standards for surgical materials (e.g. ISO 6474 or ASTM F 603).

However, it may be useful to compare the data obtained from test specimens like bending bars to the properties of hip components. For this purpose, in figure 3 the results of ball head fracture tests and of 4-point bending tests of several powder batches are presented.

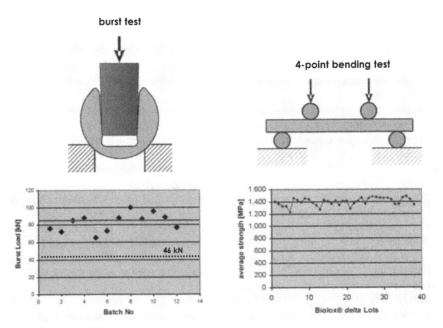

Figure 3:
Burst load of BIOLOX® delta ball heads (28 + 3,5) and strength of bending tests.

The burst tests on BIOLOX® delta ball heads (Figure 3 left) refers to a standard design diameter 28mm, taper 12/14. Each individual data point in the Figure represents the average value of a test series of at least 7 ball heads. The strength (Figure 3 right) refers to 4-point bending tests according to ASTM F 603. The strength as it is derived from bending tests represents the maximum stress in the specimen at the moment of fracture. Each individual data point represents the average of 30 specimens. As it is shown, plenty of data is available for either ball head burst tests and strength. The larger scatter in the burst tests is a consequence of the smaller number of specimens used in this test.

From these data, one is able to compare the strength of the material to the performance of the components. The average burst load is 83 kN and the average strength 1400 MPa. Usually the load acting on an artificial hip joint is expressed as multiples of the body weight (BW). A reasonable value for 1 BW is 1 kN (apprx. 100 kg). From various experiments and calculations it is derived that the maximum load which can occur in-vivo in an extreme situation (e.g. one leg balancing of a stumble) is apprx. 9 x BW. This result gives an impressive indication of the large safety margin which is provided from the use of the material BIOLOX® *delta* as a surgical material.

On this basis, the live time experiments were designed. The long term stress on the specimens was chosen such that a reasonable margin in comparison to maximum in-vivo loading is provided. Thus, for the cyclic loading tests two stress levels of 300 MPa and 600 MPa were chosen. From the comparison discussed under Figure 3 the stress level of 300 MPa is equivalent to a component loading of 18 x BW, i.e. double the maximum in-vivo load. (300 MPa / 1400 MPa ≈ 18 BW / 83 BW). Analogous, 600 MPa correspond to 4-fold maximum in-vivo load. Using these stress levels it is analysed whether the material is able to resist extreme conditions over a live-time relevant period.

Discussion of live time limiting effects

The analysis discussed in this paper refers to a combination of ageing and fatigue experiments. Any degradation of the material after long term treatment is evaluated by comparison of residual strength to the as-received state.

Ageing is a relevant issue for all zirconia containing materials. The transformation from the tetragonal to the monoclinic phase can be triggered by the so-called hydrothermal attack [3-5]. "Hydrothermal" means that this particular ageing effect only takes place in aqueous environment at elevated temperatures. It has been shown that a critical temperature range for hydrothermal ageing is around 134 – 150°C. Obviously, this temperature is not realistic for human body environment. However, today it is well accepted that the ageing in the human body environment can be simulated in an accelerated test using autoclaving conditions of 2 bar water steam and 134°C. Various authors claim that 1 hour autoclaving conditions are equivalent to 2 – 4 years in the human body [1-2]. Consequently, accelerated ageing is also required as a standard test for pure zirconia as a material for surgical implants. Usually, it is investigated whether the residual strength of the material deteriorates after ageing. The concept which is presented here does not only rely on the residual strength but also to the performance of the material at cyclic loading.

Fatigue is defined as the material sensitivity against cyclic loading. Limited fatigue resistance is usually observed when the materials ability of crack resistance is continuously deteriorating during the cycling. Even materials which offer plastic deformation and high crack resistance like metals can substantially loose their strength during cyclic loading and exhibit brittle fracture. In general, ceramics show higher fatigue resistance in comparison to metals. However, the fatigue effects of ceramics also depend on their specific crack resistance mechanisms. As it was shown under Figure 2, the crack resistance of BIOLOX® delta is rather complex. Thus, it is necessary to demonstrate whether this material may show any degradation at cyclic loading.

As a special feature of this investigation, hydrothermal ageing and fatigue are combined. According to the theoretical background one should consider if any ageing effect may also impair the fatigue resistance or vice versa.

Result of live-time experiments

The experiments were designed to simulate a combination of worst case conditions on BIOLOX® delta. The specimens were prepared according to the 4-point bending configuration as it is shown in Figure 3 (right). As discussed above, the live time limiting effects ageing and cyclic fatigue were combined in these tests.

Two stress levels (300 MPa and 600 MPa) are chosen for the cyclic loading tests. The lower stress level was applied for 20 Mio cycles, the higher stress level for 5 Mio cycles. All tests were performed in Ringer's solution. The accelerated ageing was simulated by 5 h and 100 h treatment in autoclaving conditions which is equivalent to 10 years and 200 years (!) in vivo. All specimens used for cyclic loading where proof tested prior to the cycling. Table 1 shows the test matrix including the number of specimens used.

Autoclaving	no cyclic load	300MPa, $20*10^6$ cycles	600MPa, $5*10^6$ cycles
0 h	30	6	6
5 h	30	6	6
100 h	30	6	6

Table 1:
Test matrix with number of tested samples.

Using 30 specimens is usually required for determination of strength. However, due to the time consuming experiments applying the cyclic loading it was decided to use only 6 specimens for each cyclic loading test. After the treatment, the residual strength of the specimens was determined and compared to the initial strength. Furthermore, the monoclinic phase content was measured for each treatment.

As the most amazing result the yield of specimens surviving all the tests was 100 % in all cases. Even most severe conditions (i.e. 100 h autoclaving, 600 MPa cyclic load) did not reveal any premature failure. It should be recalled that this stress level represents 4 times the highest load level at worst case conditions in-vivo. We can thus conclude that the reliability of BIOLOX® delta exceeds by far the necessary requirements for reliable surgical components.

Autoclaving		no cyclic load	300MPa, 20*10⁶ cycles	600MPa, 5*10⁶ cycles
0	Strength [MPa]	1346	1433	1284
	Monoclinic phase content	18 %	33 %	43 %
5	Strength [MPa]	1332	1248	1361
	Monoclinic phase content	22 %	35 %	42 %
100	Strength [MPa]	1234	1308	1300
	Monoclinic phase content	30 %	33 %	47 %

Table 2:
Residual strength and monoclinic phase content after diverse treatments.

Table 2 shows the results of the post – test analysis including residual strength and monoclinic phase content. There is a marginal natural scatter in residual strength which is always expected for ceramic materials. However, statistical analysis using Student's t-test did not reveal any significant deviation of all strength results.

In contrast, there is a clear tendency of an increase in monoclinic phase content both, after autoclaving and after cyclic loading. For example, the test series without autoclaving shows an increase of monoclinic phase content from 18 % in the initial state to 43 % after 5 Mio cycles at 600 MPa. It must be concluded that the cyclic mechanical loading at a high stress level (600 MPa) of almost half the strength (1,400 MPa) activated the reinforcing ability of the material. As discussed under Figure 2, a high mechanical stress triggers localized phase transformation which prevents any further crack propagation. Obviously the increased amount of monoclinic phase content does not deteriorate the strength of the material. This important conclusion is independent from the source of the phase transformation. In other words, when the phase transformation is activated either by accelerated ageing, cyclic fatigue or a combination of both, the residual strength remains on the initial level.

The reported monoclinic phase content should be discussed with respect to the composition of the material. The monoclinic phase content reported in Table 2 is related to the total zirconia. As described above, the total volume content of zirconia in the alumina matrix is 17 %. In order to assess the meaning of the zirconia content one should refer the amount of monoclinic phase relative to the total volume of the material. For example, the highest amount of monoclinic phase in a region close to the surface measured in this study is 47%. This equals a total monoclinic content of only 8% (= 47% x 17 %). Obviously, even under extreme conditions the amount of monoclinic phase in this material is well under control. In this context it is elucidative to remind that in pure zirconia an amount of 20 % monoclinic phase is allowed according to the standard ISO 13356 already in the initial state before accelerated ageing. This is an amount of monoclinic phase which is higher than the absolute limit in BIOLOX® delta which is of course equal to the zirconia content of 17 %. It is thus concluded that the specific composition of BIOLOX® delta provides inherent protection against improper phase transformation.

Conclusions

The material BIOLOX® *delta* has been exposed to extreme conditions (accelerated ageing and cyclic loading in Ringer's solution). It has been shown that even a combination of worst case conditions does not reveal any premature failure. Furthermore, it was shown that the residual strength remains on the initial level. A certain amount of phase transformation was observed during the tests. The highest amount of monoclinic phase relative to the total volume of the specimen was 47 %. The residual strength was not affected by the phase transformation.

In other studies it was shown that BIOLOX® *delta* performs extremely well in severe wear tests [6]. These results are also attributed to the reinforcing mechanism in the material. These exciting results promote the confidence that BIOLOX® *delta* offers the highest probability of long term durability in well designed artificial joint systems.

References

1. Hannink R.H.J., Kelly P.M., Muddle B.C., Transformation Toughening in Zirconia-Containing Ceramics, J.Am.Cer.Soc. 83 [3] 461-87 (2000).
2. De Aza, A.H., Chevalier J., Fantozzi G., Schehl M., Torrecillas R., Crack growth resistance of alumina, zirconia and zirconia toughened alumina ceramics for joint prostheses, Biomaterials 23, 937-945 (2002).
3. Pezzotti G. Environmental Phase Stability of Next Generation Ceramic composite for Hip Prostheses, Key Engineering Materials Vols. 309-311, 1223-1226 (2006).
4. Ohmichi N., Kamioka K., Ueda K., Matsui K. Ohgai M., Phase Transformation of Zirconia Ceramics by Annealing in Hot Water, J. Cer. Soc. Jap., 107 [2] 128-133 (1999).
5. Gremillard L., Chevalier J., Epicier T., Deville S., Fantozzi G., Modeling the ageing kinetics of zirconia ceramics, J.Eur.Cer.Soc., 24, 3483-3489 (2004).
6. Clarke I.C., Pezzotti G., Green D.D., Shirasu H., Donaldson T., Severe Simulation Test for run-in ear of all-alumina compared to alumina composite THR, Proceedings 10th BIOLOX Symposium, 11-20 (2005).

7.3 Revision Total Hip Arthroplasty with Sandwich-type Ceramic on Ceramic Liner

S.-H. Lee, J.-H. Hwang, B.-K. Kim and S.-H. Hong

Introduction

In the past, surgical techniques, implant designs, and research on bone growth factors have focused on the arthroplasty field. However, as wear and loosening became the most common causes of arthroplasty failure, many investigators have attempted to identify a new articular surface. One is the improvement of the conventional polyethylene liner, and the other is developing a new articular surface material. Among these, ceramic is the most recently developed articular material. Ceramic-on-ceramic articulation was invented by Pierre Boutin (France) in 1970. Mittlemeier-type ceramic articulation was introduced by Miller to the US and received FDA approval in 1982. Recent articles have shown the successful results of ceramic articulation during more than 10 years follow-up. Regarding the aspect of wear rate, ceramic is the most satisfactory material. Unfortunately, the hardness of alumina ceramic causes a high risk of loosening of acetabular cup [9] and consequent fracture of the femoral head and liner [3]. As this complication is related to inadequate resorption of the dynamic load on the articular surface, the new, low-stiff sandwich liner was introduced. We analyzed the short-term results of the sandwich liner in total hip arthroplasty in revisional cases.

Drawbacks

Although ceramic has many advantages, several problems can arise both intraoperatively and postoperatively. The problem of ceramic is also related to the most useful advantages of ceramic. This is acetabular loosening caused by the high degree of stiffness of the ceramic. Ceramic failure is not caused by the wear that frequently occurs in a polyethylene liner. There are several reasons for ceramic failure, the first being its stiffness on weight loading, the second one being the malposition of the acetabular cup, and the third being the improper designs of implants. Among these, the first reason is the most frequent cause of failure. Boutin et al. reported the results of ceramic liner after 15 years follow-up as having a loosening rate of 12.5% caused by the inadequacy of vibration absorption on loading and also related to its stiffness [1]. Many reports have indicated that the ideal position of the cup in a ceramic component is 30~40 degrees of inclination and that too vertical position can adversely concentrate the dynamic load and therefore loosen the ceramic [4,5]. However, the malposition of the cup is overcome by using a cementless press-fit cup.

Another large concern regarding ceramic is a surgery related problem as a chipping fracture can occur during insertion of the liner. The ceramic is stiff, and chipping fractures occur more often than femoral head fracture [8]. Proper Morse taper fitting of the femoral head can prevent malalignment of the femoral head and can therefore reduce high-contact stress and femoral head fracture.

Insertion of the femoral head through the screwing action by the surgeon is crucial in reducing the risk of femoral head breakage which is also caused by foreign particles between the femoral head and neck. Many surgeons have reported different rates of liner chipping fracture, 0.02% to 0.9% [10,11,12]. The last problem is fracture of a ceramic component. Although recent, 4th generation ceramic with its tribological superiority, has reduced this complication, clinicians must be more cautious with patients who are highly physically active and young.

Sandwich liner

Drawbacks of ceramic articulation are related to the alumina stiffness as femoral head fracture, liner breakage, and early loosening are caused by the inability of absorption the vibratory load on the articular joint surface. Therefore, the concept of low-stiffness ceramic articulation has been introduced. Theses concepts created new design, sandwich liner containing a conical alumina liner and the back side polyethylene covered liner which have advantages of high resistance to wear, effective load sharing, simultaneously. This concept was introduced in 1993 by the Lima-Lto Co. in Italy, and the CeramTec company produced this new developed sandwich liner. This liner can evenly distribute the dynamic load onto the articular surface and can minimize the any minimal vibration and contact stress. It has three advantages: (1) a remarkable decrease of coupling stiffness; (2) the ability to insert a liner with impaction; and (3) the ability to remove the liner without breakage during revisional surgery. However, this design also has some disadvantages, including the incongruence between polyethylene and metal and between ceramic and polyethylene. This geometric problem was overcome using the concept of double Morse taper (conicity = 1:10). The joint loading is therefore applied on a double Morse taper, thereby assuring steadiness to the system and without the need for a further locking system. Thanks to this geometrical solution, when loaded, the polyethylene enables an immediate arrangement of the surfaces. However, compared to the thickness of the ceramic liner, the ceramic liner itself is thin and is theoretically predisposed to breaking. D'Antonio reported clinical results of the sandwich liner with 3 to 5 years follow-up. In this study, there was no liner chipping breakage, head fracture or early loosening. Park reported 2 cases of femoral head fracture and 4 cases of liner fracture(1.7%) out of 357 sandwich liners.

Results

Other physicians have also reported successful clinical results using a sandwich liner in primary total hip arthroplasty and they reported good wear resistance and a lower incidence of acetabular osteolysis [7,13]. However, as there are no clinical results on use of the sandwich liner in revisional arthroplasty, we report the short-term clinical results of revisional arthroplasty using sandwich liner. We have performed approximately 1300 cases of ceramic on ceramic total hip arthroplasty surgeries since 1999. We have performed revision total hip arthroplasty in 142 cases using ceramic on ceramic liner and among them, we used sandwich liner in 128 cases.

Of the 128 cases, we registered the clinical data and radiological data of 103 cases (97 patients). Their average follow-up was 38.3(24~100) months. In our study, the causes of revision were 72 cases of loosening of the femoral stem and acetabular cup, 10 cases of infection, 10 cases of polyethylene wear, 7 cases of recurrent dislocation, 3 cases of periprosthetic fracture, and 1 case of liner fracture. We used a metal-backing sandwich liner in all 92 revisional cases and in 11 cases we used allogenic bone for grafting with a Kerboul plate in patients with severe acetabular defects. In these 11 cases, we used cement to keep the sandwich liner (Müller type, Lima-Lto, Italy) in place. Except in those cases where cement was used, SPH cups (Lima-Lto Co. Italy) ranging from 46~62mm were used in all cases. The size of the liners used depended on the size of the acetabular cup. From A(40.4mm), the liners were categorized as B(43.4mm), C(44.4mm), D(48.4mm), and E(54.4mm). The D-sized liners were used most frequently and compares with the primary cases in which we used B- and C-sized cups most frequently. We used distal femoral allogeneous bone to reconstruct acetabular defect which was proportional to the size of the defect area and grafted allo-bone is secured with screws which were usually two. Clinically, we evaluated the Harris hip score that increased from 58.8 preoperatively to 86.8 postoperatively. Radiologically, we checked the migration of the acetabular cup as well as loosening or osteolysis in the periacetabular area, the radioucency and ostolysis in the femoral stem.

We achieved successful results except in 24 cases. Postoperative complications included 1 cases of infection, 5 cases of early loosening of acetabular cup and femoral stem, 4 cases of recurrent dislocation, 1 case of liner breakage (Fig. 1), 3 cases of heterotopic ossification and 5 cases of periprosthetic fracture. We also have performed trochanteric osteotomy for removal of implant in 50 cases and among them, 5 cases of non-unions of osteotomy site took place.

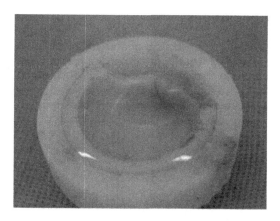

Figure1:
Breakage of sandwich liner.

Causes	Cases (Percentage)
Loosening	72 (69.9%)
Infection	10 (9.7%)
Polyethylen wear	10 (9.7%)
Recurrent dislocation	7 (6.80%)
Periprosthetic fracture	3 (2.91%)
Liner fracture	1 (0.97%)
Total	**103 (100%)**

Table 1:
Causes in revisional arthroplasty with sandwich-type ceramic on ceramic liner.

Complications	Cases (percentage)
Infection	1 (4.0%)
Early loosening of acetabula cup and femoral stem	5 (20.8%)
Recurrent dislocation	4 (16.6%)
Non-union of greater trochanter	5 (20.8%)
Liner breakage	1 (4.0%)
Heterotopic ossification	3 (12.5%)
Periprosthetic fracture	5 (20.8%)
Total	**24/103 (23.3%)**

Table 2:
Complications in revisional arthroplasty with sandwich-type ceramic liner.

Conclusions

Although the clinical and radiological results in revisional cases compare less favorably to those of primary arthroplasty with sandwich liner, we achieved satisfactory results comparable to those of the primary cases. Even though our results are short-term and are based on a limited number of cases, we accepted using sandwich liner in revisional arthroplasty as considerable option in point of wear resistance and decreasing stiffness of liner.

References

1. Boutin, P., Christel, P., Dorlot, J.M.: The use of dense alumina alumina ceramic combination in total hip replacement. J. Biomed. Mater Res. 22(12) (1998) 1203-1232.
2. D'Antonio, J.A., Capello, W.N., Manley, M.T., Naughton, M., Sutton, K.: A titanium-encased alumina ceramic bearing for total hip arthroplasty: 3 to 5 years results. Clin. Orthop. 441 (1998) 151-158.
3. Habermann, B., Ewald, W., Rauschmann, M., Zichner, L., Kurth, A.A.: Fracture of ceramic heads in total hip replacement. Arch. Orthop. Trauma Surg. 126(7) (2006) 464-470.
4. Nevelos, J.E., Ingham, E., Doyle, C., Nevelos, A.B. Fisher, J.: The influence of acetabular cup angle on the wear of "BIOLOX Forte" alumina ceramic bearing couples in a hip joint simulator. J. Mater Sci. Mater Med. 12(2) (2001) 141-144.

5. Nizard, R.S., Sedel, L., Christel, P., Meunier, A., Soudry, M. Witvoet, J.: Ten-year survivorship of cemented ceramic total hip prosthesis. Clin. Orthop. 282 (1992) 53-63.
6. Park, Y.S., Hwang, S.K., Choy, W.S., Kim, Y.S., Moon, Y.W. Lim, S.J.: Ceramic failure after total hip arthroplasty with an alumina-on-alumina bearing. J. Bone Joint Surg. (Am) 88(4) (2006) 780-787.
7. Ravasi, F. Sansone, V.: Five-year follow-up with a ceramic sandwich cup in total hip replacement. Arch. Orthop. Trauma Surg. 122 (2002) 350-353.
8. Robert, L.B., Corey, B. Harry, B.S.: Concerns about Ceramics in THA. Clin. Orthop. 429 (2004) 73-79.
9. Sedel, L., Nizard, R., Bizot, P.: Perspective on a 20-year experience with ceramic-on-ceramic articulation in total hip replacement. Semin. Arthroplasty 9 (1998) 123.
10. Skinner, H.B.: Ceramic bearing surface. Clin. Orthop. 369 (1999) 83-91.
11. Walter, A.: On the material and the tribology of alumina-alumina couplings for hip joint prosthesis. Clin. Orthop. 282 (1992) 31-46.
12. Yoo, J.J., Kim, Y.M., Yoon, K.S., Koo, K.H., Song, W.S. Kim, H.J.: Alumina-on-alumina total hip arthroplasty. A five-year minimum follow-up study. J. Bone Joint Surg. (Am) 87(3) (2005) 530-535.
13. Hwang, S.K., Jeon, J.S., Lee, B.H.: Ceramic on sandwich ceramic bearing primary cementless total hip arthroplasty(result of 2 to years follow up). J. Kor. Orthop. Assoc. 39 (2004) 679-685.

7.4 Revision Surgery of Acetabular Polyethylene Wear – cup retention or revision?

T.-Ch. Yu

Introduction

Polyethylene wear and periprosthetic osteolysis is a worrisome and frequent complication of total hip arthroplasty, at present time, it is the major problems of total hip replacement. This phenomenon is more significant in our society due to most THR cases in our daily practice are young active patients with femoral head AVN. Revision of the acetabular component (liner or +metal shell) with head segment exchange is probably the most common revision operation around the hip at this moment In this retrospectived study, we wound share our experience in the past ten years.

Materials and Methods

From 1990 to 2002 there were 126 cases undertaken revision THR due to early acetabular poly wear. The average age at revision was 51.9 years old (27 to 78 Y). The average survival time of original THR was 7.5 years (4 to 15 Y). Various types of cementless implants were included. All patients had periodic X-ray examination and OPD f/u for more than 5 years. Preoperatively, 49 cases had gross loosening with liner osteolysis around stems or cups. 27 of 49 cases received revision of insert, head and cup. 7 of 49 received revision of insert, head and stem. 15 received total revision. The other 77 cases didn't have loosening sign from X-ray and most of them had localized osteolysis. 32 of the 77 cases received revision of insert +/- head; 29 insert + cup +/- head; 4 insert + stem + head; 12 total revision. 7 cases had well fixed cup and stem but no matched liner available. We used undersized insert cemented on metal cup.

Results

The mean Harris hip score before revision was 58 and the score at final f/u was 89. One of three cemented cup insert was revised for late cup loosening. Four of 27 isolated insert and head revision cases were failed due to poly wear of new liner and acetabular component loosening and revised re-revision with acetabular metal shell.

Discussion

Wear is a feature of all biomaterials. There is not a material we know that does not wear at least some. Wear that generates small particles incites a biologic reaction. It is that biologic reaction to wear that causes bone destruction that we call osteolysis. There were two kind of bony response to wear, One is expansile and rapidly Progressive,and typically occurs with a well-fixed socket. The other is linear and slowly progressive, and typically the socket migrates into the lucent area, They are two ways of the same phenomenon. Rubash, Maloney, and Paprosky have classified the sockets in osteolysis depending on factors that probably are not very relevant today. Type I is a stable component, and osteolysis is discrete. Type II is a stable component, with the locking mechanism compromised or a malpositioned shell with discrete osteolysis. Type III, of course, is the osteolysis with an unstable socket. Types I can be treated by lesional treatment. The localized osteolysis around cup with good fixation and orientation, If no matched insert available, the undersized cross linked poly liner cemented to metal cup is another choice. Making raw of the back surface if liner with frilling some holes or other method would increase survival time of such insert we can change insert and add bone graft thru cup holes or around the periphery of the component For the prosthesis with progressive liner osteolysis or poor orientation, the revision is straightforward. The last option is to perform total3- component revision with the new generation ceramic-on cemaeric THR in young revision cases.

Tips and Tricks

8.1 Tragedy of Polyethylene Back Ceramic on Ceramic Articulation

K. Kawate, T. Ohmura, I. Kawahara, H. Kataoka, K. Tamai, T. Ueha and Y. Takakura

Introduction

A modular layered acetabular component (Alumina Bearing Surface, Kyocera, Japan) was developed in Japan for use in alumina ceramic on ceramic total hip arthroplasty. In 3933 components implanted between 1998 and 2000, 463 alumina liner fractures and dissociation (11.8 %) have been reported to the manufacturer until the end of 2006. The dissociation of the polyethylene liner from a metal shell gradually increased in recent years.

In the present study, we reported our experience of the dissociation and investigated the failure of locking mechanism between polyethylene liner and metal shell.

Materials and Methods

Between February 1998 and July 2000, 64 primary uncemented ceramic-on-ceramic total hip arthroplasties with a layered (sandwich) component (Kyocera, Kyoto, Japan) were performed in 59 consecutive patients. There were 11 men and 48 women with a mean age of 59 years (range, 21 to 74 years) and a mean weight of 55.4 kg (range, 40 to 89 kg). The pre-operative diagnosis was osteoarthritis including developmental dysplasia in 47 hips, osteonecrosis in 10, rapidly distractive coxarthrosis in 6 and rheumatoid arthritis in 1. All the operations were performed by the two surgeons (KK and TO) via a posterior approach.

The uncemented acetabular component of a titanium alloy metal shell and an alumina-bearing surface liner consisting of an alumina ceramic liner and an ultra-high-molecular-weight polyethylene shell. The ceramic liner was mechanically-fixed to the polyethylene liner and the liner was then inserted into the metal shell at surgery and held together via a locking mechanism. The locking mechanism consisted of four 0.8 mm height nail located at inside of the metal shell and 2 mm protrusion on the rim of the metal shell fitting into a locking notch of the marginal part of the circumference of the polyethylene liner. The outer diameter of the metal shell varied. The thickness of the alumina liner was 4 mm and the thickness of the polyethylene varied from only 2 mm to 9 mm depending on the size of the metal shell. The thickness of the marginal part of the circumference of polyethylene liner was 3 mm.

Partial weight-bearing was allowed on the seventh post-operative day and full weight-bearing at one and half months post-operatively.

Statistical analysis of weight and body-mass index was performed using Mann-Whitney's U test. A p value of 0.05 was considered to be significant.

Results

As of December 2006, 18 of the 64 implanted bearings have failed. Dissociation between polyethylene liner and metal shell was apparently observed in 9 hips of 8 patients. Almost simultaneous dissociation of both hips occurred in one patient (Fig. 1). In the remaining 9 hips, all acetabular bering surfaces were found to have fractured to pieces. The time to failure of locking mechanism averaged 78 months and ranged from 49 to 102 months. All failures occurred in women. Preoperative radiographs revealed osteolysis in 8 hips. The outer diameter of the metal shell was 46 mm in 4 hips, 48 mm in 2, 50 mm in 1 and 52 mm in 2. The average weight and body-mass index of the patients with failure of locking mechamism were 57 kg (range, 37 to 70 kg) and 24.3 kg/m^2 (range, 16.9 to 33.3 kg/m^2). The average weight and body-mass index of the patients without failure were 55 kg (range, 40 to 89 kg) and 23.4 kg/m^2 (range, 16.7 to 33.5 kg/m^2). No significant association was found between failure and weight, body-mass.

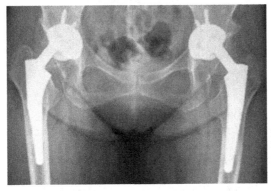

Figure 1:
Anteroposterior pelvic radiograph showing a displaced ceramic acetabular liner in both hips.

At the time of revision, the polyethylene liners had disengaged inferiorly from the metal shell and apparently entrapped by the femoral neck. Visual analysis of the acetabular polyethylene at the time of revision indicated that the marginal part of the circumference of the polyethylene liner was shaved off, and pulled out of the locking notch (Fig. 2). Scanning electron microscopy showed surface damage in the peripheral portion of the alumina inlay. Massive material excavation was observed at the area of edge loading. The superolateral portion of the alumina head was also worn.

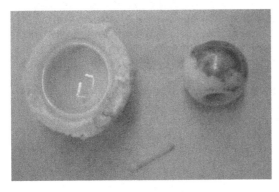

Figure 2:
Retrieved alumina-bearing surface liner showing the polyethylene rim around the locking notch worn away. The superolateral portion of the alumina head was also worn and metal transfer was observed.

Discussion

Osteolysis due to wear debris is the major long-term problem associated with total hip arthroplasty. To avoid wear debris, hard-bearing-surface total hip prosthese with improved tribological properties have been introduced into surgical practice. Ceramic surfaces have had some promising long-term results, and modern metal-backed alumina cups have been associated with very good clinical results. Concerns have been raised about the increased stiffness associated with all-ceramic and metal-backed ceramic acetabular components, which potentially leads to increased rates of migration and loosening. The design of so-called "sandwich" cup designs, with polyethylene interposed between ceramic bearing surface and outer metal shell, is to reduce the rigidity of the ceramic-on ceramic articulation and prevent impingement between rim of the ceramic liner and neck of the femoral stem. However, the ceramic layered component was withdrawn from the market because of early failures [1-3].

In all cases of the present study, the marginal part of the circumference of the polyethylene liners were shaved off, and pulled out of the locking notch. Alumina liner dissociation may be caused by a strong rotational torque because of roughening of the alumina bearing surface. Wear on the alumina component and head may be because of edge loading caused by microseparation of the bearing centers. First, the polyethylene liner circumferentially rotated in the metal shell. Then, the worn marginal part of the circumference of the polyethylene liner was torn and dissociated inferiorly.

Toni et al. reported the needle aspiration of the synovial fluid to detect ceramic particles for early diagnosis of ceramic liner fracture [4]. In case of dissociation between polyethylene liner and metal shell, the needle aspiration is possibly effective to detect polyethylene particles. Incomprehensive osteolysis, squeak and strange sensation were warning of dissociation in the sandwich cup designs.

References

1. Akagi M, Nonaka T, Nishisaka F, Mori S, Fukuda K, Hamanishi C. Late dissociation of an alumina-on-alumina bearing modular acetabular component. J Arthroplasty. 2004; 19:647-51.
2. Hasegawa M, Sudo A, Uchida A. Alumina ceramic-on-ceramic total hip replacement with a layered acetabular component. J Bone Joint Surg Br. 2006;88:877-82.
3. Poggie RA, Turgeon TR, Coutts RD. Failure analysis of a ceramic bearing acetabular component. J Bone Joint Surg Am. 2007;89:367-75.
4. Toni A, Traina F, Stea S, Sudanese A,Visentin M, Bordini B, Squarzoni S. Early diagnosis of ceramic liner fracture. Guidelines based on a twelve-year clinical experience. J Bone Joint Surg Am supl. 2006;88:55-63.

8.2 Breakage of Alumina Ceramic Head and Clinical Failure after Minor Modification of Tapered Junction

M. Ishii, M. Takagi, H. Ida, S. Kobayashi, H. Kawaji and M. Hamasaki

Introduction

Clinical application of alumina ceramic to femoral head of prostheses has been performed with possible advantage of lower friction of ceramic head / ultra-high molecular weight polyethylene (UHMWPE) or ceramic head /ceramic cup articulations, when compared to that of metal head / UHMWPE cup. Although favorable clinical results of alumina ceramic head / UHMWPE cup combination has been known, breakage of alumina ceramic head has been reported. In this study, we investigated the series of total hip arthroplasties (THAs) with alumina ceramic head, and reported breakage of alumina ceramic head combined with UHMWPE cup and critical clinical problems after tiny modification of the taper system between alumina ceramics head and metal neck.

Materials and Methods

2,410 cases of cemented THAs with alumina ceramics head / UHMWPE cup articulation (Kyocera Ltd, Japan) were performed at Yamagata Saisei Hospital, Yamagata University, and local institutions in Yamagata prefecture, Japan, since 1988 to 2005. A 28 mm sized-alumina head was also combined with titanium-alumina-vanadium alloy based Yamagata University-type femoral stem (Kyocera Ltd, Kyoto, Japan), which safety was approved by mechanical testing [8]. Neck length was controlled by three types of taper structure equipped in the ceramic head (short; -4 mm, middle; ±0 mm, and long; +4 mm). They were used with combination of four femoral stems (extra small, small, standard, large) with a taper structure compatible to that of ceramic heads. Therefore, twelve combinations for neck length control were available. This system was aimed to less economical cost due to preparation of many different sizes of the stem compatible to one size of alumina head. Series of alumina ceramic head of 26 mm in diameter with neck taper system of -4 mm, ±0 mm, and +4 mm, and that of 22 mm in diameter with -4 mm and ±0 mm sized-taper system was introduced to obtain thicker UHMWPE cup, as possible as 10 mm width of UHMWPE. The mechanical property and its safety was approved by mechanical testing of Kyocera, followed by permission of the previous Ministry of Health and Welfare, Japanese government. In the series, type of the combination of the taper system and breakage of the alumina head was investigated and analyzed.

Results

In 541 joints, 22 mm sized-alumina head was applied (±0 mm; 271, +4 mm; 270), 26 mm sized-head was in 658 joints (-4 mm; 145, ±0 mm; 290, +4 mm; 223), and 28 mm sized-head was in 1,211joints (-4 mm; 171, ±0 mm; 623, +4 mm; 417). Breakages of the head were experienced in 23 cases. All cases were in 26 mm sized-head with +4 mm of taper structure for neck length control. Incidence of breakage was 0.1 % in all series and 3.6% in 26 mm sized-head. The incidence of breakage was tremendously high up to 10.3% in +4 mm of taper structure / 26 mm sized-head.

Clinical status and information of the 23 patients (male 8, female 15) with ceramic breakage revealed mean age of the patients was 68.2 years old (50-79), and time to revision operation after primary THA was 3 years and 8months (22 months -7 years 6 months). Sixteen cases of the patients (70%) were available for further analyses on tapered junction of head and stem. EDC (Energy Dispersive X-ray Spectrometer) element analysis of one retrieved sample revealed the presence of P, Ca, and K contents at the taper structure of the alumina head, which suggested the possible interposition of tissue components of the patient between ceramics head and femoral stem, thus contributing to biomechanical stress leading to breakage of alumina head. Another three cases showed that the presence of insufficient tapered connection between alumina head and tapered femoral neck, which was found by abrasive traces of tapered femoral neck and adhesion of metal debris inside the taper structure of the ceramic head. The data indicated mal-direction between head and stem axis, thus possibly contributing to ceramic breakage, although it was uncertain wether the mal-direction occurred at initial surgery, with inappropriate insertion of the neck to alumina tapered site or after surgery, with gradual development of mal-direction. Scratched surface of the tapered site of femoral stem was marked finding of the twelve cases, indicating inappropriate fitting of the tapered junction of the system, and also contributing to the breakage.

Case presentation

Case 1: A 64 years old woman with dysplastic osteoarthritis of the right hip joint received THA with 26 mm sized-alumina head with +4 mm taper, January, 1998. She suddenly felt right coxalgia with a sound of crash during the gait examination after two years and a month of the surgery, and complained gait disturbance. Breakage of ceramic head was confirmed by X ray (Fig. 1). The broken sample retrieved at revision surgery showed presence of P, Ca, and K contents detected by EDC element analysis (Fig. 2). However, uniform metal abrasive trace was not found on the surface of the tapered femoral neck (Fig. 3). The data indicated

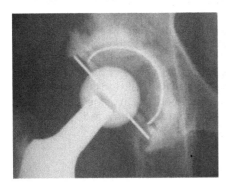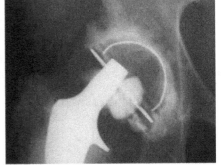

Figure 1:
Just before breakage of ceramic head.

that breakage of alumina head was probably due to abnormal fitting of the taper system, caused by interposition of host tissue. Thus, excess stress distribution has occurred in the site, leading to a small crack formation. A small crack induced a small ceramic fragment. This mechanical weak point enhanced abnormal stress distribution adjacent ceramic head and resulted in breakage of the whole body (Fig. 4).

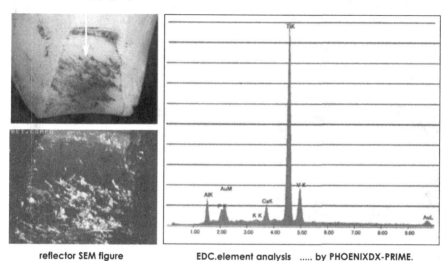

reflector SEM figure   EDC.element analysis ..... by PHOENIXDX-PRIME.

Figure 2 a,b,c:
Analysis of foreign substance.

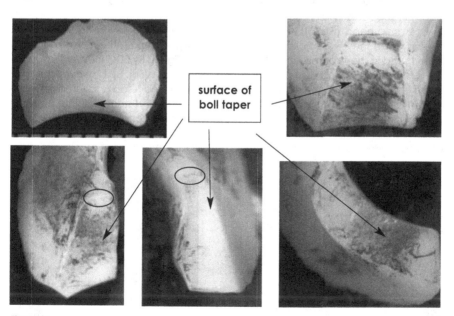

Figure 3:
Pieces of boll taper site.

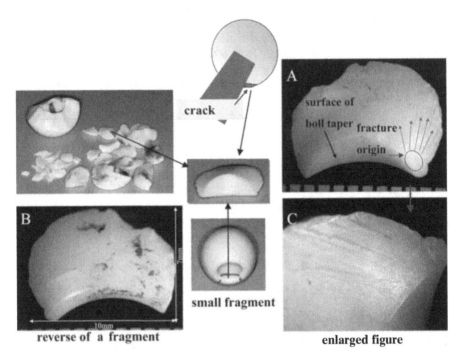

Figure 4: Crack formation. Ceramic fragments.

Case 2: A 73 years old man with dysplastic osteoarthritis of the left hip joint received THA with 26 mm alumina head with +4 mm taper, February, 2000. Three years and seven months later, he could not walk due to pain soon after he noticed peculiar noise at standing-up from the floor. X-ray analysis revealed breakage of the ceramic head (Fig. 5). A small piece of the broken alumina fragments was missing when they were collected at revision surgery (Fig. 6). The abrasive traces were found in the tapered surface of stem neck (Fig. 7). By EDC element analysis, the interposition of host tissue could not be recognized (Fig. 8). However, the axis of the traces was not paralleled with that of both alumina head and femoral neck. The data indicated that mal-direction between head and stem axis, thus possibly contributing to ceramic breakage, although it was uncertain weather the mal-direction occurred at initial surgery, with inappropriate insertion of the neck to alumina tapered site or after surgery, with gradual development of mal-direction of the corresponding axis.

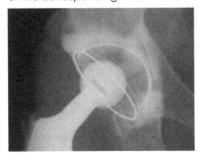
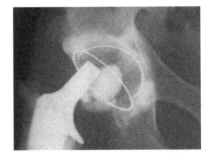

Figure 5: Just before breakage of ceramic head.

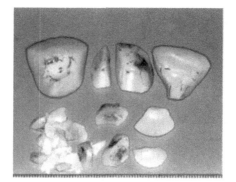

Figure 6:
Pieces of ceramic head.

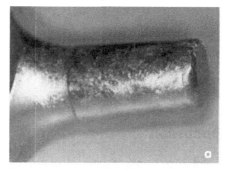

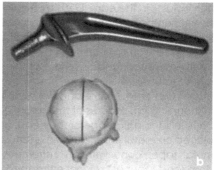

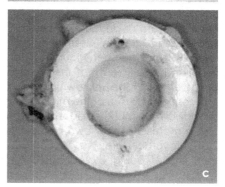

Figure 7 a,b,c:
Abrasive traces of stem neck.

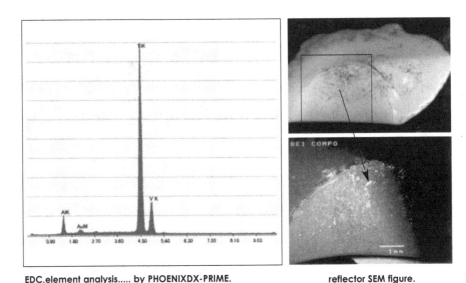

EDC.element analysis..... by PHOENIXDX-PRIME.   reflector SEM figure.

Figure 8:
EDC element analysis.

Discussion

Femoral heads made of alumina ceramic were introduced for total hip arthroplasty in the early 1970s by Boutin [1]. Due to theoretical and experimental low friction performance of alumina, they have been still clinically used. However, the series in this study showed unpredictable and poor results. Alumina ceramic is weak in tension and brittle. Especially, fracture/breakage of alumina head has been well-recognized as serious problem since early 1970s. Along with improved manufacturing, the fracture/breakage rate has decreased, but breakages are still encountered. Clarke and Willmann [4] pointed out that in general, 6 possible mishandling procedures of the ceramic head or the high precision metallic taper cone lead to a damage of the head, as follows: mismatched design of the head placed on metal taper, autoclave and shock cooling of the head, damaging the metal taper cone with an instrument, mounting a new ball on a previously damaged taper at revision, entrapped debris in the ball, and repeated usage of an original head at revision surgery. According to previous literatures, the breakage rate of an alumina ceramic ball in combination with on UHMWPE is 0.004-2.2% [2,3,5,6]. By these investigation, its rate in average was 0.1%, and it is not still a small number. Higuchi [7] reported three cases of breakage alumina head and suspected that there were some interposing foreign body, such as bone cement or the unknown biologic substances. Excessive stress distribution by interposition was one of the etiologic factors of the breakage alumina head [10]. In addition, Onishi [9] et al. reported that the interposition of the bone cement and a material of unknown biologic substances disturbed normal taper fitting, thus unfavorable stress as concentrated remarkably at the tapered site of the stem, finally leading to breakage of the head [10].

In the alumina head with taper system analyzed in this study, there seemed critical clinical problem. There was no breakage in 28 mm sized-head with -4 mm, ±0 mm and +4 mm sized-taper system, and in 22 mm sized-head with -4 mm and ±0 mm sized-taper system. Although experimental mechanical testing of the manufacture, Kyocera Ltd., reported safe and stable performance in all the series, breakage was found only in 26 mm sized-head with +4 mm taper. A +4 mm taper system in 26 mm sized-head made it possible longer neck and lateral off-set of the femoral stem, with thicker UHMWPE over 10 mm. However, shallow taper for +4 mm in the alumina head also had to limit width of margin of the alumina around the entrance of taper system. Shallow and small margin of the entrance in the taper system seemed to induce unstable connection between head and neck, leading to mal-direction and unfavorable mechanical distribution of the corresponding site, and may also to allow interposition of the tissue component of the host. The clinical results sent out a stern warning that, even with proof of warranty on safety of the alumina ceramics head with taper system, approved by the commercial testing, minor modification of the structure of alumina head easily led to clinical failure, probably based on the fragile property of the alumina ceramics.

References

1. Boutin P: Arthroplastie totale de la hanche prothese en alumine frittee. Etude Experimentale et premieres application cliniques. Rev Chir Orthop 58:229-246,1972.
2. Callaway G H, et al:Fracture of the femoral head after ceramic-polyethylene total hip arthroplasty. J. Arthroplasty 10:855-859,1995.
3. Cameron H U:Ceramic head implantation failures. J. Arthroplasty 6:185-188,1991.
4. Clarke IC, Willmann G: Structural Ceramics in Orthopaedics. In. Bone Implant Interface, ed.by Cameron, H.St Louis, Mosby, St. Louis, 203-252,1994.
5. Fritsch E W, et al: Ceramic femoral head fractures in total hip arthroplasty. Clin. Orthop.328:129-136,1996.
6. Heck D A, et al: Prosthetic component failures in hip arthroplasty surgery. J. Arthroplasty 10:575-580,1995.
7. Higuchi F, et al.: Fracture of an alumina ceramic head in total hip arthroplasty.?J Artyroplasty 8:567-571,1993.
8. Ida H, et al.: The neck length control system by alumina-ball (28mm) in Y-U total hip arthroplasty. Experimental and short term clinical studies. Bioceramics 8: 193-197, 1995.
9. Oonishi H,: Bioengineering investigation of total hip prostheses having ceramic bearing surface. Journal of Joint Surgery 17:97-107,1998.
10. Wakebe I, et al: Risk factors affecting fracture of ceramic femoral head. Orthop Ceramic Implants 16:149-153,1996.

8.3 Tips and Tricks: Fracture of a Ceramic Insert with modern Ceramic Total Hip Replacement

B.-W. Min, K.-S. Song, C.-H. Kang, K.-J. Lee, K.-C. Bae, C.-H. Cho and Y.-Y. Won

Abstract

Results obtained with ceramic bearings in total hip arthroplasty have been disappointing because of increased component loosening rates primarily caused by design issues and use of low-quality ceramic, resulting in fracture and debris generation. Although new-generation ceramics have produced a reduced incidence of fracture, concerns still persist about the fracture of ceramic liners. After investigating the underlying cause of fracture in contemporary ceramic-on-ceramic bearings, we sought to determine the incidence of ceramic liner fracture and to formulate technical guidelines for avoiding catastrophic failure. Between January 2000 and January 2005, we prospectively studied a consecutive series of 147 patients (179 hips) who had undergone primary cementless total hip arthroplasty with modern ceramic-on-ceramic articulation so that we could detect ceramic liner fracture. The mean length of the follow-up period was 3.1 years (range, 2–6.5 years). By the latest follow-up examination, delayed ceramic liner fracture had occurred in 3 hips (1.7%). One liner was chipped during insertion because of eccentric seating of the liner. Head fracture occurred in 2 hips (1.1%). Despite the improved wear characteristics of modern ceramic-on-ceramic articulations, a catastrophic failure with ceramic liner failure was still observed during short-term follow-up monitoring. This finding prompted us to define important technical aspects to be considered to minimize ceramic liner fractures.

Introduction

Contemporary ceramic-on-ceramic articulations are harder, more scratch resistant, and more hydrophilic than other bearing materials, resulting in minimized wear and reduced particle-induced osteolysis. Results obtained with ceramic bearings in total hip arthroplasty (THA) have been disappointing because of increased component loosening rates primarily caused by design issues and use of low-quality ceramic, resulting in fracture and debris generation. The greatest concern with the use of ceramics today is fracture. Although new-generation ceramics have exhibited a reduced incidence of fracture, concerns still persist about the fracture of ceramic liners [1,8,11,15,16]. After investigating the underlying cause of fracture in contemporary ceramic-on-ceramic bearings, we sought to determine the incidence of ceramic liner fracture and to formulate technical guidelines for avoiding catastrophic failure.

Materials and Methods

Between January 2000 and January 2005, we enrolled a consecutive series of 147 patients (179 hips) who had primary cementless THAs with modern ceramic-on-ceramic articulation in a prospective study so that we could detect ceramic liner fracture. We obtained approval for this study from our institutional review board. Two patients (3 hips) died and 11 patients (12 hips) were lost to follow-up monitoring before the end of the minimum 2-year follow-up period; this left 134 patients (164 hips in 82 men and 52 women) as the subjects of this study. All patients were evaluated both clinically and radiographically. They were monitored for a mean of 3.1 years (range, 2.0–6.5 years). None of the 13 patients (8.8%) who died or were lost to follow-up monitoring had required revision of the implant. At the time of THA, the average age of the patients was 39 years (range, 20–55 years) and the average weight and height were 61 kg (range, 40–90 kg) and 164.5 cm (range, 145–180 cm), respectively. The preoperative diagnosis was osteonecrosis in 105 hips, osteoarthritis in 53, rheumatoid arthritis in 2, and infection sequelae in 4. We performed all of the procedures from an anterolateral approach, with the patient in the lateral position.

Four kinds of total hip systems were chosen because the patients were young and active and had good bone quality (Dorr type A or B [4]):

1. System I, used in 35 hips, was composed of a hemispherical titanium cup (Ti-6Al-4V; Plasmacup SC, Aesculap, Tuttlingen, Germany); a slightly tapered, rectangular, collarless titanium femoral component (BiCONTACT, Aesculap); and a 28-mm modular alumina femoral head and an alumina acetabular insert (Al_2O_3; BIOLOX Forte, CeramTec, Plochingen, Germany).
2. System II, used in 47 hips, was composed of a hemispherical cementless EPF-PLUS acetabular component (PLUS Endoprothetik, Erlenstrasse, Switzerland) and an SL-PLUS cementless femoral stem (PLUS Endoprothetik). The liner had an alumina inlay packed with polyethylene (sandwich type).
3. System III, used in 34 hips, was composed of a hemispheric cementless Duraloc acetabular component (DePuy, Warsaw, Indiana) and a fully porous-coated Anatomic Medullary Locking stem (DePuy). The bearing articulation was a 28-mm modular alumina head and an alumina acetabular insert.
4. System IV, used in 49 hips, was composed of a hemispheric cementless EP-FIT PLUS acetabular component (PLUS Endoprothetik) and an SL-PLUS cementless femoral stem (PLUS Endoprothetik). The liner was the BIOLOX Forte (CeramTec).

The postoperative rehabilitation protocol was the same for all patients, who were allowed progressive weight bearing as tolerated on the third day after surgery.

Each patient was assessed clinically and radiographically before surgery and after surgery at 4 weeks, 3 months, 6 months, and 12 months and annually thereafter. Statistical analysis of the relationship between various preoperative factors and ceramic liner fracture was conducted with SPSS software (version 12.0; SPSS Science, Chicago, Illinois). The level of significance was $p < 0.05$.

Results

By the latest follow-up examination, delayed ceramic liner fracture had occurred in 3 hips (1.7%), all in men, without trauma. The ages of the patients at the time of fracture were 33, 46, and 28 years. The mean age, height, and weight of these patients did not differ significantly from those of the overall group. The mean time interval between implantation and ceramic liner fracture was 9 months. All of these hips underwent revision surgery, and the retrieved implants and surrounding soft tissues were examined macroscopically and micro-scopically. All 164 hips had radiographic evidence of bone integration at the final follow-up examination. No acetabular cup or femoral stem was revised because of aseptic loosening. Head fracture occurred in 2 hips (1.1%). Another liner was chipped during insertion because of eccentric seating of the liner.

Case 1

A 34-year-old, 67-kg man who was 164 cm tall and who had advanced osteonecrosis of the right femoral head underwent primary THA in March 2003. A transgluteal approach was used to place a ceramic-on-ceramic bearing implant (system I). The acetabular cup had a 52-mm outer diameter and a machined interior that accepted a ceramic insert (BIOLOX Forte). The metallic shell was not recessed, so that it would protect the rim of the ceramic liner. The femoral stem was cementless with a proximal porous coating (BiCONTACT). A 28-mm short BIOLOX (–3.5 mm) head was used. The cup abduction angle was 39°, and the anteversion angle was 22° (Fig. 1a). The hip was confirmed to be stable, with no neck impingement in any direction, during surgery.

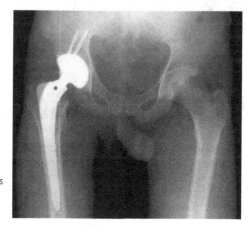

Figure 1a:
An anteroposterior radiograph of the pelvis of the patient in case 1, taken 4 weeks after surgery, shows a well-fixed cup and stem.

Postoperative progress was uneventful. Fourteen months after surgery, the patient felt crepitation without pain during hip motion. There was no history of trauma. A radiograph of the pelvis showed a comminuted fracture of the ceramic liner with fragments around the stem neck (Fig. 1b). The patient refused revision surgery. Seven months later, he felt pain, which was accompanied by increasing noise in the hip. Radiographs demonstrated increasing comminution of fragments of the ceramic liner, a well-fixed cup, and concentric placement of the ceramic head in the metal shell (Fig. 1c).

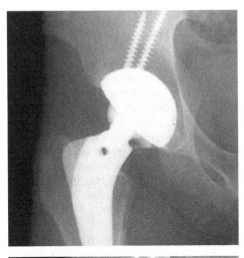

Figure 1b:
An anteroposterior radiograph of the right hip of the patient in case 1, taken 1 year 2 months after surgery, shows a comminuted fracture of the ceramic liner with fragments around the stem neck.

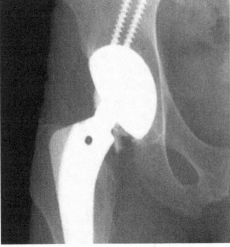

Figure 1c:
An anteroposterior radiograph of the right hip of the patient in case 1, taken 1 year 9 months later than Fig. 1b, demonstrates fragmentation and concentric placement of the ceramic ball within the metal shell.

The patient underwent revision surgery at our institution in December 2004. On arthrotomy, 4 large pieces of the ceramic liner and multiple small fragments were found (Fig. 1d). The ceramic liner was found within the metal shell, with marginal cracking in the peripheral portions (Fig. 1e). The liner and head were scratched and stained with black metal particles. There was no macroscopic wear of the ceramic liner or ceramic head. The metal shell and femoral stem were not loose, and the trunnion was undamaged macroscopically. On histologic examination, the granulation tissue excised around the cup revealed numerous foreign-body giant cells with ceramic particles. After the joint was thoroughly irrigated, a modular ceramic liner and a 28-mm BIOLOX long head (+3.5 mm) were implanted. The patient had a good recovery, with complete relief of previous symptoms.

Case 2

A 45-year-old, 68-kg man who was 176 cm tall and who had osteonecrosis of the femoral head had a ceramic liner fracture without trauma at 8 months after

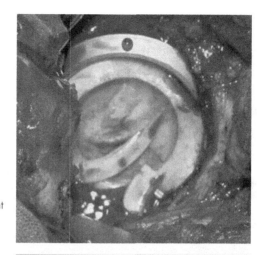

Figure 1d:
Intraoperative photograph of the patient in case 1 shows 4 large pieces of the ceramic liner and multiple small fragments.

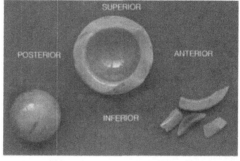

Figure 1e:
Multiple chipped fragments of the ceramic liner retrieved from the patient in case 1 are visible on the peripheral portion, especially on the anterior, superior, and inferior portions of the liner. The liner and alumina head are scratched and stained with black metal particles.

surgery (Fig 2a). System IV was used for this patient. Findings during revision surgery showed that the alumina insert was severely fractured, and a black discoloration of the alumina head was observed, with loss of its surface gloss (Fig. 2b). However, there was no evidence of alumina head fracture or recognizable damage to the Morse taper of the well-fixed stem. After extensive débridement and synovectomy to remove as much of the ceramic debris as possible, a new alumina-on-ceramic bearing was implanted; the stem and cup were left in place (Fig. 2c).

Discussion

Despite the improved wear characteristics of modern ceramic-on-ceramic articulations, we still observed catastrophic failure with ceramic fractures in a series of a relatively small number of patients with short-term follow-up. This finding prompted us to note important technical aspects that should be considered to minimize ceramic liner fractures.

Trauma, a high level of activity, and obesity may increase the risk of ceramic insert breakage by increasing the load across the joint surface [6,11]. Other factors that must be taken into account are mechanical properties of the ceramics, implant design, and surgical techniques used in implanting the prosthesis [16]. New-generation ceramic liners do not fracture at an impact force

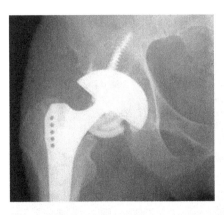

Figure 2a:
An anteroposterior radiograph of the patient in case 2, taken 8 months after surgery, shows a ceramic liner fracture without trauma.

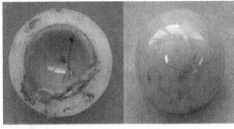

Figure 2b:
This intraoperative photograph taken during revision surgery on the patient in case 2 shows a severely fractured alumina insert and black discoloration of the ceramic head.

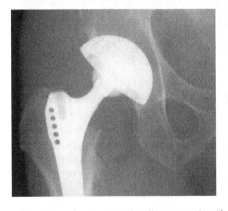

Figure 2c:
A new ceramic liner and ceramic head were reimplanted after extensive débridement and synovectomy in the patient in case 2 to remove as much of the ceramic debris as possible. The stem and cup was left in place.

of 12 kN, a force greater than most estimates of the physiologic forces to which the hip is subjected during falls or stumbling. This suggests that ceramic liner fracture caused by impact force during normal life is unlikely to occur in vivo [7]. All modern ceramic components are subjected to a burst-strength examination before sterilization and shipping.

Correct placement of the ceramic head on the femoral component taper during surgery is critical for long-term survival. The locking mechanism of the ceramic insert with conical sleeving appears to be safe and reliable, but careful technique is required to correctly position the liner. Eccentric orientation of the liner relative to the shell during impaction can result in chipping or even liner breakage. In our series, eccentric placement of 1 liner resulted in liner chipping during insertion. The importance of gaining excellent exposure to safely insert a modular ceramic liner has been emphasized to allow insertion of the shell in a nearly ideal position, exposure of the rim of the shell circumferentially, placement and impaction of the liner concentrically, and identification of any crack or chip that may occur during impaction. During implantation of the head and liner, it is also important to avoid allowing any foreign body between the cone and the ceramic head, to avoid strong impaction of the head on the cone with the hammer, and to protect the cone from damage.

Optimal position of the component is also crucial with ceramic-on-ceramic components. Malpositioning of the component may generate uncontrolled peak stress in the ceramic, which may result in fracture [1,2]. The acetabular component should be placed at an angle of ≤ 45° to optimize the distribution of forces over the greatest amount of surface area of femoral ball head and the cup. Trial liner and femoral ball heads should be used in trial reduction to avoid any potential damage to the taper, cup, and ceramic components. Placement of ceramic liner and ball by hand is a relatively easy and safe method for avoiding damage to these implants.

Another possible mechanism of ceramic liner fracture is edge-loading when the hip is flexed, as with rising from a chair or climbing a high step [17]. Edge-loading may occur with subluxation of the bearing by subluxation–relocation motion [7]. Vertical cup placement could also enhance edge-loading [12].

The alumina articular liner with an outer lining of polyethylene (sandwich type) was developed to reduce the rigidity of the ceramic-on-ceramic bearing and to prevent impingement between the rim of the ceramic liner and the neck of the femoral stem [9]. However, this design modification resulted in a thinner alumina insert, which increased the likelihood of a peripheral chip fracture and subsequent crack propagation through the brittle alumina material under impingement conditions [10]. The causes of ceramic liner fracture with a sandwich insertion are stress concentration at the rim of the ceramic liner, thin ceramic (< 4 mm), and impingement between liner rim and prosthetic heads [8,16]. The failures of the ceramic liner of the nonmodular so-called sandwich-design ceramic-on-ceramic cup were caused by high torque transmitted from the femoral head to the ceramic liner, causing dislodgment of the ceramic liner from polyethylene. Walter et al. believe that the displacement of the ceramic liner occurs during subluxation and reengagement of the head and liner during deep flexion [17].

Repeated episodes of impingement between the prosthetic neck and the edge of the ceramic liner can cause liner fracture. Squatting, kneeling, and sitting cross-legged are more common in non-Western populations. The increased range of motion required to support these positions can result in impingement and liner fracture [13,18]. Evidence of femoral neck impingement of the acetabular rim has been recognized as a common occurrence after THA, with impingement being seen in 39% of 111 retrieved polyethylene acetabular liners [18]. Orthopaedic surgeons must advise their THA patients against repeated squatting, kneeling, and cross-legged sitting to avoid impingement. Impingement also can be minimized by combining a neck with optimal geometry with a larger femoral head, optimizing the head-to-neck ratio, thus improving range of motion and decreasing the risk of impingement [14]. Computer-based studies of motion simulation show that the optimal cup position for minimizing the risk of impingement is 45° to 55° abduction and 10° to 15° anteversion [18]. Recessing a ceramic acetabular liner in a metal shell protects the liner by preventing neck impingement and edge-loading of the ceramic material [3]. However, the use of a recessed metallic shell carries the risk that wear of the femoral neck will generate metallic debris.

Despite the improved wear characteristics of modern ceramic-on-ceramic articulations, we still observed catastrophic failure with ceramic liner failure after only short-term follow-up monitoring. We therefore remain concerned that the rate of ceramic liner fracture may increase with time.

References

1. Bizot P, Larrouy M, Witvoet J, Sedel L, Nizard R (2000) Press-fit metal-backed alumina sockets. A minimum 5-year follow-up study. Clin Orthop Relat Res 379:134–142.
2. D'Antonio J, Capello W, Manley M, Bierbaum B (2002) New experience with alumina-on-alumina ceramic bearings for total hip arthroplasty. J Arthroplasty 17:390–397.
3. D'Antonio J Capello W, Manley M, Naughton M, Sutton K (2005) Alumina ceramic bearings for total hip arthroplasty: five-year results of a prospective randomized study. Clin Orthop Relat Res 436:164–171.
4. Dorr LD, Absatz M, Gruen TA, Saberi MT, Doerzbacher JF (1990) Anatomic Porous Replacement hip arthroplasty: first 100 consecutive cases. Semin Arthroplasty 1:77–86.
5. Fritsch EW, Gleitz M (1996) Ceramic femoral head fractures in total hip arthroplasty. Clin Orthop Relat Res 328:129–136.
6. Garino JP (2000) Modern ceramic-on-ceramic total hip systems in the United States: early results. Clin Orthop Relat Res 379:41–47.
7. Hannouche D, Nich C, Bizot P, Meunier A, Nizard R, Sedel L (2003) Fractures of ceramic bearings: history and present status. Clin Orthop Relat Res 417:19–26.
8. Hasegawa M, Sudo A, Hirata H, Uchida A (2003) Ceramic acetabular liner fracture in total hip arthroplasty with a ceramic sandwich cup. J Arthroplasty 18:658–661.
9. Hasegawa M, Sudo A, Uchida A (2006) Alumina ceramic-on-ceramic total hip replacement with a layered acetabular component. J Bone Joint Surgery Br 88:877–882
10. Heros RJ, Willmann G (1998) Ceramics in total hip arthroplasty history, mechanical properties, clinical results, and current manufacturing state of the art. Semin Arthroplasty 9:114–122.
11. Maher SA, Lipman JD, Curley LJ, Gilchrist M, Wright TM (2003) Mechanical performance of ceramic acetabular liners under impact conditions. J Arthroplasty 18:936–941.
12. Michaud RJ, Rashad SY (1995) Spontaneous fracture of the ceramic ball in a ceramic-polyethylene total hip arthroplasty. J Arthroplasty 6:863–867.
13. Mulholland SJ, Wyss UP (2001) Activities of daily living in non-Western cultures: range of motion requirements for hip and knee joint implants. Int J Rehabil Res 24:191–198.
14. Nishii T, Sugano N, Miki H, Koyama T, Takao M, Yoshikawa H (2004) Influence of component positions on dislocation: computed tomographic evaluations in a consecutive series of total hip arthroplasty. J Arthroplasty 19:162–166.
15. Park YS, Hwang SK, Choy WS, Kim YS, Moon YW, Lim SJ (2006) Ceramic failure after total hip arthroplasty with an alumina-on-alumina bearing. J Bone Joint Surg Am 88:780–787.
16. Suzuki K, Matsubara M, Morita S, Muneta T, Shinomiya K (2003) Fracture of a ceramic acetabular insert after ceramic-on-ceramic THA—a case report. Acta Orthop Scand 74:101–103.
17. Walter WL, Insley GM, Walter WK, Tuke MA (2004) Edge loading in third generation alumina ceramic-on-ceramic bearings: stripe wear. J Arthroplasty 19:402–413.
18. Yamaguchi M, Akisue T, Bauer TW, Hashimoto Y (2000) The spatial location of impingement in total hip arthroplasty. J Arthroplasty 15:305–313.

8.4 Minimally Invasive Two-Incision Total Hip Replacement using large Diameter Ceramic-on-Ceramic Articulation

T.-R. Yoon, C.-I. Hur, S. Diwanji and D.-S. Lee

Abstract

Background: Our experience with the minimally invasive (MI) two-incision technique over the last 4 years has shown that total hip arthroplasty (THA) can be performed safely and effectively in properly selected patients. Total hips with larger-diameter femoral heads are more resistant to dislocation. The purpose of the present study was to evaluate the short-term results of a minimally invasive two-incision THA Using Large Diameter Ceramic-on-Ceramic Articulation.

Patients and Methods: A consecutive series of 50 patients who underwent unilateral MI two-inicision THA from June 2006 to October 2006 were studied. There were 35 men and 15 women with a mean age at arthroplasty of 44.9 years (range, 23 to 73 years). There were 36 left and 14 right hip arthroplasties performed. Indications for THA were avascular necrosis of the femoral head in 29 cases, osteoarthritis in 12 cases, rheumatoid arthritis in 3 cases, femur neck fracture in 2 cases, dysplastic hips in 2 cases and ankylosing arthritis in 1 case. A modified two-incision approach was used for all procedures in lateral position. In-hospital data were collected retrospectively, and the initial postoperative radiographs were analyzed. Twenty-eight patients received 36 mm diameter femoral heads, while 22 patients received 32 mm diameter heads.

Results: All patients could mobilize in the following days after surgery. There was no case of intraoperative complications such as intraoperative fracture, nerve palsy, or vascular injury. Postoperatively there was no dislocation or deep vein thrombosis. All femoral stems were inserted neutral or within 5 degree valgus. In all patients, leg length discrepancy was within 5mm difference. The average ROM of hips at last follow-up was significantly improved compared with the preoperative values.

Conclusion: Short-term results of a minimally invasive two-incision THA using large diameter ceramic-on-ceramic articulation were excellent.

Introduction

Although total hip arthroplasty remains the cornerstone of surgical treatment of degenerative joint disease, dislocation continues to be a relatively common complication of the procedure, second in frequency only to late prosthetic loosening [23]. Approximately 80 % of all dislocations following total hip replacement occur in a posterior direction, with a reported prevalence of 0.7 to 5.5 % following primary surgery and 5 to 20 % following revision [14]. The contributing causes to total hip dislocation are reported to include femoral component stem design [29], acetabular component orientation [1,22], surgical approach [24], soft tissue laxity [28], femoral component head size [8], and patient factors [12].

Minimally invasive total hip arthroplasty is an alternative to traditional total hip arthroplasty as it offers the patient a smaller incision, less rehabilitation time, and better functional recovery. The benefits of the two-incision total hip arthroplasty over the traditional or mini-single procedures include faster physical therapy and rehabilitation with immediate weight bearing. The dislocation rate is theoretically less with this procedure and patients can resume activities of daily living such as return to work, driving, and recreational activities much sooner. But, this two-incision technique is a technically demanding procedure.

It is generally appreciated that the range of motion of the artificial hip prior to impingement increases with an increase in the diameter of the femoral head because of the corresponding increase in the ratio of the head and neck diameters. However, with the increasing recognition that osteolysis is a major cause of long-term failure of total hip replacements, many authors have advocated the routine use of femoral heads of smaller diameter to reduce the volumetric wear rate when polyethylene liner is used. With the advent of alternative bearings, such as a metal-on-metal or ceramic-on-ceramic articulation, the use of larger femoral head size may provide increased stability while not compromising the wear properties.

This study was undertaken to determine the short term results of a modified minimally invasive two-incision total hip replacement using large diameter ceramic-on-ceramic articulation.

Materials and Methods

Patient Demographics

A consecutive series of 50 patients who underwent unilateral MI two-inicision THA from June 2006 to October 2006 were studied. There were 35 men and 15 women with a mean age at arthroplasty of 44.9 years (range, 23 to 73 years). There were 36 left and 14 right hip arthroplasties performed. Indications for THA were avascular necrosis of the femoral head in 29 cases (58 %), osteoarthritis in 12 cases (24 %), rheumatoid arthritis in 3 cases (6 %), femur neck fracture in 2 cases (4 %), dysplastic hip in 2 cases (4 %) and ankylosing arthritis in 1 case (2 %). A modified two-incision approach was used for all procedures in lateral position. In-hospital data were collected retrospectively, and the initial postoperative radiographs were analyzed. Twenty-eight patients (56 %) received 36 mm diameter femoral heads (Fig. 1), while 22 patients (44 %) received 32 mm diameter heads (Fig. 2). Mean body mass index (BMI) was 23.0 (range, 16 to 29). Mean patient weight and height was 64.7 kg (range, 40 to 88 kg) and 167.4 (range, 148 to 186 cm), respectively. Mean radiologic follow-up period after the index operation was 8.7 months (range, 6.3 to 10.9 months). All operations were performed by single surgeon (TRY) using the modified MI two-incision approach. Anesthesia method was epidural in 23 cases (46 %) and general in 27 cases (54 %).

Implant

All patients had placement of a cementless acetabular shell with porous coating. Acetabular components inserted were truncated alumina ceramic acetabular components, a ceramic head (BIOLOX®, Osteo AG, Selzach, Switzerland) and ceramic liner. Acetabular cup diameter was 44 mm in 3 cases (6 %), 46 mm in 6 cases (12 %), 48 mm in 13 cases (26 %), 50 mm in 6 cases (12 %),

52 mm in 15 cases (30 %), 54 mm in 7 cases (14 %). All cementless femoral stem inserted was M/L taper® stem (Centerpulse Orthopaedics, Baar, Switzerland).

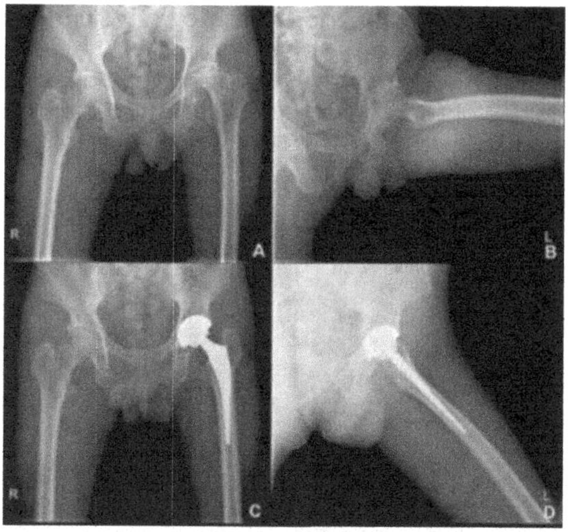

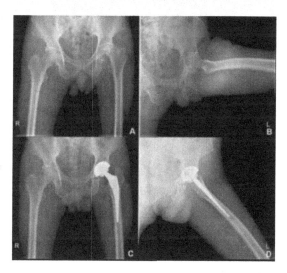

Figure 1:
(A, B) Preoperative anteroposterior (AP) radiograph and femoral head lateral radiograph show a patient with avascular necrosis of left hip. (C, D) He was operated with a 36mm ceramic femoral head articulating with ceramic insert. In the last follow-up, he can put on a Budda position and walk without any discomfort or limping.

Figure 2:
(A, B) Preoperative anteroposterior (AP) radiograph and femoral head lateral radiograph show a patient with avascular necrosis of left hip. (C, D) He was operated with a 32mm ceramic femoral head articulating with ceramic insert. In the last follow-up, he can also put on a Budda position and walk without any discomfort or limping.

Surgical Technique

Landmarks for the skin incision such as the tip, anterior and posterior border of the greater trochanter and trochanteric (vastus) ridge were identified. The first incision was made over the anterolateral aspect of the hip ranging from 6-8 cm. The incision started from the point approximately one finger breadth posterior to anterior border of trochanter and just distal to trochanteric crest, extending cranially and anteriorly at an angle of 30 degrees to the long axis of femur. The incision roughly aimed at a point on iliac crest 3 cm posterior to the anterior superior iliac spine (Fig. 3). Subcutaneous tissue and fascia lata were divided in the anterior border of the gluteus medius was palpated at its insertion on the greater trochanter. Intermuscular dissection between the gluteus medius and tensor fascia lata was done, carefully ligating lateral circumflex femoral vessels. After anterior joint capsule was incised, femoral neck was osteotomised and femoral head was removed.

For better visualization of the acetabulum, one or two Steinmann pins were inserted at the posterosuperior side of the acetabulum to retract the gluteus medius. Additionally, two or three curved Hohmann retractors were placed around the acetabulum, usually anteroinferiorly, posteroinferiorly and inferiorly (Fig. 4). After exposing the acetabulum as shown in Figure 4, reaming was performed.

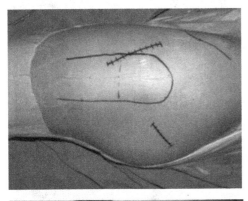

Figure 3:
Photograph showing landmarks (greater trochanter, vastus ridge, anterior superior iliac spine) and sites of anterolateral and posterolateral skin incision.

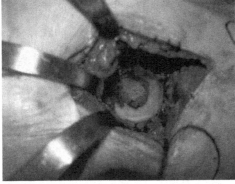

Figure 4:
For better view of acetabulam, one Steinman pin and three curved Hohmann retractors are placed around the acetabulam.

The posterior skin incision was then placed over the posterolateral aspect of hip. The hip was flexed to 90 degrees and 4 to 6 cm incision was made over the greater trochanter. After dissection through the muscle fibers of gluteus maximus, the fat layer separating gluteus maximus and medius was exposed. The piriformis, which was the landmark for the intermuscular dissection, was identified after excising the fat (Fig. 5). The intermuscular dissection between fibers of piriformis and gluteus medius led to joint capsule. Under direct visualization joint capsule was incised on the posterosuperior side of the hip joint. A starting reamer was introduced in to the femoral canal. After preparing the proximal femur with rasp, size of femoral component was determined under fluoroscopy and femoral component was inserted (Fig. 6). Femur was then brought anteriorly with traction, external rotation and extension of the hip. With hip in external rotation and bone hook around the neck, trial femoral head was inserted through anterior incision. After trial reduction was performed, leg length and range of motion of hip joint were evaluated by both clinically and under fluoroscopy (by comparing the level of the lesser trochanters with obturator foramina). The appropriate size final femoral head was inserted and joint was reduced. In case of tight soft tissues, sometimes it may not be possible to reduce the joint after insertion of a large femoral head component. In that situation, we first put the femoral head in to the acetabular cup and then engage the trunion in to the head with traction and gentle manipulation. Leg length and range of motion was checked again. Negative suction drain was placed and the posterior joint capsule, the anterior joint capsule, fascia lata and subcutaneous tissue were repaired and the skin was closed (Fig. 7).

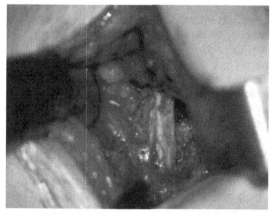

Figure 5:
This photograph shows piriformis as a landmark for intermuscular dissection between gluteus medius and piriformis.

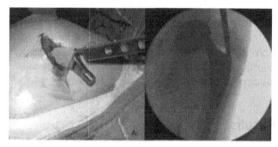

Figure 6:
(A) Through the posterior incision, femoral stem is inserted and (B) final evaluation of its position is made with fluoroscopy.

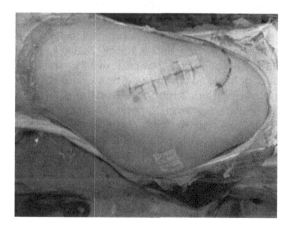

Figure 7:
Immediate postoperative photograph showing the postoperative incision wound of minimally invasive two-incision total hip replacement.

Postoperative protocol included abduction pillow between two legs to prevent dislocation, and elastic stockings and limb mobilization to prevent deep vein thrombosis. Quadriceps strengthening exercises were started on the same day and sitting by the side of the bed was also allowed on the day of surgery if patient was comfortable. Mobilization was recommended with tolerable weight bearing on postoperative day one, if patient's general condition is allowed. All the patients were discharged home when they were safely able to mobilize with an ambulatory aid.

Clinical Evaluation

All hips were evaluated preoperatively and at last follow-up using the Harris hip score and WOMAC score. Patients specifically were asked about episodes of instability or dislocation that could have been treated elsewhere. Other studies investigated were range of motion of hips, hospital stay, operation time, fluoroscopy time, blood loss by checking the hemoglobin and hematocrit changes and intraoperative or postoperative complications. In the immediate postoperative period, patients' rehabilitation processes were checked. For some patients who were unable to return for a last follow-up visit, the hip function were evaluated by telephone interview.

Radiographic Evaluation

A complete radiographic follow-up series, including preoperative, postoperative, and last follow-up radiographs, was available for 50 hips. All radiographic measurements were made by two investigators (CIH, DSL) other than the senior investigator who did 100% of the surgeries. Radiographic exams included an anteroposterior and frog lateral view of the hip. These views determined acetabular anteversion angles and allowed a assessment of the component position. The latest follow-up radiographs were assessed and compared with the original postoperative radiographs to determine component orientation, evidence of bony ingrowth, possible component migration, fracture, dislocation, and/or mechanical failure.

Results

The average time of clinical follow-up and examination was 8.7 months (range, 6.3 to 10.9 months). Hemoglobin level was changed from preoperatively 11.7 (range, 8.8 to 15.5) to 10.2 (range, 6.9 to 12.8), postoperatively. Hematocrit levels were changed from 35.2 % (range, 26.3 to 46.8 %) to 30.6 % (range, 21.4 to 39.1%). Mean operation time was checked 71 minutes (range, 48 to 91 minutes). Mean intraoperative fluoroscopy exposure time was 6 seconds (range, 2 to 11 seconds). The average Harris Hip Score (HHS) and WOMAC scores at last follow-up were significantly improved compared with the preoperative scores (83 and 47 points versus 3537 and 93 points, respectively). Also, the average ROM of hips at last follow-up was significantly improved when compared with the preoperative values (Table 1). Two cases would squat down because of ankylosing spondylitis in one and CVA sequela in one. Four cases could not take Buddhist position because of multiple fractures in two, ankylosis spondylitis in one and CVA history in one. No case developed hip dislocation and needed further surgery.

	Preoperative Hip ROM	Postoperative Hip ROM
Flexion	95.5°	113.1°
Internal rotation	2.2°	22.3°
External rotation	28.8°	56.7°
Abduction	21.7°	38.8°
Adduction	14.0°	24.9°

Table 1:
The average ROM of hip at last follow-up was compared with preoperative values.

Radiographically, the median acetabular shell abduction and anteversion were 36° (range, 27 to 48°) and 17° (range, 5 to 32°), respectively. There was no evidence of cup migration. There was no fracture of the femoral component. Average stem position was valgus 1.9° (range, varus 2.3° to valgus 4.8°). In all cases, the stem position was within the valgus or varus 5°. There were no complications intraoperatively or postoperatively.

Postoperatively, the average amount of hemovac drainage was 740cc and average transfusion was 384cc. All patients could ambulate on the first postoperative day with tolerable weight bearing. Rehabilitation proceeded with initial walker ambulation postoperative 1.6 days and then, crutch ambulation was started within the 6.5 days, and ambulation without any support was possible after mean 9.3 days postoperatively. Climbing up the stairs without assistant device was possible within 29.5 days on average, postoperatively.

Discussion

Wear at the articulation as a result of the increasing demands in active and young patients remains a significant clinical challenge. Age and activity level are among the most important predictors of wear after THA. Despite the improvement of implant, wear and osteolysis resulting in failure of the THA remain significant concerns. Ceramics were introduced in total hip replacement to address the problems of friction and wear that were reported with metal-on-polyethylene articulations. This very hard and wettable material can limit wear debris production and provide longer lifetime of the artificial hip after implantation. Recent studies have reported the efficacy of using ceramic-on-ceramic or metal-on-metal bearing surfaces, particularly in high-demand patients. The alumina-on-alumina combination currently is being recognized as one of the best answers to wear debris-induced osteolysis and is best used in young and active patients [15].

However, one of the most publicized limitations of ceramic articulation is implant fracture. The fracture rate of ceramics was 13.4% for implants manufactured before 1990, fracture rate has decreased and now ranged from 0.2% to 5.7% due to development of technology [9,16,17,18]. D'Antonio and Capello [11] reported no case of ceramic articulation fracture in over 950 THAs in their large prospective study series. Some authors described that the principle causes of ceramic fracture were related not to the material or manufacturing but to surgical techniques [31]. The limitations for the use of this material are an extra small socket [3], the need for a small head [5], and osteoporotic bone [6]. In our study, all cases used ceramic-on-ceramic articulation and no cases developed implant fracture until this short period of follow-up.

Dislocation is a common complication after THA [23] and can severely disrupt a patient's quality of life. Early dislocation is a frequent problem following primary THA. The prevalence of early dislocation following primary arthroplasty has been reported less than 1% to 5% [19,27]. Late dislocation, occurring many years after THA, is an increasing problem [30] and, in one study the prevalence increased by 1% every 5 years with a 22 mm femoral head [2]. The patient risk factors for dislocation after primary THA have been reported to be age 75 years or older, preoperative diagnosis of femoral neck fracture or nonunion, chronic neurologic disorders and a prior history of alcohol abuse [4,20,25,26]. The major factors of prevention of dislocation are proper orientation of both the acetabular and femoral component. Therefore, the use of larger femoral head to hip arthroplasty adds to improve hip stability, and increase hip ROM and therefore lower the incidence of dislocation [7,10]. The cause of dislocation is often secondary to impingement. The type of impingement depends on the size of the femoral head. With 22mm femoral heads, impingement between components occurs, most often between the femoral neck and the acetabular component [10]. With femoral head larger than 32mm in diameter, bony impingement symptoms commonly occur between the proximal femur and pelvis. This is because the head to neck ratio increases as the size of the femoral head increases, which allows a greater arc of curvature before the neck can make contact with the acetabulum at the extremes of motion. The jump distance (the distance the head must travel to disengage from the socket) is higher with a larger femoral head, which is more stable against dislocation. Thus, the larger femoral head adds substantially more stability to the hip reconstruction [7,10]. In our study, no case developed hip dislocation even they were allowed for squatting and all cases except two cases could squat.

The use of large diameter femoral heads in THAs with metal on polyethylene articulation is limited because of wear. Studies have shown a higher volumetric polyethylene wear rate with conventional UHMWPE articulating with a larger diameter femoral head [21]. The issue of increased wear must play a major role in the decision making process. Historically using a larger head and thinner polyethylene liner may not have been optimal because this patient has a higher risk for revision surgery/liner exchange during his/her lifespan. However, a larger femoral head is an attractive choice when stability is a critical factor and wear is not a major concern such as ceramic-on-ceramic articulation. In our study, we could not estimate the effect of large diameter femoral head regarding the wear and osteolysis because of short follow up duration.

The benefits of minimally invasive two-incision total hip arthroplasty include a smaller incision and minimal soft tissue injury than with the traditional posterior approach, therefore use of minimally invasive decreases hospital stay and permits quicker recovery. In our study with the use of two-incision minimally invasive THA, the patients' recovery was much quick and stability was better which was proved by increased ROM and possibility of squatting position in most patients. Also, there was no dislocation with this procedure and patients could resume activities of daily living such as return to work, driving, and recreational activities much sooner [13]. We believe that two-incision technique, because of its complete muscle-preserving technique is the most advantageous approach to date for better functional recovery if the surgery is performed by experienced surgeon.

Our data suggest that 32 and 36 mm femoral heads with ceramic-on-ceramic articulation notably reduce the prevalence of early dislocation after primary THA, especially in combination with the modified two-incision minimally invasive THA approach when compared to historical controls. To date, no patient with a larger femoral head in primary THA has undergone revision for recurrent dislocation in our institute.

Conclusion

A minimally invasive two-incision THA using large diameter ceramic-on-ceramic articulation is excellent method that prevents dislocation, has good functional and clinical results and faster recovery.

References

1. Barrack RL, Butler RA, Laster DR, Andrews P (2001) Stem design and dislocation after revision total hip arthroplasty: Clinical results and computer modeling. J Arthroplasty 16:8-12.
2. Berry DJ. Von Knoch, Schleck CD, Harmsen WS (2004) The cumulative long-term risk of dislocation after primary Charnley total hip arthroplasty. J Bone Joint Surg Am 86:9-14.
3. Boehler M, Knahr K, Salzer M et al (1994) Long term results of uncemented alumina acetabular implants. J Bone Joint Surg Br 76:53-59.
4. Boettcher WG (1992) Total hip arthroplasties in the elderly: morbidity, mortality, and cost effectiveness. Clin Orthop Relat Res 274:30-34.
5. Boutin P (1972) Arthroplastie Totale de Hanche par Prothese en Alumine Frittee Rev Chir Orthop 58:229-246.
6. Boutin P, Blanquaert D (1981) Le Frottement Al/Al en Chirurgie de la Hanche-1205 Arthroplasties Totales. Rev Chir Orthop 67:279-287.
7. Burroughs BR, Hallstrom B, Golladay GJ, Hoeffel D, Harris WH (2005) Range of motion and stability in total hip arthroplasty with 28-, 32-, 38-, and 44-mm femoral head sizes: an in vitro study. J Arthroplasty 20:11-19.
8. Bystrom S, Espehaug B, Furnes O, Havelin LI (2003) Femoral head size is a risk factor for total hip luxation.: a study of 42,987 primary hip arthroplasties from the Norwegian Arthroplasty Register. Acta Orthop Scand 74:514-524.
9. Capello WN, Dantonio JA, Feinberg JR, Manley MT (2005) Alternative bearing surfaces: alumina ceramic bearings for total hip arthroplasty. Instr Course Lect 54:171-176.
10. Crowninshield RD, Maloney WJ, Wentz DH, Humphrey SM, Blanchard CR (2004) Biomechanics of large femoral heads: what they do and don't do. Clin Orthop Relat Res 429:102-107.
11. D'Antonio J, Capello W, Manley M, naughton M, Sutton K (2005) Alumina ceramic bearings for total hip arthroplasty: five-year results of a prospective randomized study. Clin Orthop Relat Res 436:164-171.
12. DeWal H, Su E, DiCesare PE (2003) Instability following total hip arthroplasty. Am J Orthop 32:377-382.
13. Duwelius PJ, Berger RA (2005) Minimally invasive total hip arthroplasty: the two-incision approach. Curr Opin Orthop 16:5-9.

14. Eftekhar NS (1993) Dislocation and instability. In: Eftekhar NS(eds) Total Hip Arthroplasty. Mosby, St. Louis CV, pp 1505-1553.

15. Hannouche D, Hamadouche M, Nizard R, Bizot P, Meunier A, Sedel L (2005) Ceramics in total hip replacement. Clin Orthop Relat Res 430:62-71.

16. Hannouche D, Nich C, Bizot P, Meunier A, Nizard R, Sedel L (2003) Fractures of ceramic bearings: history and present status. Clin Orthop Relat Res 417:19-26.

17. Hasegawa M, Sudo A, Uchida A (2006) Alumina ceramic-on-ceramic total hip replacement with a layered acetabular component. J Bone Joint Surg Br 88:877-882.

18. Ha YC, Kim SY, Kim HJ, Yoo JJ, Koo KH (2007) Ceramic Liner Fracture after Cementless Alumina-on-Alumina Total Hip Arthroplasty. Clin Orthop Relat Res 458:106-10.

19. Katz JN, Losina E, Barrett J, Phillips CB, Mahomed NN, Lew RA, Guadagnoli E, Harris WH, Poss R, Baron JA (2001) Association between hospital and surgeon procedure volume and outcomes of total hip replacement in the United States Medicare Population. J Bone Joint Surg Am 83:1622-1629.

20. Lachiewicz PF, Soileau ES (2002) Stability of total hip arthroplasty in patients 75 years or older. Clin Orthop Relat Res 405:65-69.

21. Lee PC, Shih CH, Chen WJ, Tu YK, Tai CL (1999) Early polyethylene wear and osteolysis in cementless total hip arthroplasty: the influence of femoral head size and polyethylene thickness. J Arthroplasty. 14:976-981.

22. Lewinnek GE, Lewis JL, Tarr R, Compere CL, Zimmerman JR (1978) Dislocations after total hip-replacement arthroplasties. J Bone Joint Surg Am 60:217-220.

23. Mahoney CR, Pellicci PM (2003) Complications in primary total hip arthroplasty. Avoidance and management of dislocations. Instr Course Lect 52:247-255.

24. Masonis JL, Bourne RB (2002) Surgical approach, abductor function, and total hip arthroplasty dislocation. Clin Orthop Relat Res 405:46-53.

25. Morrey BF (1992) Instability after total hip arthroplasty. Orthop Clin North America 23:237-248.

26. Muratoglu OK, Bragdon CR, O'Connor D, Perinchief RS, Estok DM 2nd, Jasty M, Harris WH (2001) Larger diameter femoral heads used in conjunction with a highly cross-linked ultra-high molecular weight polyethylene: a new concept. J Arthroplasty 16(suppl 1):24-30.

27. Phillips CB, Barrett JA, Losina E, Mahomed NN, Lingard EA, Guadagnoli E, Baron JA, Harris WH, Poss R, Katz JN (2003) Incidence rates of dislocation, pulmonary embolism, and deep infection during the first six months after elective total hip replacement. J Bone Joint Surg Am. 85:20-26.

28. Robbins GM, Masri BA, Garbuz DS, Greidanus N, Duncan CP (2001) Treatment of hip instability. Orthop Clin North Am 32:593-610.

29. Turner RS (1994) Postoperative total hip prosthetic femoral head dislocations: Incidence, etiologic factors, and management. Clin Orthop 301:196-204.

30. Von Knoch M, Berry DJ, Harmsen WS, Morrey BF (2002) Late dislocation after total hip arthroplasty. J Bone Joint Surg Am 84:1949-1953.

31. Weisse B, Zahner M, Weber W, Rieger W (2003) Improvement of the reliability of ceramic hip joint implants. J Biomech 36:1633-1639.

8.5 MIS and the Demands on Bearing Couples

S. Junk-Jantsch and G. Pflüger

We started to tackle the issue of minimally invasive hip surgery in our clinic in March 2004. The first problem was to look for the ideal approach for performing minimally invasive hip arthroplasty, for alternative implants and for a reproducible procedure that could rapidly become routine practice. Based on the impressions gathered during numerous periods spent abroad, we undertook an attempt for our department to define minimal invasiveness in hip surgery. What we wanted in introducing this procedure into the routine of the department, in terms of both our demands and our expectations were the following:

Definition:

Minimally invasive means minimally traumatic and involves making the portal smaller and retention of all the muscle attachments in order to ensure immediate post-operative and final sufficient gait profile.

Our wishes:

To retain the anterolateral approach between the tensor fasciae latae muscle and the glutaeus medius and minimus as well as operating in a supine position, retaining the usual landmarks.

Our requirements:

Not to accept any compromises with regard to optimal positioning of the implant, as well as to achieve the planned leg length and the offset. To continue using the cementless prosthesis model used by us (Bicon threaded cup and Zweymüller stem), characterised by excellent long-term results 28 years after implantation (X-ray 1).

Our expectations:

Improved cosmetic results thanks to the reduction in size of the skin incision, preservation of the muscle attachments with consequent faster mobilisation and rehabilitation, shorter hospitalisation time and increased patient satisfaction.

We have applied this procedure for our purposes as follows:

The anterolateral approach in a supine position according to Watson–Jones [7] has been retained in a modified version. The skin incision has become considerably smaller (Fig. 1), the muscle attachments of the glutaeus medius and minimus muscles are preserved, which does not cause any problems for adjusting the cup if the resection of the neck of the femur is sufficient and the retractors are accurately positioned (Fig. 2a, b). Broaching of the femur is carried out in external rotation, adduction and hyperextension of the leg (Fig. 3). This manner of proceeding requires sterile washing and draping of both legs and the technical pre-requisite that it must be possible to tilt the leg section of the operating tabledown.

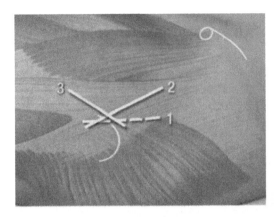

Figure 1:
Skin incision:
MIS: 7-13cm Ø 9.3cm
Conventional: 9-25cm Ø 18.9cm.

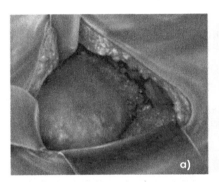
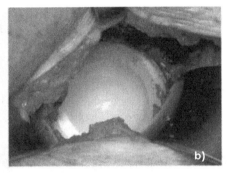

Figure 2a, b:
View of the acetabulum with three Hohmann retractors (a) and inserted Bicon-Plus cup (b).

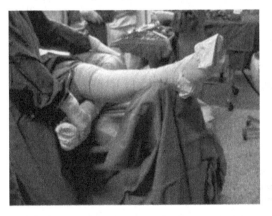

Figure 3:
Femoral positioning: external rotation, adduction and hyperextension table tilted down.

The key to success lies in extensive release of the joint capsule [4,5,6], which has been standardised by us (Fig. 4). Step-by-step mobilising of the proximal femur enables a tension-free entry portal for the stem rasps and the original implant. The instrument set has been modified. Alongside the very helpful double-offset handpiece (Fig. 5) for the rasping process, these rasps can also be used, with standard or lateralised necks, as test prostheses for simulating optimum joint stability, the offset and the planned leg length rapidly, using reduction manoeuvres that entail little trauma [6].

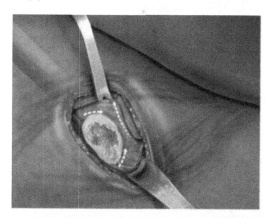

Figure 4:
Femural/capsule release in trochanteric fossa optional partial release of the piriformis tendon.

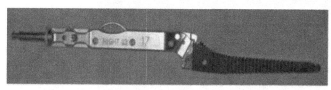

Figure 5:
Modified Instruments.

One step that in our opinion is particularly innovative was achieved by modifying the design of the Zweymüller stem (Fig. 6). Following elimination of the trochanteric wing proximally but retaining the proven meta-diaphyseal anchoring. The new stem is easier to implant using the minimally invasive technique; it preserves and protects the greater trochanter bone and protects the soft tissues, thus considerably lowering the risk of intra-operative and postoperative damage to the trochanter or soft tissues. This is illustrated very clearly by the comparison between the old and the current pathway of the rasp and the diagrams of the loss of substances in the trochanter region (Fig. 7). Nothing has been changed with regard to the proven metaphyseal and diaphyseal anchoring .

Statistics:
We have been implanting this modified SL-MIA stem since December 2005.

Overall, we have recorded abundant data concerning this modified approach with retention of the muscle attachments on 1000 implanted prostheses, of which all of 342 with the new SL-MIA stem. The mean age of the patient s was 68.5 (range, 43-92), ratio of men to women 1:2, mean BMI 26.4 (17.7-38.5). Increasing experience with this procedure now enables us to use the minimally invasive procedure in almost all cases of primary hip replacement, and more and more frequently even in difficult initial situations. The following presentation provides an overview of the implants and bearing couples used in 1000 cases of hip prosthesis operations. We have analysed a large quantity of pre-operative, peri-operative and post-operative data. In this context, the new SL-MIA stems were found to be particularly interesting, and with regard to which it has been shown that the elimination of the trochanteric wing has not led to any drop in quality as far as concerns positioning of the stem and primary stability.

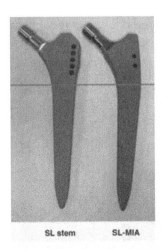

SL stem   SL-MIA

Figure 6:
Zweymüller SL-Plus stem and SL-Plus MIA stem.

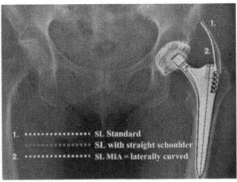

1. ···············SL Standard
   ·············SL with straight schoulder
2. ···············SL MIA ≈ laterally curved

Figure 7:
Theoretical model of pathway of rasp.

Axial migration and formation of proximal radiolucent lines during the course of the first few months following surgery were measured and compared with the results achieved with the SL-PLUS stem. The angle of inclination following implanting of the cup was also measured, paying particular attention to the optimum implanting criteria demanded by the manufacturer CeramTec for ceramic-ceramic bearing couples.

Table 1 shows the stem sizes used, indicating a ratio of 2:1 for the standard versus lateralised variant (Table 2). Table 3 shows the head diameters used. All of 41.32% of the cases were treated with size 32 heads. If a head diameter of 32 had been available to us for ceramic-ceramic pairing, this proportion would have been roughly 20 % higher. This indicates a noticeable tendency towards larger head diameters, with a benefit in terms of stability and post-operative range of motion of the joint. Table 4 shows the cup sizes of the conical Bicon-threaded cup used. Sizes 2 (46 mm), 3 (49 mm) and 4 (52 mm) were used in 90% of cases, that is to say preferably the smaller implants. In our opinion it is better to medialise the cups only to the extent that a stable bony anchoring ring is present and to stop reaming of the cone in the hard sub-chondral sclerotic layer of the acetabular socket. The original hip center should be achieved. Table 5 shows the bearing couples used. The proportion of ceramic-ceramic amounts to approximately 20%. We use this form in younger patients, setting at this time the age of 70 as the upper age limit. The proportion would have been higher, however, if there had been a ceramic inlay at our disposal also for the size 2 cups.

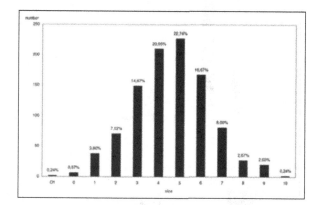

Table 1:
Distribution of stem sizes implanted in the SL-Plus and SL-Plus MIA cohorts. MIS-THR: stem-sizes 01/2005-04/2007 (n=1000).

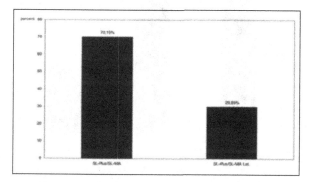

Table 2:
In 1/3 of the implantations a lateralized stem was used. MIS-THR: SL-stems standard: lateralized in % (n=1000).

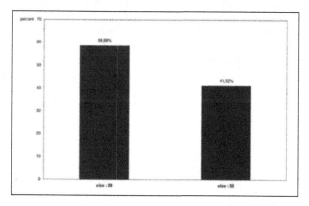

Table 3:
MIS-THR: head-sizes in % (n=1000).

It can be seen from this presentation that metal-metal bearing couples have not been used any longer. We used to implant MM bearing couples the years from 1994 to 1999, mainly in younger patients in view of the low wear rates, in the hope that the survival period would be as long as possible and complication-free. We subsequently discontinued using this form of bearing couple and summarised our negative results in an interdisciplinary presentation [5a].

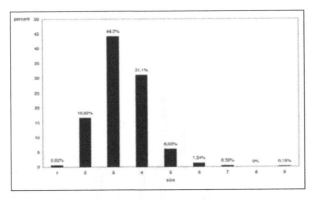

Table 4:
Predominantly smaller sizes
of the BICON conical cup
were used.
MIS-THR: cup sizes in %
(n=1000).

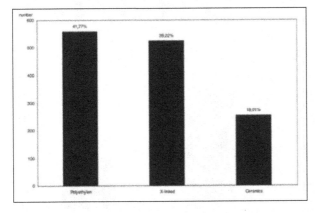

Table 5:
MIS-THR: inlays (n=1000).

In the early years between 1994 and 1996, a Zweymüller stem prosthesis with a high carbide gliding surfaces was implanted (Fig. 8) followed until 1999 by the Zweymüller stem with its low-carbide bearing couples alloy (Fig. 9). Between 1994 and 1999, 781 hip endoprostheses with metal-metal bearing couples were implanted in 708 patients. The proportion of MM hips amounted to slightly over 20% (Fig. 10) of the total during the years of full availability. These values are comparable with the proportion of ceramic-ceramic couples implanted, currently chosen in our department mainly for younger patients. Following an initially normal post-operative course, within a period of time ranging from 5 to 30

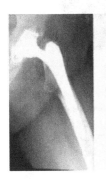
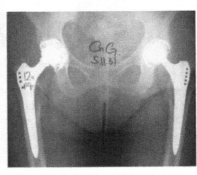

Figure 8:
Female, 74 years,
Alloclassic MM High Carbide.

months radiological modifications on the cup and in the region of the proximal femur were found in a considerable number of patients, with areas of lysis, coupled with resumption of pain in the hip (Fig. 11) and followed by revision-operation. A follow-up study of the 781 implanted MM couples was started in 2004 (Fig. 12). The result was a re-operation rate of 9.9% (Fig. 13). The statistical figure of 9.9% corresponds to 47 revisions and is shown in Figure 14. In almost half of the cases replacement of the ball-head and inlay was sufficient, while 23.4 % of them exhibited loosening of the cup and 10.6 % loosening of the stem. In 17% of cases both components were replaced. Apart from the revisions, we were particularly worried by those cases with lysis areas that were already visible radiologically, or those in which nothing particular was noticeable in the X-rays but in which pain in the hip had resumed, and for which we have to expect re-operation (Fig. 15).

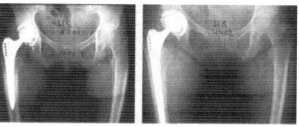

Figure 9:
Female, 67 years,
SL Plus MM Low Carbide
→ SLR Plus CC.

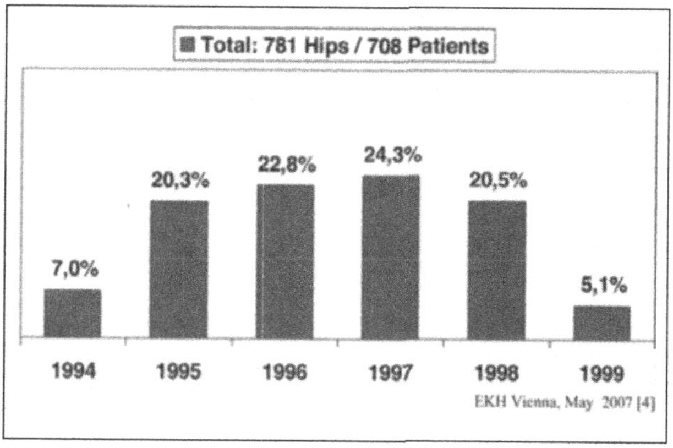

Figure 10:
Metal-Metal Implantations,
1994-1999.

Total: 781 Hips / 708 Patients

7,0% — 1994
20,3% — 1995
22,8% — 1996
24,3% — 1997
20,5% — 1998
5,1% — 1999

EKH Vienna, May 2007 [4]

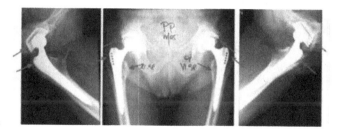

Figure 11:
Male, 68 years,
SL Plus MM Low Carbide.

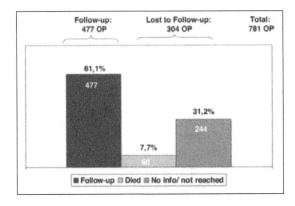

Figure 12:
Metal-Metal Implantations:
Follow-up 2004.

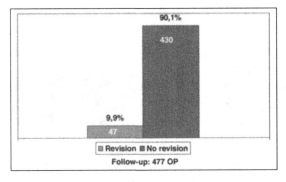

Figure 13:
Follow-up Results.

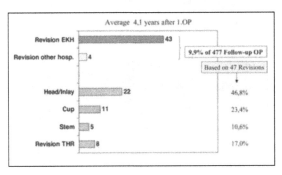

Figure 14:
Follow-up Results:
Number and Type of Revisions.

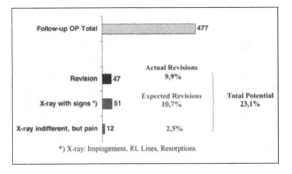

Figure 15:
Revisions: Actual and Potential.

Critically speaking, this results in 23.1% of unsatisfactory post-operative outcomes. In all cases of re-operation, massive accumulation of fluid in the region of the trochanteric bursa and enormous thickening of the joint capsule were found, but not the typical profile of metallosis. All the explants were subjected to thorough analysis. The samples of intra-operatively taken joint fluid and fresh blood were analysed (histology, analysis of metal in the tissues, wear, etc.). Low and high-carbide bearing couples can produce a hypersensitivity reaction [1,2,3,8], markedly less frequently with high-carbide alloys. Alongside widespread perivascular lymphocyte infiltrations, thickening of the endothelium of the veins, fibrin exsudation and accumulations of macrophages with drop-like inclusions were found as well as eosinophile granulocytes and mast cells. It is unfortunately not possible to identify pre-operatively patients who could develop a hypersensitivy reaction. Because of this unforeseeability, we have implanted no more MM bearing couples since 2000, and we are also of the opinion that the boom in resurfacing prostheses in younger patients should be observed with great caution.

Evaluation and analysis of the THR of (n=342) Bicon threaded cup and SL-MIA stems:

The measured angles of inclination of the implanted cups are shown in Table 6, forming two collectives in which the dark strokes correspond to the PE-ceramic and X-linked PE-ceramic bearing couples (n=252), while the light strokes correspond to ceramic-ceramic couples (n=90). To make the data easier to compare, the comparison is indicated in the form of percentages of the absolute figures. Looking at the overall satisfactory values, there are no cups in the ceramic-ceramic group at a steeper angle than 54° and 81% are in the ideal range between 40 and 49°. In knee surgery we have been supporters and users of navigation for 8 years now. Up to now our impression of navigated hip surgery had not been convincing enough to use it as a routine procedure for all primary implants. Positioning of the sensors for navigation is not yet as minimally invasive as would be desirable, and the choice of the optimum anteversion of the cup has not yet been defined.

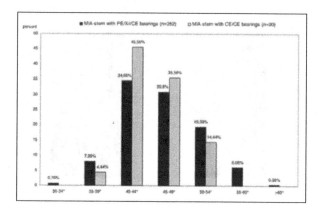

Table 6:
THR-socket inclination angle.

The radiological measurement and evaluation of the stem positioning of the new SL-MIA stem (n=236) is provided in Table 7, as well as a comparison with 50 measured SL-PLUS stems. The minimally invasive implanting technique was used for both groups. The result confirms our practical experience. Due to the elimination of the trochanteric wing, with the smaller portal with retention of the muscle attachments of the glutaeus medius and minimus the risk of forcing the implant into a varus position is considerably lower with the MIA-stems (24% in the SL-Plus group versus 7.4% in the MIA group). The risk of later subsidence of the stem due to the fact that the proximal part has been made smaller has also been discussed repeatedly. Table 8 shows, once again in a comparison between the two models, that there are no reasons for such scepticism. The new stem exhibits a trend towards better the same results. Minor axial migration of 2 to 3 mm has been measured twice as frequently on the old stems as on the new modified implant. The comparative evaluation of formation of a proximal radiolucent line for the two stems is equally favourable. This aspect has already been described and illustrated in publications on several occasions and is due to the meta-diaphyseal anchoring of the stem with a certain moment of oscillation in the proximal part. There is no evidence of any effects on stability. Notwithstanding, we are pleased to say that the occurrence of radiolucent lines in the first post-operative year has been observed to a lesser extent with SL-MIA stems than with SL-Plus stems (Table 9).

	SL-Plus n = 50	SL-MIA n = 236
Neutral (+/- 3%)	76 %	92,6 %
Varus position	24 %	7,4 %
Valgus position	0 %	0 %

Table 7:
Evaluation of monitor-targeted a.p. radiographs in standing position.
Stemposition SL-Plus/SL-MIA.

	2-3 mm	> 3 mm
SL-MIA stems (n=133):	6,02 %	1,50 %
SL-Plus stems (n=133):	11,29 %	0 %

Table 8:
Axial Migration.

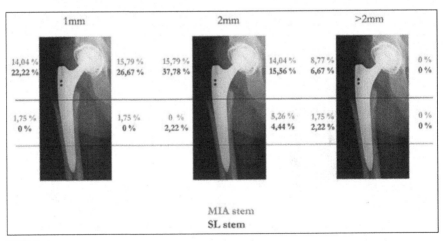

	1mm		2mm		>2mm	
	14,04 % 22,22 %	15,79 % 26,67 %	15,79 % 37,78 %	14,04 % 15,56 %	8,77 % 6,67 %	0 % 0 %
	1,75 % 0 %	1,75 % 0 %	0 % 2,22 %	5,26 % 4,44 %	1,75 % 2,22 %	0 % 0 %

MIA stem
SL stem

Table 9:
Radiolucent lines MIA stem (n=57)/SL stem (n=45) 6-12 months postop.

Summary

Minimally invasive hip implantion with a smaller skin incision, a non-traumatic procedure, protection of the soft tissues and retention of the muscle attachments responsible for a sufficient gait profile has become our gold standard.

The approach by means of an anterolateral portal in analogy to the Watson-Jones approach in a supine position has been perfected by us and illustrated in publications [7]. Following adaptation draping, of the patient's position and of the instrument set and after carrying out the extensive and accurate capsule release, the adjustments for both cup preparation and stem preparation by direct vision and using the habitual landmarks for guidance can be carried out without disruptions.

The clinical results referred to the immediate post-operative period, the first post-operative weeks and the later period are impressive thanks to retention of the functions of the pelvico trochanteric muscles and make rehabilitation far easier for patients. Positive post-operative Trendelenburg signs have become rare in our precise documentation of the results. This is confirmed by the progress of the Harris Hip Score (Table 10), which already rises from an average pre-operative score of 41.6 to 71,6 at the time of discharge, reaching 94,5 by post-operative week six and 95,2 by post-operative week 12.

The design of the Zweymüller stem was further adapted to improve bone saveing and soft-tissue protection. The meta-diaphyseal anchoring has not been altered and this improvement is best provided by the elimination of the trochanteric wing. The radiological results confirm our own impression that the modified design should not entail any loss in terms of quality and indeed, to the contrary, that it leads to recognisable advantages in terms of positioning and easier implantation.

We have stopped implanting metal-metal bearing couples due to our own negative experiences. For younger patients the ceramic-ceramic bearing couple with the lowest wear rates is the method of choice. We would also like to see ceramic inlays and inlays with larger inside diameters for the smaller cups, too, so as to enable us to follow the significant trend towards larger head diameter in order to improve stability and mobility.

	SL-stem (n = 150)	SL-MIA (n = 150)
preop:	ø 45,7	ø 41,6
10 th day postop:	ø 71,3	ø 71,6
6 weeks postop:	ø 94,5	ø 94,5
3 month postop:	ø 95,0	ø 95,3
6 month postop:	ø 96,5	ø 96,2

Table 10:
Harris Hip Score:
SL-stem versus SL-Mia.

References

1. Lohmann CH: Can Metal-Metal Total Hip Arthroplasty induce Hypersensitivity reactions? Proceedings CeramTec Meeting, JA d'Antonio, M Dietrich (Eds.), Steinkopff, Darmstadt, pp33-37, 2006.
2. Lohmann CH, Nuechtern JV, Willert HG, Junk-Jantsch S, Ruether W, Pflueger G: Hypersensitivity Reactions in Total Hip Arthroplasty, Orthopaedics, in press 2007.
3. Lohmann CH, Pflüger G, Yazigee 0, Junk-Jantsch S, Schmotzer H, Becker A, Morlock M, Willert HG: Low Carbide vs. High carbide - Is there a Difference in Tissue Response and Clinical Predictability? In: 25 Years of Cementless Arthroplasty, Santore R (ed.), in press.
4. Pflüger G, Junk-Jantsch S, Schöll V: The anterolateral approach in supine position for minimally invasive implantation of hip endoprostheses, Interact Surg (2006) 1: 21-25, Springer 2006.
5. Pflüger G, Junk-Jantsch S, Schöll V: Minimally Invasive Total Hip Replacement via the Anterolateral Approach in the Supine Position, Int. Orthopaedics, in press.
5a. Pflüger G, Junk-Jantsch S, Koppelent R, Results of a 5-10 Year Follow-Up Study of Hip Replacements with Metal-Metal Bearings, Radiological Findings, Interdisciplinary presentation, 2005.
6. Schöll V, Frank M, Junk-Jantsch S, Pflüger G: Kraftanalysen mittels Raspelversuchen mit modifizierten Raspelsystemen für MIS-Hüftendoprothesen, MOT, in press.
7. Watson-Jones R : Fractures of the neck of the femur, British Journal of Surgery, Vol. 23, Issue 92, p. 787-808, 1936.
8. Willert HG, Buchhorn GH, Fayazzi R, Flury T, Köster G, Lohmann CH: Aseptic Loosing of Metal/Metal Endoprostheses is Associated with Lymphocytic Reactions - Signs of a Delayed Type Hypersensitivity Reaction Type IV. Journal of Bone and Joint Surgery (Am), 87A(1):28-37, 2005.

8.6 Computer Navigation: Improving Outcomes with Hard on Hard Bearings

R. G. Middleton, C. Olyslaegers and T. W. Wainwright

Background

The design and manufacture of ceramic implants has improved significantly over the last decade. Consequently the use of ceramic-on-ceramic bearings in total hip replacement has become increasingly popular with over 150,000 components having been implanted in Europe [1]. This increased use and uptake of the ceramic-on-ceramic combination can be thought to reflect the low wear rates that it has exhibited as a bearing couple [2-4]. In addition to these lower wear rates; ceramic-on-ceramic bearings have a subsequent reduced incidence of osteolysis, the possibility to be used in smaller cups without increasing wear, and the absence of any metal ion production.

The reduced incidence of wear and subsequent osteolysis which ceramic-on-ceramic implants offer is related to the high scratch resistance and wettability of the material [5]. This wear rate has been shown to be 4000 times lower than that of metal articulating against polyethylene [6] and should be considered alongside the established notion that osteolysis induced by polyethylene wear debris remains the long-term complication of the conventional metal-on-polyethylene total hip replacement.

Metal-on-metal articulations share this advantage of low wear and have been reported as exhibiting a wear rate of almost two orders of magnitude less than conventional bearings [7]. However, metal-on-metal bearings generate raised systemic metal ion levels, which may have possible adverse effects in the long-term. Whilst short term studies have found no casual association between increased metal ion levels and carcinogenesis or metal hypersensitivity the unavailability of evidence has led the United Kingdom Department of Health to release a statement on the biological effects of wear debris [8]. In this the panel concluded that increased metal ion levels "gave rise to concern because this may present a potential risk of carcinogenicity in humans".

Ceramic-on-ceramic bearings have exhibited good long-term results [3] and appear to have notable advantages over other alternate bearing combinations. However, a ceramic bearing has its disadvantages and can offer limited intra-operative options. Elevated liners cannot be used to prevent dislocation and achieving correct leg length without impingement can be difficult in the absence of variable offset. Such limitation to component options is of significant importance to surgeons because it means greater surgical precision and accuracy is required. It has been established that ceramic-on-ceramic couples provide less dislocation stability in sub-optimal implant positions compared to metal-on-polyethylene [9].

Preventing dislocation is of major concern in total hip arthroplasty and dislocation remains the second most common complication of the procedure after late prosthetic loosening [10]. Using an elevated rim acetabular liner has been demonstrated to improve stability following total hip replacement [11] and malorientation of components has been shown to be the cause of approximately one half of all dislocations [12]. Therefore, when using a ceramic-on-ceramic bearing couple surgical accuracy can be considered imperative.

Surgical accuracy can be improved by the use of computer navigation. Of particular relevance to the ceramic-on-ceramic total hip replacement procedure is the decreased variability and increased accuracy of acetabular cup positioning which has been widely demonstrated when using imageless navigations systems [13, 14]. The application of computer navigation to ceramic-on-ceramic total hip replacement is further strengthened by the findings of Sugamo et al. [15] who report excellent mid-term results of using computer navigation to implant a cementless ceramic-on-ceramic bearing in 59 hips. When compared with the control group the navigated group demonstrated a reduced dislocation rate and increased precision of acetabular component orientation.

Our Experience

We feel that surgical accuracy and pre-operative planning for ceramic-on-ceramic bearings can therefore be considered critical to optimise patient outcomes. This situation can be thought of as similar to that found in the hip resurfacing procedure where the risks of notching, oversizing the femoral head and impingement have been overcome by the use of computer navigation.

Our unit has a three-year experience of using computer navigation in the clinical setting. This has involved the development of operative techniques for using both fluoroscopic and imageless computer navigation for the hip resurfacing procedure. In our series of 30 hips we have found both forms of navigation to be safe and successful at helping to achieve optimal component positioning. We have observed no complications and found no increase to operative time once the initial learning curve of using and setting up the equipment has been overcome [16].

The Future

We believe that applying the concept of computer navigation to the ceramic-on-ceramic total hip replacement procedure is of particular benefit. Ceramic-on-ceramic bearing couples have demonstrated excellent wear characteristics in comparison to other alternate bearing surfaces. However, the wide spread uptake of the combination is currently limited due to the absence of elevated liners and offset options. Computer navigation offers a solution to this problem by affording the surgeon increased pre-operative planning and intra operative surgical accuracy so that optimal component alignment may be assured.

References

1. Sandhu HS, Middleton RG (2005) Ceramic-on-ceramic. Ann R Coll Surg Engl 87: 159-162.
2. Sedal L (2000) Evolution of alumina-on-alumina implants: A review. Clin Orthop Relat Res 379: 48-54.
3. Hamadouche M, Boutin P, Daussange J, Bolander ME, Sedal L (2002) Alumina-on-alumina total hip arthroplasty: a minimum 18.5-years follow up study. J Bone Joint Surg Am 84: 69-77.
4. Yoo JJ, Kim YM, Yoon KS, Koo KH, Song WS, Kim HJ(2005) Alumina-onalumina total hip arthroplasty. A five-year minimum follow up study. J Bone Joint Surg Am 87: 530-535.
5. Sedal L (1997) The Tribology of hip replacement. In: Kenwright J, Duparc J, Fulford P, eds. European Instructional Course Lectures, vol3 London: The British Editorial Society of Bone and Joint Surgery p25-33.
6. Dorlot JM, Christel P, Meunier A (1989) Wear analysis of retrieved alumina heads and sokets of hip prostheses. J Biomed Mater Res 23: 299-310.
7. McMinn DJW, Daniel J, Ziaee H (2005) Metal-on-metal. Ann R Coll Surg Engl 87; 159-162.
8. Statement on biological effects of wear debris generated from metal on metal bearing surfaces: Evidence for genotoxicity (2006) Committee on mutagenicity of chemicals in food, consumer products and the environement, Department of Health, United Kingdom. HYPERLINK "http://www.advisorybodies,doh.gov.uk/com/hip.htm" www.advisorybodies,doh.gov.uk/com/hip.htm
9. Bader R, Steinhauser E, Zimmermann S, Mittelmeier W, Scholz R, Busch R (2204) Differences between the wear couples metal-on-polyethylene and ceramic-on-ceramic in the stability against dislocation of total hip replacement. J Mater Sci Mater Med 15(6): 711-8.
10. Bartz RL, Noble PC, Kadakia NR, Tullos HS (2000) The effect of femoral component head size on posterior dislocation of the artificial hip joint. J Bone Joint Surg Am 82; 1300-1307.
11. Cobb TK, Morrey BF, Ilstrup DM (1996) The elevated-rim acetabular liner in total hip arthroplasty: Relationship to postoperative dislocation. J Bone Joint Surg Am 78; 80-86.
12. Daly PJ, Morrey BF (1992) operative correction of an unstable total hip arthroplasty. J Bone Joint Surg Am74; 1334-1343.
13. Nogler M, Kessler O, Prassl A, Donnelly B, Streicher R, Sledge JB, Krismer M (2004) Reduced variability of acetabular cup positioning with use of an imageless navigation system. Clin Orthop Relat Res 426; 159-163.
14. Kalteis T, Handel M, Herold T, Perlick L, Baethis H, Grifka J (2005) Greater accuracy in positioning of the acetabular cup by using an image-free navigation system. Int Orthop 29; 272-276.
15. Sugamo N, Nishii T, Miki H, Yoshikawa H, Sato Y, Tamura S (2007) Mid-term results of cementless total hip replacement using a ceramic-on-ceramic bearing with and without computer navigation. J Bone Joint Surg Br 89; 455-460.
16. Sandhu HS, Middleton RG, Wainwright TW, Serjeant SA (2005) Durom hip resurfacing with Medtronic computer navigation – Initial Experience. Submitted Poster Presentation. CAOS Meeting, Helsinki.

Printed in the United States
By Bookmasters